{ THE STEAMER PARISH }

UNIVERSITY OF CHICAGO GEOGRAPHY RESEARCH PAPER, NUMBER 244

Series editors:

MICHAEL P. CONZEN
CHAUNCY D. HARRIS
NEIL HARRIS
MARVIN W. MIKESELL
GERALD D. SUTTLES

Titles published in the Geography Research Papers series prior to 1992 and still in print are now distributed by the University of Chicago Press. For a list of available titles, please see the end of the book. The University of Chicago Press began publication of the Geography Research Papers series in 1992 with number 233.

{ THE RISE AND FALL OF MISSIONARY
MEDICINE ON AN AFRICAN FRONTIER }

The Steamer Parish

Charles M. Good Jr.

THE UNIVERSITY OF CHICAGO PRESS
Chicago & London

CHARLES M. GOOD JR. is professor emeritus of geography at the
Virginia Polytechnic Institute and State University. He is the author of *The
Community in African Primary Health Care* and *Ethnomedical Systems in Africa*.

The University of Chicago Press, Chicago 60637
The University of Chicago Press, Ltd., London
© 2004 by The University of Chicago
All rights reserved. Published 2004
Printed in the United States of America

13 12 11 10 09 08 07 06 05 04   5 4 3 2 1

ISBN (cloth): 0-226-30281-4
ISBN (paper): 0-226-30282-2

Library of Congress Cataloging-in-Publication Data

Good, Charles M.
    The steamer parish : the rise and fall of missionary medicine on an
African frontier / Charles M. Good, Jr.
        p.   cm.—(University of Chicago geography research paper;
no. 244)
    Includes bibliographical references and index.
    ISBN 0-226-30281-4 (cloth : alk. paper)—ISBN 0-226-30282-2
(pbk. : alk. paper)
    1. Universities' Mission to Central Africa—History.
2. Missionaries, Medical—Africa, Central—History—19th
century.   3. Boats and boating in missionary work—Africa,
Central—History—19th century.   I. Title.   II. Series.
    R722.G66   2004
    610.69′096—dc22

                                        2003016362

⊗ The paper used in this publication meets the minimum requirements of
the American National Standard for Information Sciences—Permanence
of Paper for Printed Library Materials, ANSI Z39.48-1992.

{ FOR MY SON, ALEC SHEPARD GOOD }

Contents

Illustrations

TABLES

FIGURES

Preface

Health services in postcolonial Africa owe a substantial debt to the pioneering, sustained efforts of Christian medical missions in the colonial era. Urban and rural populations in Malawi and many other countries continue to extensively rely on church-related hospitals and health centers. Typically these institutions are staffed by a mix of African and expatriate professionals. Today, with most public sector health services in dire straits, Protestant and Catholic affiliated institutions commonly represent the only accessible and reliable places where Western-type health care of decent quality is available.

This book offers a case study and critique of the medical agenda of the Universities' Mission to Central Africa (UMCA), which operated in Malawi from about 1885 to 1964. It is written with an interdisciplinary audience in mind, and from the perspective of historical-medical geography. I examine how this high-church Anglican mission, directly inspired by David Livingstone, conceptualized its health care responsibilities to Africans, and how effectively it fulfilled its goal to provide medical services to remote rural populations in the vast region of Lake Malawi and its borderlands. The book contributes to the existing literature by tracing how a mission "field" and medical services actually originated and evolved in place and time. It also recognizes that missionary medicine was not introduced into a medico-religious vacuum. Facilitated by the innovation of steamer transport, the mission introduced a cluster of new social institutions, cultural norms and symbols, and religious and political ideas. These exogenous influences had markedly varied effects upon the local African peoples and landscapes in the mission's sphere. Whereas the book appropriately values missionary efforts in the colonial context, it also offers a critical analysis of the UMCA's achievements and underachievements in relation to Malawians' health and social welfare.

The "Steamer Parish" idea rapidly materialized once the UMCA's pioneer missionaries on the Malawi frontier persuaded the mission's London headquarters that steamboats offered a viable technological solution to exploiting the region's opportunities for evangelism. The mission's decision to use steamboats, built in Britain and reassembled on Lake Malawi, as a means to build and service a chain of missions spread across four hundred miles was seen as a brilliant solution to its transportation and communication needs. The steamers *Charles Janson* and *Chauncy Maples* performed both tactical and strategic roles in the development of the mission field. Paradoxically, the UMCA's expanding spatial concept of itself brought the missionaries into a growing dependency on the steamers. Yet in the long run many factors detracted from the steamers' value to the mission's general program, and to its medical work in particular. Breakdowns, lack of spare parts, and repair time reduced the steamers' reliability and availability, and often disrupted sailing and mission services.

While certainly a "success" on many counts, the UMCA also had to confront numerous practical and social issues that reduced its effectiveness as an agent of evangelism, education, and in particular, progressive medicine. They included chronic financial constraints, the mission's social philosophy, two world wars and depression, and changing leadership and policies that eventually deeply antagonized African political sensibilities.

The study of medical missions opens windows onto a fascinating range of theoretical and substantive issues that span the social sciences and humanities. This book traces the process of mission expansion and of African-European and European-Muslim relations. It examines issues relating to cultural contact and frontiers. These themes systematically lead to the question of how missions, as agents of landscape and social change, exemplify geographies of "generic" imperialism. Since this book focuses primarily on missionary medicine, before undertaking the analysis of health conditions and changes in the colonial period it was necessary to develop baseline evidence and review what is known about the health of precolonial Malawians.

I evaluate colonial policies, including taxation and impelled labor migration, as well as mission policies and collaborations with government, that affected African health. Significantly, the missionaries immediately encountered African medico-religious institutions that had endured for generations. Tensions between African customs and Euro-Christian values proved salient and persistent features of cultural diversity and conflict in the mission system. One result was a growth of medical and cultural-religious pluralism, rather than replacement of the indigenous medico-religious regime with a mission version of Western medicine.

Where and why the mission located its hospitals and dispensaries created important issues of space management that ultimately influenced its medical outreach and effectiveness. Questions about curative treatment vs. health promotion and prevention eventually gained importance in response to international developments. In time, race and class issues snowballed, and reached a tragic impasse during the years of the Central African Federation. Finally, I present evidence and draw conclusions about the mission's overall influence on African health and social change during its colonial tenure. The findings reveal significant continuities with Malawi's ongoing struggle today to strengthen its medical and public health services.

The research for this book is based on visits to former UMCA hospitals and mission villages; intensive study of primary documents in the Malawi National Archives, Zomba; and multiple visits to the main UMCA archives on deposit at Rhodes House Library, Oxford. "Go Ask the Old Men," in chapter 7, presents a series of conversations I had at Malindi with four elderly men, Christian and Muslim, about their connections to and reflections on early contacts with the UMCA's medical mission.

Readers will see that *Central Africa* (1883–1964), a journal edited and published several times yearly in London, is an invaluable source of primary and secondary materials used in the book's preparation. *Central Africa* was the UMCA's primary voice for communicating mission activities and news to Anglican parishioners and patrons in Britain, as well as among its missionaries in Malawi, Tanganyika, and Northern Rhodesia. It is filled with human interest stories and accounts of daily life. It is also an important record of the social calendar of the Anglo-Catholic church both in Britain and Malawi, and mirrors the concern of this branch of the Anglican Communion with ecclesiasticism, including hierarchy, ritual, liturgy, and raiments. The journal's pages apparently edit out some of the more controversial details of mission policies and practices.

Central Africa gives much space to social and financial issues, including missionary perceptions of African cultural practices (often contrasted with English ways); the running of hospitals; interest in African welfare issues; fundraising at home and church-giving among Africans; the perennial shortage of resources; mission-government relations in the colonial state; and the ongoing concern that Africans integrate "Christian values" into their daily living patterns. The latter was complemented by the missionary compulsion to exact strict church discipline when Africans "failed" to meet the missionaries' desired standards of African comportment. *Central Africa* reflects paternalistic sympathies for Africans, and often presented the missionaries as protectors of African interests in the new environments brought on by taxation, male labor migration, world wars, and harsh treatment of workers by white settlers. Overall, the journal provides a remarkable record of mission endeavor spanning more than eighty years. Considering its undeniable cultural and political exclusivity—it is written by and for Europeans—*Central Africa* represents a balanced attempt to document the mission's experiment, guided by a British sense of fair-mindedness.

Acknowledgments

This book is grounded in field and archival research in Malawi, England, and the United States. It has had a large claim on my energy for several years, during which time many individuals and organizations have given valuable assistance. The National Geographic Society generously provided the basic financial support with two grants (1989–91). I am particularly indebted to Professor Harm J. de Blij for the encouragement and guidance he offered when he served at the NGS. Professors Donald E. Vermeer and John M. Hunter also made significant contributions to my efforts to obtain funding. I also appreciate each of them for the intellectual stimulation, professional support, and friendship they have given me throughout my academic career. Additional funding was received from the National Science Foundation, Grant No. SES-9025009, and from the College of Arts and Sciences Small Grants Committee at Virginia Tech (1989–90), and through a Virginia Tech Summer Humanities Fellowship in 1993.

I was honored by Malawi's National Research Council with permission to conduct both field studies and archival research. Mr. Charles B. Malunga, Director of the Malawi National Archives in Zomba, and his assistants Joel S. Thaulo and Victor L. Khonde, provided many days of enthusiastic and tireless support in helping me to locate and copy essential mission and colonial government records. Augustius C. Msiska, Africana Librarian, at

Chancellor College, gave me invaluable access to journal and special papers and contacts. Bishop Benson Aipa of the Diocese of Southern Malawi opened the doors for me to work in former UMCA mission centers such as Malindi and Mponda's station. No words can adequately describe the wonderful hospitality and support I received from Mr. H. M. Kangunga, Chief Clinical Officer at St. Martin's Hospital, Malindi. The Reverends Stanley Mandala and David Oneika, Priests-in-Charge at Malindi in 1989 and 1990, respectively, also invited me into their homes and gave access to key individuals, including Archdeacon Chikokota, Shannon Bango, Chief Makwinja, and Chief Chiwaya. These elders met with me on the lakeshore at Malindi and graciously shared their memories of early contacts between Africans and the UMCA's medical mission. The late Agnes Chiwaya, medical secretary and organizer at St. Martin's, offered much useful information and remained a special friend after I left Malawi. Mr. Chegwengembe, Superintendent of St. Luke's Hospital, Malosa, shared with me information about the post-missionary era hospitals and health centers in the old UMCA diocese. The staff at St. Anne's Hospital, Kota Kota, graciously allowed me to observe them at work. I am also grateful to Professor Owen Kalinga, then Head of the Department of History at Chancellor College, Zomba, and his wife Margaret, for their warm hospitality and guidance when I first arrived in Malawi. Dr. Chrissie Chawanje, at Virginia Tech during the 1990s, graciously cross-checked a number of facts for me during a Malawi home visit.

In England, Rhodes House Library, Oxford, houses the main UMCA archives. I received expert professional assistance from the archivists during my research there in 1989 and 2002. In London, Mrs. Catherine Wakeling, Archivist at the United Society for the Propagation of the Gospel, unselfishly offered and delivered outstanding professional assistance in my efforts to track down old UMCA photographs and financial records, and to obtain authorizations to reproduce various materials.

I am indebted to Dr. John Orr Dwyer, a historian and educator based in Atlanta, and Professor Jim Newman, a geographer and Africanist at Syracuse University. Both graciously responded to my request for a critical early reading of the manuscript. Later, upon learning from then-editor Penny Kaiserlian that I had submitted the manuscript to the University of Chicago Press, Michael Conzen and Marvin Mikesell recommended it for publication in the Geography Research Paper Series. Senior editor Christie Henry gave me outstanding guidance, from the manuscript's initial review through the final stages of evaluation. Jennifer Howard, editorial associate for sciences; Claudia Rex, senior production editor; and Michael

Cowden supplied excellent technical support. Two anonymous outside reviewers provided helpful commentaries. Brandon Herrington prepared the two computer-based maps. I owe much to Richard Allen, the copyeditor. His concern for clarity of expression and meticulous attention to detail has made a significant contribution to this book. Finally, I offer special thanks to my wife, Laurie Good, for caring about the project with me over several years of fieldwork and writing.

Abbreviations

ALC	African Lakes Corporation
BCA	British Central Africa
BELRA	British Empire Leprosy Association
BSAC	British South Africa Company
CCAP	Church of Central Africa Province
CA	*Central Africa: A Monthly Record of the Universities' Mission to Central Africa*
C.J.	*S.S. Charles Janson*
C.M.	*S.S. Chauncy Maples*
CSM	Church of Scotland Mission
DC	District Commissioner
DMS	Director of Medical Services (Nyasaland Protectorate)
DO	District Officer
DRCM	Dutch Reformed Church Mission
FCSM	Free Church of Scotland Mission
MO	Medical Officer
PEA	Portuguese East Africa
PHAM	Private Hospital Association of Malawi
SDA	Seventh Day Adventist
STI	Sexually-transmitted infections
UMCA	Universities' Mission to Central Africa
USPG	United Society for the Propagation of the Gospel
WF	White Fathers
WHO	World Health Organization

{ THE STEAMER PARISH }

CHAPTER ONE

Christian Medical Missions and African Societies

Christian missions profoundly aided Europe's imperial expansion into Africa. In what was colonial Nyasaland and is Malawi today,[1] an English geographer asserted without risk of rebuttal that "the first steps for occupation, civilization and development of our colonies were taken by the Church" (Sharpe 1912, 1). Missionaries also brought to Africa elements of the diverse technologies that symbolized industrial and scientific progress at home, including locomotion and medicine. With such tools available, they promoted their own mission societies' evangelistic aims, and less intentionally supported the secular goals and achievements of empire. It was also true that the missionaries' initial success with technological applications in the pioneer era was no guarantee that the same tools would remain potent means of sustaining progress as they envisioned it.

Arguably, the most profound influence of Protestant missionaries in Malawi and elsewhere in tropical Africa did not come from their theological persuasiveness. Rather, the stronger impacts came from their uses of basic technology and science, and their provision of elementary and religious education for willing Africans. Today, the remaining elders of Africa's last colonial generation can recall the efforts that many missionaries also made to instill in them British (or French, Portuguese, etc.) cultural values. Such ideals included a preference for reserved over emotional behavior, knowing one's place in society, "making do," and charity beyond one's immediate family. Many younger, postcolonial Africans can also readily identify the numerous indirect influences of the missionary period on their own lives.

I began work on this topic because I was intrigued by the often-shrill critiques of medical missions that began to emerge in liberal and critical studies in the 1970s. One of the basic charges leveled by critics, exemplified by a World Health Organization official, is that missionary medicine focused primarily on curative activity to the exclusion of preventive services. Instead, missions used medical services as a deliberate tool to evangelize and win souls for Christ. The underlying assumption was that the emphasis on "soul" work had little bearing on health. Another alleged pitfall was that missionaries were historically predisposed toward "certain medicosocial tasks," such as care of leprosy patients and the blind. Having concentrated on hospital practice rather than community outreach, they had contributed to "highly fragmented and uncoordinated health services" that persist even today (Akerele et al. 1976). Furthermore, missions had failed to train sufficient numbers of African health workers, and branded traditional healers as evil rather than collaborating with them (ibid.).

The criticisms cited above generally have some factual basis to them.[2] However, it is also evident that they often ignore historical context, and are overgeneralized and one-sided. They fail to acknowledge the significant work carried out by many unselfish and far-sighted individuals and organizations. The critiques imply that Africans derived little health benefit from their interactions with medical missionaries, including those to whom they imparted medical skills.[3] Also overlooked is the fact that medical missionaries often desired and campaigned for more and better quality services than their institutional resources could produce. The case study developed in these pages illustrates the enervating limitations and frustrations of missionary medicine. Such texture and balancing of viewpoints is possible only by giving careful attention to the primary historical records that document the unfolding of events in time and space within the entire mission sphere.

Finally, only blinding ideology could prevent one from acknowledging that, collectively, medical missions laid the essential foundations and "spearheaded" the future development of biomedical services and public health.[4] In 1965, the churches provided 40 to 50 percent of all hospital beds in Malawi, for which the new government, "getting a bargain," provided an annual subsidy of US$85,000.[5] Most of these hospitals were located in remote areas, although the pattern of individual mission spheres meant that some parts of the country had received few if any medical facilities in the colonial period. Since independence in 1964, the Private Hospital Association of

Malawi (PHAM), which is sponsored by the Christian Council of Malawi, has worked closely with the government to raise the country's level of health services and welfare. Today PHAM oversees some 23 hospitals and about 115 Health Centres (including dozens of outlying health posts), that provide slightly over 6,000 beds.[6]

This book tells the story of the rise and fall of the London-based Universities' Mission to Central Africa (UMCA). Eventually a far-flung enterprise in East and Central Africa, the UMCA, headquartered in London, was resurrected in 1875 following its disastrous first effort in Malawi in the early 1860s. Once again the mission acted on David Livingstone's earlier challenge to the church—to go to Central Africa to help suppress the slave trade and open the region to Christianity—delivered when he visited Oxford and Cambridge universities in 1857. When the expansion process had run its course, the UMCA had planted a series of "fields" that included the Dioceses of Zanzibar, Likoma/Nyasaland, Northern Rhodesia, Masasi, and South West Tanganyika. The Diocese of Nyasaland also included a slice of Portuguese East Africa adjacent to Lake Malawi (colonial Lake Nyasa) and was thus spread over three colonial territories (fig. 1.1).

There is more than a hint here that the UMCA bargained on a strategy of spreading its resources thinly. This study reveals the extent to which the Nyasaland mission, aided by modern technology and a modicum of government support, penetrated, claimed, and changed African societies and environments in the Lake Malawi region (fig. 1.2). I trace this historical-geographical process beginning with the last years of Malawi's precolonial isolation from Europe, and continue through the colonial era to independence in 1964.

Winning souls was the paramount purpose of these men and women who went to the mission fields. Mostly English and high church, they committed much, and in some cases all, of their adult lives to work in the mission's dioceses. UMCA clergy were mostly Oxbridge-educated English missionaries. To fulfill their calling, the clerics together with the mission's women nurses and teachers voluntarily gave up their considerable home comforts and privileges, including their incomes. Malawi was over four hundred miles away from a seacoast and five thousand miles from the mission's London headquarters. Extremely remote even within tropical Africa, Malawi in the last quarter of the nineteenth century continued to be a turbulent region wracked by destructive slave raiding. Life was brutal for many African communities as they sought to stay a day ahead of the slavers. While the missionaries received limited and often faltering support from London, as a practical matter they supported themselves. They relied heavily on self-grown solutions and

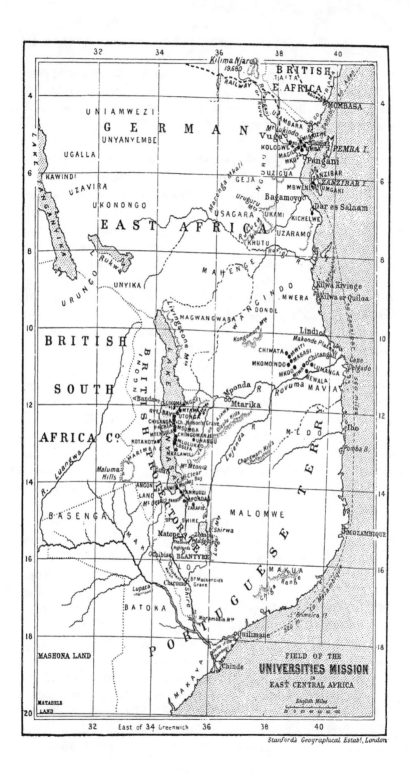

FIELD OF THE
UNIVERSITIES MISSION
IN
EAST CENTRAL AFRICA

Stanford's Geographical Establ., London

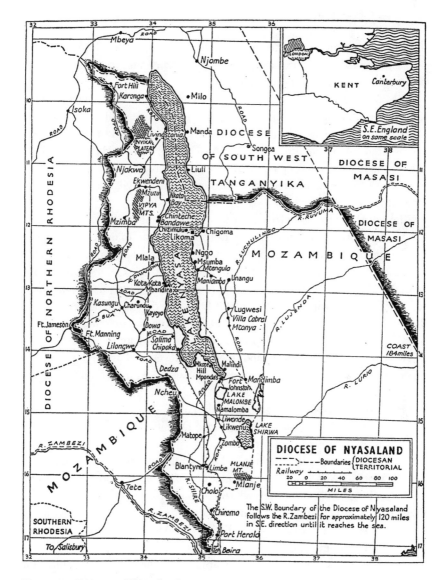

Figure 1.2. Diocese of Nyasaland, c. 1952.
(Source: Blood (1962). From the archives of the USPG.)

◁ **Figure 1.1. Field of the Universities' Mission in East Central Africa.**
(Source: Palmer and Ashwin (1900), 8. This illustration and all others from the USPG archives are reproduced with the kind permission of the United Society for the Propagation of the Gospel, London.)

innovations, ranging from steamer repairs, to coping with exhausting work patterns due to severe shortages of mission workers, and to finding ways to promote maternal and child health.

In Malawi, the UMCA missionaries depended extensively on technology they imported. From 1885, steam navigation proved essential to the mission's primary activities along the coast of Lake Malawi. Mission steamers played an essential role in creating the UMCA's Diocese of Nyasaland. By World War I, the diocese encompassed an area that spanned four hundred miles from north to south, and included portions of Tanganyika and Portuguese East Africa.

Immense health risks led to a huge loss of life among the early missionaries in Malawi. Slowly, conditions for the Europeans began to improve. By 1900, knowledge of disease prevention was increasingly available, particularly for malaria and blackwater fever. The latter condition is a sequel to subtertian, or malignant falciparum malaria, apparently induced by quinine, in which red blood cells are rapidly destroyed. Only the freed pigment passes through the kidneys. The altered cells remain blocked in the kidney's fine tubes. The urine is blackened and its flow practically stops (Wingate 1976, 68).

Nevertheless, persistent, debilitating illness, fever, and stress, the latter felt especially among the women, kept many missionaries from contributing as fully as expected.

By 1900, the UMCA began a small-scale, laborious effort to set up rudimentary medical services for Africans. Despite the enormous need for treatment of endemic health problems (e.g., thousands of all ages suffered from painful and debilitating tropical ulcers), for decades only small clusters of Africans who lived near the mission's far-flung stations had access. In the early years, dread of the white-skinned, costumed missionaries and their medical procedures kept many Africans from attending, or revisiting, UMCA hospitals and dispensaries. Few if any Africans were denied treatment on religious grounds.

Used separately and in tandem, steam and medicine soon became vital instruments in the mission's quest to impose its will, indelibly, on hundreds of thousands of unsuspecting people in the vastness of south-central Africa. Its foremost goal emerged from a collective imagination: the dream of shaping a productive mission field peopled by African Christians.

Initially, Western medicine was viewed almost exclusively as a tool to support evangelization. How effectively the UMCA missionaries adapted steam power and medicine to serve their ambitions offers a fascinating case study of innovation, struggle, and vulnerability. My aim here is to describe and interpret how the mission, aided by Western technology and ambivalent support from the colonial government, altered human relationships, influenced African health, and changed places and environments in the Lake Malawi basin. A recurring theme in this story is how the UMCA's distinctive institutional rules, style, and resources both encouraged and constrained the missionaries' fields of vision and actions.

With little or no formal collaboration, the UMCA, Scottish Presbyterians, Roman Catholics, and other mission societies moved ahead with measures that they hoped would prepare Africans in Malawi to adopt many presumably superior values of European civilization. Such acquiescence would diminish if not eliminate what the missionaries viewed as the undesirable and least progressive elements of African life that conflicted with a Christian design for living. But the missionaries' aspirations set up a paradox that became a two-edged sword, since, in British eyes, their race, class and culture prevented Africans from becoming anything except Africans.

In the broad frame, at least, the missionaries could normally count on at least tacit support from the colonial government. After all, the missions were willing to commit resources to building up the very institutions the government professed to need but declined to supply, such as education and basic medical services. Thus in Malawi, and many other parts of the colonial world, missions acted as convenient proxies for areas of government responsibility. While the protectorate government in Malawi was in principle not against education and medicine for its African wards, schools and dispensaries were not built unless subsidized by African taxation.

Africans were expected to be humble, cooperative, and eager to learn in the face of superior European tutors, values, and institutions. This agenda was pressed upon Africans "for their own good," and to shine light on the mythical African darkness. In time, it became clear to some missionaries and officials that outsiders could not easily manipulate many aspects of the life of the mind among Africans, such as cosmology and spiritual practices such as ancestor veneration and witchcraft beliefs. In attempting to drive it underground, colonial practices may have reinforced the debilitating social forces of witchcraft.

Social structure and labor proved less resistant to changes wrought in the struggle between European and African lifeways. Routinization of taxation and the resulting out-migration of men in search of jobs forced fundamental adjustments in work patterns and jeopardized healthy family relations. The changes impinged on the holistic and kin-group values that undergirded African social and spiritual life, and affected reproductive and demographic

patterns. New and deep fault lines in household labor and other social relations emerged, causing Africans to undergo major adjustments in patterns
of subsistence farming and cash crop production.

In its sphere, the UMCA offered useful but much limited opportunities
for Africans in formal education, employment, and paramedical training
and dispensary work. At least thirty years passed before the mission began
to view health care as part of its mandate, rather than simply a tool for
evangelization. Debates persist about the nature and scope of opportunities
Africans had to train for careers in health care, and thus also the extent of
the UMCA's accomplishments in this domain.

POWERING MISSION EXPANSION

Steam

The introduction and sustained use of technologies such as steam, medicine,
and electricity offered many opportunities for missions to impress Africans
with Western prowess. It was essential to find the means to encourage in "the
African" a sense of mystical agency and awe through European technology.
This might also hasten a wider receptivity to evangelism. Technology enabled and reinforced missionary efforts to contact people in remote areas. It
helped them carve out viable physical and psychological places on the new
cultural and political frontier inhabited by Africans and empire-builders.
Whether by design or accident, the innovations brought by missionaries and
others from the industrializing world were not benign. They contributed significantly to the reconfiguring of social and spatial relations in tropical Africa.

In most places, Africans looked on in awe and even fear at the steamboat
and other newly arrived exemplars of the Industrial Revolution, including the magical syringe. In each case, how the innovations actually worked
was rarely visible or self-evident to local people. The imported technologies
embodied radical ideas and processes such as germ theory, machine propul-
sion, and life-enhancing techniques such as anesthesia and powerful drugs
derived from aniline dyes. In a relatively short time, these and other non-
military technologies began to have practical applications in transport and
helped to stimulate new (not always beneficial) opportunities for employment, trade, technical training, exchange, education, and improvements in
health care. Such technologies also stimulated the intensification of human
relations with their environments, as in firewood collection for the steamers and labor migration. Steam engines, medicine, and the Gatling gun

also served as powerful allies in the frequently violent imposition of Pax Britannica.

Overall, steam navigation provided unprecedented efficiency of travel to and within several of Africa's large river basins including the Zambezi, Congo, Niger, and Senegal. The continent's great lakes, including Malawi, Tanganyika, Kivu, and Nyanza (Victoria) also offered opportunities for long-distance trafficking by steamers. While steamer transport never came close to achieving its full potential, as the UMCA's experience reveals, its use was remarkable considering that the vessels were built in Europe.

Depending on the African destination and route, the new iron or steel-clad steamers were sometimes disassembled into hundreds of parcels and reassembled twice, en route to an African destination. Transport to the final assembly and launch site inland was usually accomplished in three phases, in the British case beginning with shipment from a shipyard in London or Glasgow to Africa on an ocean steamer. On arrival at the mouth of a river such as the Zambezi in Mozambique, which was the initial route to UMCA territory in Malawi, a crew then sailed it to the next head of navigation or confluence of rivers, such as the Shiré. Again, the steamer was disassembled, and in Malawi African porters then had the arduous task of carrying the vessel inland. This feat required movement of hundreds of heavy packages around five waterfalls. The distance around the falls to the point of final reassembly on the Shiré was fifty miles.

Steamers provided a unique conduit for the spread of new ideas to Malawian societies. They helped shrink distance by moving more people and goods faster and farther, simultaneously opening up new avenues of thinking and behavior. Effects were felt in many spheres, including customary gender and authority relations, people's mental maps, and economic and environmental relations on land and water.

Diverging Methods: Missionary Medicine Meets African Healing

By World War I, the "missionary" variant of Western medicine had acquired considerable influence on African modes of health care in some of Malawi's more accessible areas. However, contrary to its original goal of replacing local medicine and "heathen" healers with missionary medicine, the UMCA witnessed the powerful bond and hold of African religion and traditional healing. Inadvertently, the missionaries helped to fuse strands of Western medical practice into the repertoire of African therapies.

The confrontation of African and Western missionary therapeutic systems encouraged medical pluralism. But unlike Western medicine, with its debt to the mind-body dualism of Cartesian philosophy, African religious and health care practices remained closely connected and not compartmentalized. African healing was deeply embedded in spirituality, and remained that way. At the same time, missionary medicine enabled African healing to develop into a more eclectic ethnomedicine that could incorporate Western medical practices. In time, Africans acted on their new choices of medical treatment, such as injections, antiseptic applications, and surgery. The striking efficacy of the drug-filled syringe was unmatched, and among Africans it soon achieved an exalted status as the most popular of all missionary therapies. Those who came to appreciate the value of the imported medicine, which was part art and part science, also realized that its therapy focused primarily upon the physical body. For Africans, this approach created an artificial body-mind distinction and left aside the traditional frameworks for understanding mental and spiritual health.

Healers and religious specialists, notwithstanding their diverse ethnic traditions, crosscut practically all spheres of African social and cultural life in Malawi, as was the case throughout the African continent. Their specialized roles encompassed life crises such as birth; transition to adulthood; interpretation of perceived personal, community, and environmental experiences; ritualized protection of adults, children, the unborn, people, crops, houses, and domestic animals against witchcraft and sorcery; and the circumstances of death, including responsibilities to spirits of the departed.

Few if any UMCA missionaries viewed African healing as a valid institution, with the possible exception of certain aspects of herbalism believed to be benign or unconnected to the supernatural. Most could not accept the fact that missionary medicine had to compete against African ideas and practices. In this light, it is no surprise that the UMCA missionaries had limited success in marginalizing the bedrock philosophy of African healing.

In the long run, "missionary" medicine did make limited political and therapeutic inroads into African healing. In addition to procedures already noted, Africans gradually accepted elements of first aid and a smattering of hygiene practices (boosted by instruction in mission schools). Such measures contributed substantially to the increasingly eclectic variety of choices available within the widening scope of indigenous medical pluralism. At the same time, it must be remembered that for many decades the great majority of Africans had little if any access to mission health care, nor to opportunities for instruction in Western health education.

In their pioneer phase the missions in colonial Malawi established hundreds of stations and outstations, along with schools, churches, and a number of hospitals and dispensaries. By the turn of the twentieth century the relative isolation of mission stations from each other, and of the missionaries from contact with their families and friends at home, had lessened in some areas. Evangelism, Anglican ritual and rules, and related activities had been introduced into diverse African ethnic communities and habitats. Missionaries, now including a small body of African faithful, preached against indigenous behaviors and beliefs, such as "the witchdoctor" institution and the heathen pursuit of polygamy. Such attitudes and practices were often misunderstood and caricatured by both the missionary and secular European communities. (In truth, Africans also gained amusement from the Europeans' own typically unexamined mores and behavior, including the UMCA's self-imposed rule of celibacy.) A serious attempt on the part of the missionaries to understand the cultures they confronted would threaten the established mode of power sharing between individuals and among groups. An illustration of this control phenomenon was the enthusiasm of the missionaries and other Europeans to call the African men who worked for them "boys," virtually as a natural right and without examining their assumptions. Social Darwinism would not be easily displaced. In the late nineteenth century, Europeans generally believed that Africans occupied a low position on the scale of human development and possessed inferior cultures. British protagonists, secular and often religious, viewed African peoples "as the merest adjuncts to the central conflict with the continent. At most, the Africans are but the passive objects of British endeavors. As subjects to be governed, ignorant people to be taught, heathens to be converted, patients to be treated, they almost always belong to the faceless, nameless category of the 'natives'" (Hammond and Jablow 1992, 169).

As missionaries soon discovered, powerful African, or "pagan" religious beliefs, and influences from Islam presented formidable obstacles to achieving their goals. For Africans, there would be no easy acceptance and assimilation of the most unyielding missionary values and ideology. In bold contrast to the universalism and exclusiveness of most forms of missionary faith and ideology, African religiosity in Malawi seemed to express greater holism and less compartmentalization than was the typical experience of Anglican parishioners in England. For Africans, there was really no escape from the spiritual web in which they lived. A pervasive influence, religion contained the major sources of social control, including how to cope with the spirit world and the universal belief in witchcraft. For Africans, there could be no separation of attitudes about health and disease from religious beliefs. Cartesian partition of body and soul was generally alien to African religious sensibilities.

African resistance to Western forms of Christian practice was powerfully demonstrated in missionary assumptions and ultimatums. Africans were expected to discard many of their own customary institutions and practices, and replace them with European designs for living. They often emphatically rejected such demands as too intrusive. Acquiescence to European and missionary demands would be disruptive and undermine the social order. Well-known resistant institutions included polygyny, female circumcision, use of alcohol, separate domiciles for spouses, and reliance on indigenous healers. On the other hand, Africans saw literacy and formal education as instrumental to their own upward mobility. In this they also gave fundamental aid to colonial administrations that could not have survived without African clerks and other literate personnel (Isichei 1995).

I now focus on four ideas that help to frame this story: the geography of imperialism, the African frontier, medical missions, and the role of technology.

THE GEOGRAPHY OF IMPERIALISM

Missionaries tended to believe that their motives lay on a higher plane than those that drove government and commercial interests. It would be remiss and unfair not to recognize that most missionaries tried to live their lives according to the ideals they espoused. Countless missionaries gave of their own resources, time, and lives in following the evangelical call. Some, such as the UMCA's William P. Johnson, were truly remarkable human beings who exhibited extraordinary courage and endurance against great odds. In British territories and many others, it was the missionaries who provided important educational and medical resources that the colonial state chose to ignore for so long. In the process they introduced significant benefits to select groups of people within African societies.

While guns, floggings, and use of forced labor (*thangata* in Malawi) were surely uncharacteristic of missionaries, on occasions some did choose to stand by and watch injustices occur. In Malawi, comparatively well-known cases in which missionaries resorted to violence include the UMCA's military support of the Manganja people in their struggle against cruel Yao slavers (1861), and the Church of Scotland's atrocities in the name of justice and order in Blantyre (1879) (Hanna 1956; Rotberg 1965).

Missionaries had many reasons to seek help from others in order to gain and keep control of converts and allies. There is also much evidence that the generally uninvited incursions of missions into African lands and society, and their methods of appropriating and maintaining control of indigenous resources, frequently involved subterfuge and other tactics (see, for example, Olumwallah 2002, 106–23; H. Johnson 1967). In this sense it is no exaggeration to say that they fit into the imperialist agenda, and gained from a loose interdependence with administrators, traders, military forces, and other secular agencies of colonialism.

A geography of imperialism necessarily involves new spatial processes triggered by what Meinig (1982) calls "the encroachment of one people upon the territory of another." To uncover the geographic significance of imperialism, it is necessary to probe beyond ideological motivations to describe and analyze when, where, and by what means areas and peoples have been changed. Beginning in the sixteenth century, European imperialism involved direct assaults made on other peoples' territories and wealth. By 1914, the European powers, notably Britain, France, and Russia, controlled about 85 percent of the earth's land surface. Yet history repeatedly shows that imperialism was not a European invention. Imperialism has been commonly identified with other major realms of cultural expansion where strong invaders have encountered weaker societies. Examples include the Islamic empire created by the Arabs beginning in the seventh and eighth centuries and later the Ottoman Empire. As mission institutions reveal, the consequences of imperialism reach far beyond simply imposing a different system of production and distribution in another place.

A comprehensive approach to uncovering the influences of imperialism begins with an acknowledgment that it is a generic phenomenon that has operated throughout history. Evidence of its imprints on societies, cultures, and landscapes can be deciphered through close study of processes that changed life for populations in places and regions (Meinig 1982). For instance, how did missions organize the lands and peoples they came to dominate? What changes did these actions produce among the subjected peoples and places? In this light, a comprehensive interpretation of mission imperialism hinges on identifying and understanding the physical, social, and cultural traces of missionary encounters, and the consequences of unequal relationships with local peoples in specific places.

Meinig's concept of generic imperialism focuses attention on the political, social, cultural, economic, and psychological domains of confrontation, restructuring social and economic life, and locational and ecological change. Medical missions offer a compelling case of how the new human geographies are expressed in each domain (Good 1991).

Imperial domination occurs when local peoples' authority is subordinated to the coercive or, more accurately in the case of mission societies,

manipulative power of the intruders. To accomplish their style of domination foreign missionaries and their indigenous agents negotiated with
local authorities including African kings and Arab slave traders in parts of
Eastern and Central Africa. They formed tentative alliances with the locals
and moved into strategic positions within zones targeted for occupation (Sim
1897; Oliver 1952). In Malawi, such zones and places included safe harbors
such as islands in Lake Malawi deemed safe from bands of Ngoni marauders and slavers. Other advantageous places for the missionaries included
lakeshore coves where the steamers could safely drop anchor, and places
with greater population concentrations and thus potentially fertile ground
for evangelization.

The ability to place exotic trade goods in the hands of local African chiefs
and other authorities, and to exploit their differences, proved invaluable to
the negotiating success of European missionaries. Mission societies pushed
hard to open and secure supply lines, often with the assistance of foreign
traders or other de facto agents of colonialism. Early on missionaries also
felt pressure from colonial officialdom to give precedence to treaty making
("the work of Empire") with neighboring chiefs (Hammond and Jablow
1992, chap. 3).

A gradual influx of missionary and lay personnel, material goods, and
new information brought both dramatic and subtle changes to lifestyles in
Central Africa's lake region. New linkages between people and places began to form, including land and water transportation routes and a small
but growing commerce on the lake. Even distant mission stations and communities discovered small if fragile bonds of interdependence. In time, even
remote, rear outposts and mission stations on the frontier became more or
less connected. For example, in the late 1870s the pioneer Presbyterian mission, situated on the western coast of Lake Malawi across from the UMCA's
zone on the eastern side, was known to have superior medical capabilities.
Some UMCA missionaries, urgently in need of emergency care, made often-
hazardous journeys across the lake to receive treatment from the renowned
Dr. Robert Laws. The field stations naturally also became dependent to
varying degrees on metropolitan center(s) of missionary support such as
London, and thus also with imperial and ecclesiastical authority managed
from afar.

Missions often experienced frustrating delays involving months or years.
Almost invariably the UMCA missionaries experienced shortfalls in operating budgets and "development" capital. Forced relocations of planned
head-stations and outstations occurred, sometimes due to the resistance of
hostile local authorities or supply problems. They suffered failed schemes

and, in the early decades, a crushingly high mortality from malaria and blackwater fever. Serious physical debilitation and stress frequently caused men and women to be invalided to Britain, some of whom were never allowed to return to the mission field.

Obstacles aside, within a short time, and certainly by the 1880s in tropical and southern Africa, chains of mission stations had become significant markers of change in the local African landscape. These religiously motivated settlements linked remote, scattered interior regions and peoples, and sometimes connected them with coastal towns (Christopher 1984; Good 1991).

New Social Relations

Refugees, freed or purchased slaves, orphans, the blind, lepers, barren women, and the destitute—marginalized and "socially displaced" adults and children—typically formed the earliest social foundation of a mission's work. Experience varied geographically, of course. It is noteworthy, however, that many initial relationships between missionaries and Africans probably served to *diminish* inequality between adults and children who had been displaced and marginalized vis-à-vis the general population.

Africans and missionaries alike confronted each other's stark differences of race, social patterning, and cosmology. Most British missionaries seemed to know their place in the social system of the African frontier. Motivated by the call of the Great Commission to spread the Gospel world-wide, and by personal needs, they drew support from a powerful sense of their own national character and imperial responsibility. Coming from a strongly hierarchical society, the English missionaries, at least, disembarked on African soil greatly influenced by their own experience of rigid class relations as natural and proper. Their palpable sense of cultural superiority was supported by what they viewed as the inferior, noncompetitive, non-surplus-oriented character of African economies. To them, African achievement paled when viewed against the fruits of "the prevailing emphasis in Victorian society on material progress and production" (Kubicek 1990, 27) in Europe.

Africans practiced hospitality, and under peaceful conditions they exhibited a strong capacity to accept strangers into their midst. Whatever benefits came with it, the yoke of imperialism was burdensome and often humiliating. Africans often proved unsuccessful when they needed to define and establish their own positions vis-à-vis Europeans and other whites in the new, evolving social order.

Notable and sometimes dramatic acts of peaceful resistance and violent defiance certainly did occur on a variety of fronts in Malawi and many other regions. Examples include dramatic gestures such as the wholesale evacuation of a mission's hinterland by the resident African population (mostly adult males; Mufuka 1977), as well as seizure of the leadership of a mission by the local indigenous population (Gray 1990).

Among the more influential acts of resistance was the short-lived but long-remembered armed rising in 1915 led by John Chilembwe. With assistance from a white American missionary, Chilembwe studied theology in Virginia for a year. Most European planters and administrators already viewed him as a dangerous radical who stood against their natural right to exploit Africans. They were correct in the sense that he was committed to eliminate the cruelties, and if possible the perpetrators, of the harsh forced labor system practiced by Malawi's small but influential planter class. After his return home from Virginia, he was killed leading his followers in a desperate armed raid on the planters' homesteads. Chilembwe's death solidified his growing reputation as one of Africa's pioneer nationalists. For their part, the UMCA and most other missions chose to rationalize the grievances that Chilembwe represented.

In Malawi and elsewhere, the early missionaries generally defined and sought to control the upward social mobility of Africans who stayed connected with mission activities. Missionaries exercised a strong hand when they delimited the places and defined acceptable times for contact with Africans. In this way they successfully elevated themselves to positions within a dominant class essentially defined by the powers of race and resource control. Occasionally, exceptionally independent social thinkers emerged such as William Percival Johnson, the UMCA's heroic pioneer explorer and missionary, who spent fifty years in Malawi. Johnson was an extraordinary linguist whose life-long habit was to live in remote areas with, and in the manner of, his poor African followers. He was usually admired, and sometimes just tolerated, but never emulated by his missionary colleagues. His remarkable, seminal role in the UMCA's story is developed more fully in coming chapters.

In Malawi and British Africa generally, rigidly segregated spaces for Africans and European residential and family life grew increasingly commonplace, as the two groups became more familiar with each other. The latter change was often explained in terms of prevailing European beliefs about disease transmission, particularly the need to create "sanitary" spaces to combat the spread of malaria (Howard 1904). However, as the record will show, such social separation was conspicuously not a feature of the early pioneer years.

Mission stations stimulated the formation of new social geographies, ranging from interpersonal to interethnic relations in both new and well-established places. Conditioned by ecclesiastical-political authority, race, and culture, the emerging social relations included diverse elements such as churches, schools, and hospitals. In some localities missionary values dictated radical changes in African patterns of spousal cohabitation, and such developments could have pronounced effects on long-term demographic patterns (Greeley 1988). The presence of European women and children at many Protestant missions also added to the hybrid social structure of stations (Beidelman 1982, 13, 69–71, 224; Isichei 1995; Miller 1994, 59–64, 68). Beidelman, who writes about the Church Missionary Society in Tanganyika, asserts that this factor produced "a new and less flexible domestic colonialism" preoccupied with "the sexual accessibility or vulnerability of wives, with corresponding notions about the felt need for spatial and social segregation" (1982, 13).

Whether they came as missionary wives, unattached, or in religious orders, the arrival of European women in missions provided a new and direct opening to African women (Gray 1990). Missions that insisted on celibacy, such as the Anglo-Catholic Universities' Mission to Central Africa (UMCA), and the Roman Catholic White Fathers and White Sisters, also had to cope with sexual tension and repression among themselves as well as with Africans of the opposite and same sex (Beidelman 1982, 69–71; Hyam 1990).

Cultural Change

Sustained contact also brought culture change in both the host and missionary communities. Useful examples include acceptance of exotic medical practitioners, often-passionate demands for Western schools, and relations between the sexes. Other dimensions of adaptation and change—accomplished through addition, subtraction, and synthesis—embraced elements of material culture such as clothing, transport, and building construction. New relations of production, consumption, and exchange gained increasing importance in everyday life, including the use of a single currency and growth of a cash economy. Language, marriage, and descent-group authority also experienced pressures for uncontrolled change.

Cultural exchange on the African-missionary frontier was "always asymmetric" (Meinig 1982). Beidelman, a staunch critic of the missionary modus operandi, argues that they possessed a pronounced "cultural arrogance" and "represent[ed] the most naive and ethnocentric, and therefore the most thorough-going, facet of colonial life" (Beidelman 1982, 5). Whereas administrators and settlers also required subjected natives and often resorted to psychic domination, they generally had more modest goals. In contrast,

> missionaries invariably aimed at overall changes in the beliefs and actions of native peoples, at colonization of the heart and mind as well as body. Pursuing this sustained policy of change, missionaries demonstrated a more radical and morally intense commitment to rule than political administrators or businessmen. While missionaries deliberated about the results of their policies, in their repeated protestations that they pursued only sacred ends they underrated the impact of their deeds. (6)

Acculturation on the African-European frontier was selective, and its elements spread unevenly at different rates. Pressures for change typically weighed heaviest on the African populations most involved with and nearest to a mission. Impacts of the uninvited culture upon indigenous and other African groups represented in the mission field proved unbalanced and complex. Missionaries and their most loyal converts, in cooperation with colonial authorities, frequently attempted to coerce adaptation, as in efforts to denigrate and suppress polygyny, female circumcision (but not male circumcision), erotic and protest dances, and the influence of traditional healers and other ritual authorities (Good 1987). Missionaries also frequently demanded the rejection of African cultural forms that stood unopposed by Christian doctrine, and they sometimes pushed hard for a plainly absurd substitution of European for African practices (Irvine 1958).

Mission stations developed their own subcultures and typically became "islands of Christian conformity" vis-à-vis the wider and more differentiated colonial society (Beidelman 1982, 21). For their part, the Africans did not simply act as passive onlookers. Many adopted one set of behaviors inside the station and another on the outside. In time the "Mission Africans," often independent-minded folk to begin with, learned to read, write, and employ their new social and technical skills. They became an upwardly mobile, advantaged class in the emerging colonial system, differentiated and sometimes estranged from their unconverted family members and neighbors. Often they risked ostracism and even physical harm by refusing to conform to important tribal customs deemed un-Christian by their denomination (Leys 1926; Good 1991, and field notes).

In Malawi, upward mobility was more likely realized among mission Africans who came up through the Presbyterian system, with its work ethic and achievement values, than through the UMCA's. Extraordinary efforts by African converts greatly facilitated the popular spread of Christianity. In every part of Africa leading personalities emerged to create movements within as well as outside mission religion. These activities often bore a direct relationship to felt spiritual needs and desires of African individuals and societies as they confronted the general crisis of cultural contact and modernization.

New African religious impulses arose, sometimes meteorically, in response to the contradictions of colonial racial domination and privilege. Sometimes their political methods were passive, with the aim of maximizing distance from discrimination imposed by European churches. In other cases, such the 1915 Chilembwe uprising in Malawi, violent conflict followed the failure of peaceful strategies adopted by Africans to redress the deep grievances of a whole class of exploited Africans. Many small groups of Africans also appropriated and transformed certain Christian rites and symbols that acquired special political significance in forms such as prophecy and healing (Ranger 1982). Gray argues that Africans' openness to Christianity and general tolerance of religious diversity represent greater evidence of a healthy and flexible theological pluralism, than of syncretism with its "easy bridges back to nativism" (1990, 71–75).

On the other hand, the European missionary's need to maintain cultural identity was crucial to his or her self-image and mental health. Observing his countrymen during his travels in South Africa, James Bryce observed that "they are as much Englishmen in Africa as in England."[7]

Economic Change

Effective penetration of African territory by missionaries stimulated new economic relations and channels of population movement and exchange. Missions generated both positive and negative influences on local economies, affecting both villages and regions and stimulating new wants and expectations (Fountain 1966). In colonial Malawi, the stations of the Dutch Reformed Church Mission (DRCM) each had their own store and weekly markets, and the mission introduced its own currency (Pretorius 1972). The UMCA's two steamers stimulated a small amount of goods transport, buying and selling, and passenger transport as they sailed among the many tiny ports that emerged along the shores of Lake Malawi. As discussed below, the UMCA and some other mission societies remained passively opposed to encouraging African participation in the colonial economy. In contrast, the Free Church Scottish Presbyterians in Malawi actively supported labor migrancy, entrepreneurship, and upward mobility. Unlike most other missions, they often vigorously opposed the harsh labor policies of the protectorate and its white settlers (Sindima 1992).

Cole's (1960) analysis suggests that the missionary relationship to economic development may be seen as a series of stages. He asserts that missions exerted disproportionate influence relative to other social agencies operating in the same areas and periods. This was particularly the case "before the days of easy travel or of motion pictures or scientific journals." Cole argues that between 1700 and 1960, "missionaries coursing out of the nations of advanced economies and advanced civilizations may still be awarded the distinction of giving . . . greater stimulus toward economic development over a larger portion of the earth's surface than any other aggregate—and doing so with a system of communication ill adapted to that purpose" (1960, 127). In contrast, evidence from Malawi reveals how mission policies could also promote economic dependence and underdevelopment (McCracken 1977).

Psychological Imperialism

As imperial agents, missionaries relied upon a variety of psychological strategies to gain the allegiance of the "host" peoples. They summoned respect, approval, loyalty, and even fear by manipulating various symbols of authority, power, and prestige. Spatial expression of such objectives required conscious management of landscapes to project and optimize the visible and audible character of ecclesiastical places. Mission authorities designated new sacred and profane spaces (categories traditionally recognized in all African societies) and integrated them into the main stations and outstations.

Missionary use of traditional African building construction in the early years gave way to innovative adaptations of local materials used in both new vernacular and monumental architecture. Missionaries endowed sites on land they acquired from the indigenous people with churches and even grand cathedrals built in a European national or hybrid style. The UMCA's massive Likoma Cathedral, on Likoma Island in Lake Malawi, provides a spectacular, and enigmatic, example of religious and political place-making (fig. 1.3). Other significant elements of mission landscapes included religious icons, cemeteries, hospitals, schools, and official residences and gardens. The Church of Scotland mission headquarters at Blantyre in Malawi (1876), and especially its magnificent, mortarless and earthquake-resistant Church of St. Michael and All Angels, is a dramatic example of such site development.

For both Europeans and Africans, the materials, style, and scale of structures provided physical and symbolic evidence of the power and reach of ecclesiastical and imperial authority. Visible and potent distinctions in race,

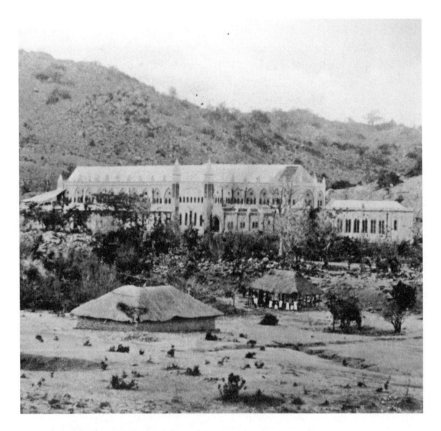

Figure 1.3. Likoma Cathedral.
(Source: The National Archives of Zimbabwe.)

culture, and class took the form of walls and gates; residential, recreational, and public spaces; separate sick places as seen in the placement of hospitals and dispensaries for Africans and Europeans; and clothing (Meinig 1982). Imperialism does reveal itself overtly and subtly in many different places, institutions, and under different guises, in both material and nonmaterial landscape features.

AFRICAN FRONTIERS

Frontiers exist in several dimensions. Often they are viewed as the leading edges of contested territories or physical zones that expand or contract in favor one group or another. Frontiers are also places of mind, where political, cultural, and economic ideologies and systems compete for preeminence. As Deveneaux (1978) observes them in African history, frontiers form "a meeting point, and area of interaction between different and sometimes conflicting concrete realities and philosophies" (68). Generally, frontiers do not represent fixed boundaries; rather, they mark "the moving fringes of an expansionist society" with missionaries, settlers, capitalists and other "frontiersmen" in the vanguard (75, citing Hancock 1942, ix).

During the last quarter of the nineteenth century the cultural diversity among the indigenous peoples of south-central Africa was undergoing unprecedented challenges from outside forces. These unsettling influences often led to growing insecurity and conflict, and to the displacement of African communities. Outside pressures on Africans came from slave traders and raiding, competing European imperial and territorial actions, and Muslim and Christian proselytizers. Territorial and psychological frontiers developed where these forces met, and the frontiers expanded and contracted with shifting alliances of convenience and competing claims to authority over people and space. The moving, discontinuous Afro-European frontier was highlighted by efforts to establish trade and military outposts, and eventually a number of permanent European settlements and plantations. Overall, Africans initially put up little effective resistance to European-driven developments. As for the European missions in Malawi, life was often complicated by the persistent slave trading in their midst and its connections to what they saw as Islam's stubborn expansion. Threat of attacks by African slavers, and the hostility of Muslim chiefs who wanted no part of the missionary agenda, caused the Christian foreigners continued anxiety.

In Deveneaux's analysis of the frontier, science and technology rank highest on the list of most significant Europeans contributions. D. Headrick (1981, 1988) underscores the validity of this interpretation. The development and transfer of innovations such as quinine, cordite, and steamboats, he asserts, not only powerfully influenced the timing and locations of European expansion; such advances actually motivated imperialist schemes (1981; 1988, 3–48). Kubicek (1990) also argues that the Victorian state leaned heavily on an uncritical acceptance of technology. Its willingness to transfer steamboat technology to West Africa led to a waterborne conquest that made the extension of formal colonial control in West Africa "inevitable" by an otherwise indifferent British government.

Christian missionaries served as "the foremost innovators" of technological change, including literacy. Practically every mission station introduced some new forms of technology (Gray 1990). At the same time, it is the African cultural elements that have prevailed and have "molded the success" of those elements of Western technology and Islam transplanted into Africa (Deveneaux 1978). One must certainly add Christianity to this accounting of alien cultural institutions "molded" by local forces (Gray 1990).

Cosmology, Culture, and Healing

African philosophy and religion was long ignored or negated by European scholars. Today, it is more widely appreciated that the powerful hold of African cosmology and spiritual life was underestimated as a frontier force capable of defending itself against European attempts to impose core changes from without.

In the case of African healing, the bonds of religion and traditional therapeutic systems were indivisible. Despite the growing presence of Western medicine and Christian teaching, African concepts of causation and ways of experiencing illness and misfortune remained predominantly and firmly anchored in African metaphysics. Ultimately, these powerful indigenous systems of thought, ritual, and behavior served as a kind of "cultural shield" against a too-rapid accommodation of European religious and secular culture.

African communities in Malawi generally incorporate several types of "traditional healers," including diviners, village and market herbalists, and diviner-herbalists. (I write in present tense because these traditional institutions retain much vitality today.) Other specialists include spirit healers, villages midwives (mature or elderly women), and faith healers. The latter belong to African independent, or healing churches, that have grown up outside the main denominations, such as Zion Christian Church (ZCC) and the African Apostolic Church of John Maranke (AAJM).[8] Devout Muslim teachers may also act as diviners, including the practice of geomancy (kupiga ramli, Arabic and Swahili) (Cox 1952; Trimmingham 1964, 124).

In Malawi generally, sing'anga (pl. asing'anga, ChiChewa) is the term used for all types of traditional healers. While their functions and skills often overlap, the most important distinction among healers is whether or not they practice divination, or possess some other ritual authority. Diviners, male and female, are medico-religious specialists. Through divination (maula, Nyanja; chisango, Yao) they have power to diagnose the source(s) of affliction in an individual or group,[9] and may recommend a course of action to the sufferer. These practitioners, often inaccurately grouped together and pejoratively labeled "witchdoctors," act as custodians of ritual and as intermediaries with God (Malungu), powerful ancestral spirits, and other sources of spiritual energy.

Much of a diviner's energies and time go into the treatment of physical, psychosomatic, and psychiatric illnesses. He or she really embodies many different qualities. Since the cultural explanation of "dis-ease" is tied to magico-religious concepts, the *sing'anga* is often engaged in "warding off evil influences." He or she is thus intrinsically linked to witchcraft and sorcery, and has a major role in the social control of these institutions (Morris 1989, 46). As Morris observes, the *sing'anga* "acts as an oracle, giving advice on some future venture or journey, or helping to discover the whereabouts of some stolen article. In articulating the social tensions within a community he often has a judicial role, serving to highlight community problems and conflicts, and thereby assisting in their eventual resolution" (Morris 1986, 376).

Herbalists empirically diagnose diseases and treat their patients with preparations made from numerous medicinal plants and occasionally other natural substances (*mankhwala*) (Morris 1989). Diviner-herbalists combine divining with the use of herbs. It is fair to say "herbalism and divination are inextricably linked in the Malawian therapeutic context" (Morris 1986, 376). Traditional midwives may also be ritual specialists and herbalists, and primarily treat infants, young children, and women.

Diviners, herbalists, and midwives are numerous and generally close at hand,[10] living and working in ways often identical to those of other villagers. They act as the primary guardians and conveyors of society's received religious cultural traditions. They have a responsibility to treat, as appropriate, the physical and psychosocial ills of individuals and the wider community. They attend to the ritual and spiritual needs of the living generations, the afterlife with ancestors, or shades, and those yet unborn. People consult one or more types of healer for appropriate rituals and for authoritative counsel in coping with the quandaries, misfortunes, and fears of daily living. Variously using physical, psychic, and kin-group therapies, healers shoulder responsibility to help ensure the ritual protection, reproduction, and survival of infants and young children, families, lineages, farms, livestock, and other economic and social assets. Any of these things could be at risk to an antagonist's ill-will, possibly identified as a witch or demon (*mfiti*), an angered ancestral spirit (*ufiti*), or depraved living persons such as night-time eaters of decaying human flesh (*wafiti*).[11]

Belief in human agency, and particularly in witches and the practice of witchcraft, and in sorcery, is a pervasive and often harmful mindset to which people customarily resort to explain much of the illness, misfortune, and death that accompany daily living. Bewitchment is a condition of the mind-body produced by apparent but unverifiable actions and projected thoughts of another person or agency. In Malawi, most witches are reportedly perceived as women, who are viewed as the "more emotionally and so-cially organized" of the sexes. Such women are thought to harbor and use inherent powers to harm people, or to perpetrate other antisocial actions. In contrast, sorcerers are thought to be primarily men, and are character-ized as "more rational" and operationally independent (Peltzer 1987, 153). They use poisons,[12] and "black" magic to harm or terrorize their victims. Both witches and sorcerers are known as *afiti* (sing. *mfiti*) in ChiChewa, the national language from 1968, and in ChiNyanja.[13]

The poison ordeal (*mwavi;* the poison used came from the *mwavi* tree, *Erythrophloem guiniense*) was a traditional form of jurisprudence. Adminis-tered by a ritual specialist, it was used to determine guilt or innocence in serious disputes. It was widespread in Malawi at the time of initial mis-sionary contact, although the practice apparently diminished after it was banned by the colonial government in 1911 (King and King 1991, 25). Dr. W. Elmslie, a Scottish missionary in Ngoniland from 1884 to 1924, wrote that "the number killed by the muave cup cannot be estimated." The UMCA's Archdeacon Johnson noted that a person charged with witchcraft had to drink the poison directly, whereas on lesser charges it might be given to a dog or fowl to determine guilt or innocence (Johnson 1922, 124).

In Malawi and most of Africa, decisions about choices and courses of therapy in a time of illness are usually not made by the individual(s) most directly concerned. Instead, some form of what Janzen calls a "therapy management group"—the close kin, friends, and significant others near the patient—has the prerogative to initiate treatment and collaborate with healers to devise a strategy for treating the problem. The composition of this group varies with the nature of the affliction, including its seriousness, longevity, and social and ritual implications. Sometimes the ill person does not attend a divination rite. Rather, it is a group of close kin who consult the diviner. Treatment may include both traditional and Western-type therapies (Janzen 1978; Morris 1989, 51; Good 1987; see also Devisch 1993; Shaw 2002). In Malawi, as discussed later, matrilineal descent and Islamic practices illustrate the importance of the social controls in therapy decision-making.

African religious beliefs and healing systems in Malawi remain viable to-day. They are inseparable, evolving elements of local cultures and their moral codes. Their customary, ultimate aim is to ensure the integrity and continu-ity of the lineage, which requires individuals and kin groups to give proper ritual care and respect to ancestral spirits (*mizimu*), to nonrelated, less power-ful spirits (*mashawe*), and to various nature spirits that are part of the natural environment. Many religious rituals also relate to different stages in the life cycle, including birth, adolescence, marriage, and death. For example, among the ChiChewa-speaking peoples of Malawi, Zambia, and Mozambique, the *nyau* secret societies sponsor *gule wamkulu,* a ritual "big dance," in which male spirit dancers (*vinyao*) wear animal or human masks (*nyau*). Traditionally, these dances occur as part of funeral ceremonies. They are synchronized with the agricultural slack season and the final stages of beer brewing. Today *nyau* are also staged on national holidays and as cultural shows.[14]

Spirit worlds play major roles in traditional Malawian religious beliefs and health-related practices (Nelson et al. 1975). Veneration of *mizimu,* including the most prestigious ancestral spirits of particular families, is accomplished through prayers and sacrifices offered by a lineage group head. Such practices can keep evil spirits responsible for sickness and other misfortune from entering a household. This ongoing communication with the spirits of departed ancestors serves to reinforce the idea of the family as a closely-knit kin group. Spirit veneration also "encourages conformity because ancestors serve as models that, at least theoretically, are not to be surpassed. Even among Christian[s] . . . few would deny that ancestral spirits are still influential" (103).

Divination can provide an acceptable explanation of why an event such as abnormal illness (sudden, dysfunctional, or chronic) or other misfortune occurs. Witchcraft can also support social mores, "since it particularly acts against the moral code[s] which are likely to bring about . . . acts of sorcery or accusations of witchcraft. In Shona society [Zimbabwe] a man who commits incest, for example, is regarded as a witch" (Chavunduka 1978, 78).

Naming or confirming a perpetrator, sorting out what had transpired through divination, and most importantly *why,* often makes the witch-finding of *asing'anga* a socially disruptive process complete with prospects of retaliation from the those alleged to be suspects. In the old days "wizards or witches, if convicted, are either burnt alive, sold into slavery, or simply expelled from the place" (Johnson 1922, 129).

Bewitchment can produce both somatic illness and spiritual turmoil in a person, and infect his or her wider social relations. The fear it causes sometimes kills. It is generally not a condition that the bewitched individual can manage alone. This observation is no less applicable today than it was before the powerful influences of modernity began to affect social life. In 1941, a UMCA study reported that "buying protection against witchcraft is now on a par with buying insurance against burglary in England" (Munday 1941, 101). Over thirty years later it was still appropriate to emphasize that the sweeping social and economic changes, and malaise, associated with modernization have "reinforced the belief in witchcraft because it seems to deal with forces that are not fully understood" (Nelson et al. 1975, 104). As the Comaroffs contextualize it today, "witches are modernity's prototypical malcontents. They provide—like the grotesques of a previous age—disconcertingly full-bodied images of a world in which humans seem in constant danger of turning into commodities, of losing their life blood to the market and to the destructive desires it evokes. . . . These desires are eminently real and mortal" (Comaroff and Comaroff 1993, xxix).

The existence of witchcraft and sorcery reflects the persistence of a strong, culturally conditioned undercurrent of fear in society. Such terror prospers in today's commodified compost heap of human envy, greed, insecurity, and desire for revenge. Occasionally such terror can be transformed into mass hysteria that sweeps through a village or school.

The perpetrators or "petitioners" of witchcraft are socially connected to the "victim," but need not be near in space. Fear is thus the fuel of witchcraft, and it can be manipulated for evil or good, depending on whether the vantage point is that of the "victim" or the intended "beneficiary."

On balance witchcraft can "cause" unfavorable events in someone else's life, or alternatively improve one's own position or status. For example, a jealous woman may be accused of avenging her own infertility and insecurity by "causing" some negative event to infect the psyche of someone such as a co-wife, or her sister-in-law. The event suffered by the "targeted" woman might be a miscarriage or even the death of an infant. Husbands and wives may seek help through divination and bewitchment to "bring back" a straying spouse.

A Struggle of Competing Orthodoxies

Terence Ranger (1975), desiring to dispel old stereotypes of African and missionary responses to one another, provides insightful generalizations about the various forms of confrontation that occurred in terms of time, place, and social context. He challenges the commonly held stereotype that encounters between indigenous African and European Christian systems of religion and healing necessarily confounded cultural communications. Ranger asserts, and the present study confirms, that a more complicated reality existed. African beliefs and practices were far from being inalterably opposed or incompatible with the purposes and offerings of Christian medical missions.

While Ranger's general point is irrefutable and invaluable, the strength of traditional African religion and health-related practices introduces still greater complexity. Probably the most remarkable feature about the cultural and territorial confrontations provoked by missionaries and other colonial Europeans was the resilience of African religious belief systems against this unprecedented incursion of outside influence. This view is buttressed by the well-known observation that sub-Saharan Africans generally rely on a human- and spirit-centered religious ontology, in which God is simultaneously immanent and impersonal. Deveaneaux (1978) draws upon the seminal work of Mbiti (1971) and others, and argues that this medico-religious focus provides an integrative force in African life that permeated and conditioned all thought and behavior, including responses to external challenges.

In time, missionary practice of Western medicine could justifiably claim measurable success in the treatment of certain diseases, including the use of techniques such as antisepsis, injections, and surgery. Africans might visit the dispensary or hospital, and eventually most who had access did just that. Yet missionary and secular medical authorities generally proved far less successful at neutralizing traditional African conceptions of illness etiology and therapeutic practices, including the use of traditional medico-religious specialists. Also important, as this study will reflect, is that mission societies displayed widely different interests, capacities, and success in their attempts to "capture" and benefit Africans through Western medicine.

Resort to African healers, and thus much of traditional African religion and medicine, was widely believed by missionaries to be antithetical to Christian values. Some individual missionaries developed a slightly more benign view of herbalists, whom they believed were practitioners of "white," or good, medicine. In contrast, diviners and ritual specialists were seen as purveyors of "black" or harmful medicine because they manipulated minds, called forth many kinds of spirits, and trafficked in evil potions and superstition.

Missions also often took distinctive positions in their attitudes and policies toward other features of African cultures. Significant controversies emerged among Protestant and Catholic missionaries concerning their tolerance level for indigenous practices, even as these institutions themselves underwent adaptation and change in response to other forces of colonialism. Prominent targets of concern and debate included polygyny, cohabitation outside marriage, drinking of alcohol, rites of passage that included erotic dancing (Londsdale 1968; Welbourne 1971), and local adaptations of Christian ceremonies such as spiritual healing (Ranger 1982). In general, Catholic missionaries in Malawi developed a reputation for greater leniency and more accommodation than did the Protestants in matters such as polygyny, drinking, and dancing.

It is inaccurate to argue that African religious concepts and traditional therapeutic practices remained immune to Christian ideas and missionary biomedicine. Some current scholarship asserts that many Africans appropriated Christianity because it offered them powerful new symbols (e.g., Satan) and resources to rely on in the perennial struggle to explain and combat the forces of evil. Most individual and group experiences with disease, epidemics, famine, infertility, broken relations, and unexplained death were, at a minimum, interpreted as brushes with evil (Gray 1990).

This book is a step toward understanding how African societies in Malawi and beyond adapted missionary and government medical services to their own needs in the new colonial environment. High hurdles to understanding the African side of the "medicine and change" equation remain. The availability of elderly folk who witnessed some part of the colonial period, and who can capably recall it, is nearly depleted. There is a shortage of scholars, African and expatriate, to collect and interpret oral history.

As Kenyan historian Osaak Oumwalla observes, in many places the written documentation left by missionaries, administrators, and other Europeans is plentiful. Yet those materials rarely embody African voices, and usually little can be gained from them about how colonialism changed the cultural production of knowledge in the indigenous population. Ultimately, it must be recognized that "the wider world [was] is not external to the local community; it is at the heart of the community's internal processes of differentiation" (Olumwalla 2002, 12).[15]

Until more African sources are found and heard, at least half of the story of how the introduction of biomedical services and foreign technologies affected colonial Africans' daily lives, social space, and cultures will remain in obscurity. The same principle also operates to restrict understanding of the reciprocal influences of African change on the institutions and actions of missions and other colonial agencies. I merely begin to address these some of issues in chapter 7 (see section headed "Go Ask the Old Men": Tapping Personal and Institutional Memory).

Colored postcards published by the UMCA and other mission societies offer powerful insights about the early missionary ethos—how they saw themselves in relationship with Africans and how they desired to be portrayed to the public at home. One such card, "The Healer," by Harold Copping, shows a European doctor on one knee outside his tent in an African village (fig. 1.4).[16] Wearing a pith helmet and spectacles, he attends an adolescent boy who sits on the ground in a weakened condition, supported from behind by his bare-breasted mother. The boy's father, whose newly bandaged arm indicates that he has already been treated, and an older child, look on in rapt attention. A life-size image of Christ, as the Great Physician, stands close behind the doctor, diffusing holy light over the scene. The doctor's black medicine bags lay open on the ground exposing

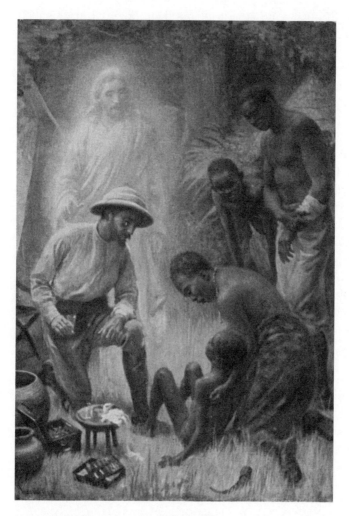

Figure 1.4. "The Healer," by Harold Copping.
(Source: Council for World Mission, London.)

numerous vials of medicines and small tools. An antelope horn lies a few feet away, visible but removed from prominence. The horn seems intended to symbolize the poverty and futility of magical native healing in the face of European curative medicine. This emotive scene shows emergent scientific medicine undergirded by the power of the Holy Spirit. It aims to reinforce the legitimacy of missionary healing as an all-powerful process and subtly conveys the European sense of cultural superiority.

Such postcards portrayed a variety of mission ideals and activities, and were sent home to encourage financial and moral support from the faithful in Britain. Simply stated, their main themes converge on the paramount notion that Africans needed missionaries, and would otherwise remain "degenerate." Was Africa not overburdened by hopeless suffering, and also a "patient," acutely in need of healing through Christian evangelism and the example of a European "civilizing" mission? What more was needed to justify the self-invited entry of missions, as generic and de facto agencies of imperialism, into Africa?[17]

Matched against the empiricism of scientific medicine, Europeans viewed indigenous African medicine as interesting and sometimes even awe-inspiring in its mysterious and pervasive grip on people's thought patterns and behavior. It did not take long for missionaries to realize that indigenous medico-religious institutions placed tough obstacles in the way of Euro-peanized Christian evangelism. African medicine in Malawi and elsewhere was holistic in theory and practice, serving as the irreducible mind-body hub of the social order. While the concept of natural, God-given illness was well known, few health-related events happened according to the new European concept of probability. Most illness and accidents could be connected to webs of human agency and supernatural forces that conditioned and sanc-tioned personal and social behavior. Bewitchment, broken rules or taboos, and other ritual offenses figured prominently in illness causation. Treat-ment ranged from divination (*kuombeza ula*) and the varied use of powerful, God-sent plant medicines, to confession and group therapy.

Thoughtful missionaries and others who tried to understand indigenous medical systems recognized that they faced an extraordinary cultural force that was slightly pervious yet basically unyielding in its core institutions and values. As late as 1952, the UMCA's Canon Cox wrote at length to *Central Africa* readers about the ongoing need to warn African Christians that the church forbade them to consult with a diviner (*mwene ula*) when they became sick. The "worst evil" was the diviner's common suggestion to a client that he or she had been bewitched. Invoking bewitchment meant, from a mission interpretation, that "he constantly revives old enmities," sometimes even splitting villages through his accusations, in contrast to "the Christian law of love and forgiveness" (*CA* 70 [1952]: 99–107).

Missionaries tended to treat local medicine as the "dark" side of African life, as a primitive and pervasive feature that Christianity might one day neutralize and reduce to a mere side-show. In hopes that it could be de-centered, indigenous medical practice was best kept at a physical and psychic distance. Europeans were much less preoccupied with herbalism than with the mystifying, more obviously supernatural aspects of traditional healing, such as divination, veneration of the ancestors, "witch-finding," antisorcery practices, and ritual protection of newborns, homesteads, crops, and fields. Both missionary and secular colonial authorities viewed and feared this holistic religious dimension of healing as "pagan," and a real or potential threat to European authority. Typically, a diviner was (appropriately) seen as "a man or woman of ability and with a wide knowledge of the affairs and especially of the quarrels of a very large district" (*CA* 70 (1952): 101). Their roles gave them access to social control through "stirring up" quarrels, antiwitchcraft rituals, and *mwavi* (poison) ordeals. Most traditional diviners wielded considerable influence in their own communities, and some were respected and feared well beyond their own districts. This remains true today.

African *materia medica* was based on an extensive variety of plants, and to much lesser extent animal products, collected in the fringing vegetation around compounds, and in fields and forests. African therapies depended greatly on these plants, which were prepared for external application or ingestion, for relief of physical symptoms as well as for ritual and supernatural purposes. In practice, knowledge of plants, appropriate combinations of plant derivatives, specific therapeutic uses, and dosages showed considerable variations according to the healer, the place, and ethnic group. What was known of the specifics of claimed pharmacological actions and values of herbs was mostly retained in the memories of practitioners. This indigenous technology and ritual did not circulate widely. When it was passed down it was done orally and privately, most commonly to a younger apprentice.

In colonial times some European doctors, as is true of some African medical doctors today, privately admitted that they believed certain African therapies they had heard about in the course of their work seemed to have benefit, such as herbal teas, inhalation treatments, and massage. Occasionally, stories circulated about the favorable pharmacological action of a certain plant-based remedy on fevers, digestive disorders, swelling, and other maladies. Many concoctions appeared harmless. Others definitely had harmful effects, including certain treatments for eye infections such as conjunctivitis and, of course, known poisons. Also, some Western-trained medical personnel sporadically sent mentally ill, "psychosomatic," terminal, and other refractory cases *to* traditional healers.[18]

Herbalists posed little threat to missionary medicine or public order, to the extent that they did not practice divination or other magico-religious observances deemed incompatible with Christian or European values. Occasionally, "good" herbalists might receive a nominal stamp of approval from European medical workers, based on the latter's personal experiences or hearsay. Few scientific studies of African medicine, based on experiment and observation, were made anywhere during the colonial period.

During the colonial era African medicine continued to function "in the sunshine" and often underground as well. Secretive practices emerged in response to efforts by missionaries and the colonial state to suppress, if not eradicate, what mystified Europeans called witchcraft.[19] While witchcraft was (and is) a pan-African belief system with regional variations, objectively no one had ever actually seen it. Yet all Africans knew that its consequences could be deadly. Attempts to eradicate witchcraft beliefs and practices had to confront a deeply institutionalized fear system that is grounded in the art of secrecy and control of the believer's mind (Good 1987).

In time, Africans grafted numerous Western medical and health practices onto their indigenous therapeutic systems, resorting to them as they perceived a need. Most Africans used their own therapies[20] and mission medicine, or other available therapies, serially or concurrently. To the consternation of medical missionaries, intentional efforts to Westernize African ideas of causality and to Christianize certain African practices generally proved ineffective (Ranger 1981). A significant result of the contact between the missionary and African frontiers of knowing was the emergence of an evolving medical pluralism (Good 1987). The UMCA and other missions also witnessed another form of African cultural therapeutic strength in the broad appeal of African separatist churches. These were syncretistic institutions spawned by alienation from conventional mission dogma. Their formation was sometimes reinforced by the European practice of segregation of themselves from Africans in Christian worship. Separatists gained converts because they offered customary means of individual and community healing that the foreign churches overlooked.[21]

THE IDEA OF MEDICAL MISSIONS

I WAS SICK AND YE VISITED ME. . . . INASMUCH AS YE HAVE DONE IT UNTO ONE OF THE LEAST OF THESE MY BRETHREN, YE HAVE DONE IT UNTO ME.

Matthew 25:36, 40

THE MEDICAL MISSIONARY SHOULD BE A REAL MISSIONARY. HIS PRIMARY COMMISSION IS TO PREACH THE GOSPEL, NOT TO HEAL THE SICK.

Mercy and Truth (1897)[22]

Science, Medicine and Missions: Change with Convergence

Ask a thoughtful person today about the purposes and activities of foreign missionaries in colonial Africa and it is almost certain that medical care (together with evangelization and education) will rank among the top three roles mentioned. In fact, for a long time the reality was quite different. In most missionary circles there was little notice or acceptance of a connection between medicine, healing, and evangelization until the closing decades of the nineteenth century. Certainly there was no mandate to do more than evangelize.

Today, with the potential of modern medicine more obvious, it may be difficult to appreciate the perspective of Victorian Europeans on health matters. For instance, why did the pioneer mission societies delay giving medical work a high priority? One report asserts that no more than thirteen European medical missionaries existed worldwide in 1852. From 1851 to 1870 the Church Missionary Society (CMS) did not encourage applications from people with medical training. In fact, of the 307 new missionaries recruited during this period only seven were doctors (C. Williams 1982, 271). Explanations of this situation point to evidence that "preaching was the authentic medium of mission" throughout most of the nineteenth century (Warren 1967, 93). Public acceptance of this form of evangelization effectively restrained any concerted effort that might attempt to bring medical work into the mainstream of missionary endeavor. Warren's critique is most penetrating when he asserts that the prevailing ethos surrounding mid-Victorian health care was tinged by a callousness toward physical suffering and ignorance of its treatment. Disease and illness might also reflect degrees of consequences (sin and guilt) brought on by the individuals' transgressions and guilt.

In mid-Victorian Britain, at least, the medical profession was not well organized and enjoyed little prestige. A "fierce confrontation" had developed between British herbalists schooled in Thomsonian medical botany and orthodox medical doctors. The competition was fueled by shifts in patient attitudes, including a greater acceptance of vegetable substances thought to be less toxic, and a growing disapproval of toxic organic and inorganic medicines. Holism was gaining popularity, stimulated in part by disdain for doctors who tended to neglect the patient as a person. Geographically, herbalism was most strongly concentrated in the Industrial Midlands and the North, with a secondary focus south of Birmingham (Brown 1985). Doctors' status and prestige rested on shaky ground. Their tenuous position probably helps to account for the fact that the Church Missionary Society, which was among the very first to introduce substantial medical activities, generally required that doctors be ordained before they could serve (Warren 1967).

The first permanent medical work by Protestant men and women missionaries in West Africa began in the 1860s, although a large percentage of them—including all the American Baptists—were either killed by disease or invalided home. The Baptists' leader, Rev. Tom Bowen, was strongly wedded to miasmatic theories. Bowen believed, for example, that establishing settlements on hilltops was hazardous because winds carried malaria upslope. He also thought malaria was attracted to and absorbed by water, and that low-lying riverbanks were relatively healthier places. Unfortunately, Bowen's ideas of disease ecology proved responsible for numerous poorly located and thus disease-prone mission stations (Bowen 1857, cited in Schram 1968). His miasmatic legacy, the rise of herbalism, and the "pre-microbial" tools of orthodox practitioners offer a glimpse of the pluralism that characterized the medical world of missionaries and Europe generally in the late nineteenth century.

Popular notions about the proper roles for mission societies dramatically changed during the second half of the nineteenth century. The revolution in thinking and practice that ushered in the biomedical era was crucial in moving the wider missionary establishment to make a long-term commitment to some minimal level of medical care for Africans.

A "decisive turn" toward a scientifically oriented concept and practice of human medicine did not occur until the last quarter of the nineteenth century. This change was powered by a "leap forward" in medical knowledge that stimulated a radical recasting of professional and lay images of medicine's nature, scope, and possibilities (Janssens 1971). Germ theory, the idea of specific etiologies, and the specialist sciences of bacteriology, epidemiology (including the critical role of biological vectors), and surgery exploded onto the scene. These developments brought power shifts that propelled scientific professionalized medicine, and society at large, into an era of "curative confidence."[23]

Meanwhile, tropical medicine, together with sanitary engineering and military medicine, was finding increasingly prominent niches (Curtin 1989). The field's rapid emergence owed as much to the build-up of empires as to the spectacular growth of the biological sciences. People such as Patrick Manson, a key player in the development of the malaria-mosquito hypothesis in 1894, and author of *Tropical Diseases: A Manual of the Diseases of Warm*

Climates (1898), and Ronald Ross (his study of malaria in birds in India confirmed the Manson hypothesis in 1897–98)[24] brought instant credibility to tropical medicine (Chernin 1992). In addition to malaria etiology, incremental, practical advances occurred in understanding and controlling bubonic plague, relapsing fever, sleeping sickness, cholera, yaws, rinderpest, onchocerciasis, and other diseases. Numerous medical research laboratories opened in Africa in the 1890s, including Boma (1894), St. Louis (1897), Dar-es-Salaam (1897), and Leopoldville (1899). By 1930, another fourteen had been founded (Janssens 1971). Medical science also became engaged in the production of new and increasingly effective drugs, although Africans seemed to have had little access to them for decades. This era was further distinguished by the opening of Britain's first university schools of tropical medicine at Liverpool, Edinburgh, and London.

Outsiders generally viewed tropical African environments—outside the true highlands—as places of hyper-unhealthiness, where insidious disease agents lay in wait for innocents and fools. Few reflected on the host of ways in which imperialism and colonialism promoted unprecedented population mobility and mixing, upsetting natural systems and the balance of human-environment relations (Ford 1971; Kjekshus 1977; Good 1978). In certain missions, some of the ruling patriarchs fell back on "stick-in-the mud" conservatism and continued to dispute the value of doctors in missions at all. Yet by the 1890s it was widely recognized that mission societies could not ignore the opportunities and social expectations inherent in the rapidly growing prestige and possibilities of scientific medicine. At the same time, benevolence in the forms of altruism, good works, and compassion for the lives of those less fortunate was gaining popularity in Victorian society. Its impetus came on the one hand from the puritan stream, not infrequently Scottish, and increasingly from other Europeans, believers or not, who valued the ideal of Christian charity (Williams 1982). The popularity of benevolence as a spiritual act increased as beliefs in the eternal damnation of the heathen diminished. Williams argues that in this process "the compulsion to save the 'perishing heathen' had been replaced by the desire to spend a useful life improving the lot of fellow humanity—a task for which the doctor was eminently suited" (279).

The Medical Missionary Society had formed in London in 1878. By the 1870s many mission societies had begun to recruit nurses for the field. At the start of this "Nursing Era" tropical diseases and their remedies remained poorly understood, but they still demanded palliative treatment, at least. Primary responsibility for the care of fevers, dysenteries, and "sanitary" diseases and prevention techniques (e.g., food and water handling) became the province of skilled nurses, whose efficiency had recently been demonstrated in the Crimean War (Anderson 1956).

As the Victorian Age drew to a close it was clear that missionaries could not long remain isolated from or immune to medicine's growing professionalization. Armed with university qualifications, "medical men" now rose quickly to positions of unprecedented authority within missionary societies. By 1914 the doctor and his cadre of nurses and native assistants was practically a universal feature of mission landscapes. At home and in the mission field, faith in scientific medicine grew in proportion to its sometimes-startling accomplishments, the reproduction of doctors, and its widening prestige, thanks largely to media exposure. Competing therapies felt the squeeze as epidemiology, surgery, and biomedicine in general started to acquire unprecedented popularity at home. By World War I, medical pluralism was considerably less diverse, at least in terms of social practice and identity, in Western Europe and North America than a generation earlier. With the arrival of missionaries, just the opposite process was occurring in Africa and other colonial spheres.

In this new spirit of scientific medicine, the raison d'être of medical work emerged as a subject of serious discussion among influential insiders and professionals in the surging mission movement. The topic spawned lively, often hair-splitting position papers over philosophical and procedural points, over whether a medical missionary's first obligation was to practice medicine or to evangelize. The debates spanned medical missions from Africa to China and stretched over several decades. For many this issue of balance was never fully resolved even after several decades of experience with medical work (Allen 1927).

It is important not to lose sight of the continuity that characterized the development of medical missions. Speaking to medical students at a conference in London in 1900, Dr. Herbert Lankester referred to nineteenth-century medical missionaries as the missionary army's "heavy artillery" (Lankester 1897, 250). While acknowledging the late growth of institutionalized medical missions, he cautioned against forgetting they had a lineage. At least from the late eighteenth century, "generations of missionaries carried out a form of pillbox ministry, gravely administering draughts, lancing excrescences and proceeding by trial and error" in such places as Calabar, the Pacific, India, and the Central Africa of Livingstone (Walls 1982, 287, n. 11, citing Lankester). Nevertheless, these primitive "pillbox" ministrations by missionaries who lacked professional credentials in scientific medicine inevitably lost credibility in missionary circles as qualified nurses and doctors became more numerous (Walls 1982).

The Medical Missionary: Visions of Purpose

It was commonly believed that a missionary doctor could expect to labor hard for Africans' trust and confidence in his hospital methods and treatments; to expect quick acceptance would be unrealistic. Many obstacles and vested interests confounded medical work. Locked in a struggle for cultural dominance, some missionaries such as the CMS's Robert Keable militantly pursued scapegoats: "the Mohammedan teacher, the medicine man, and the witch doctor," he said, unite to discredit the missionary and to ridicule his motives, and dissuade people from going to him (Dale 1925, 241).

The rush to embrace scientific medicine in the late nineteenth century helped to shape and define the credibility of medical missions. If Williams's interpretation is correct, mission leaders did not so much pioneer a new connection between healing and souls as "succumb to the pressures from the enthusiasts and to the mounting consensus of a society which was increasingly convinced that it should alleviate physical suffering, as it was doubtful it possessed any eternal truths" (Williams 1982, 285). At the same time, strong beliefs and internal tensions over how to interpret the theological foundations and limits of medical work continued to check any tendency for the mission doctor to misinterpret and overplay his professional role. In 1893 the UMCA's Charles Smythies, Bishop of Nyasaland, viewed the model medical missionary as a doctor who "uses all his medical knowledge for a missionary end; whose aim is to use the great influence which his profession gives him to draw his patients to the love of God; who longs not only for the healing of bodies but for the salvation of their souls" (*CA* 11 [1893]: 51).

Paradoxically, there was also a growing sense of awe in the new medicine's observable power to draw Africans into the missionary orbit, thereby creating opportunities to lead them from "darkness into light." Smythies recognized this condition and its implications for medical education, observing candidly:

There are some mission fields in which only doctors seem to be able to gain any great influence. There is a fantastic hatred to Christianity, which can only be broken down by sympathy shown for sufferings of the body, to which all are liable, together with the power to alleviate them. It seems as if it is only through medical work, which is sure in the long run to be welcomed, that an opening to the hearts of these people can be found. (*CA* 11 [1893]: 51)

In 1885, when the UMCA returned to the Malawi mission frontier to stay, the society had already determined that the medical missionary was a professional whose time and skills had arrived. A "very great" need for doctors was becoming a standard plea in the Nyasa and Masasi districts. Recruitment of committed personnel for the mission field was now opened to include individuals who lacked the financial means and completeness of training to serve as doctors. They could now avail themselves of "Medical Missionary Studentships" offered by the Society for Promoting Christian Knowledge (SPCK). Tenable for up to four years, these awards carried an annual stipend of £150. The terms under which an individual might qualify for a SPCK studentship reflected a growing consensus among British mission societies about the integral nature of evangelism and medical work. To do one and neglect the other was in effect a misappropriation and dubious application of one's medical and ministerial calling. It was intended that qualified applicants would be drawn from:

1. Medical men, who having completed their predoctoral education, are willing to go through the training needed for ordination and, after being ordained, to go out to exercise their medical skill and experience as missionaries among the heathen.

2. Clergymen who are willing to go through the needful training for the medical profession, and, after obtaining their diploma, to go out as missionaries as those described under class No. 1.

3. Medical men who, having completed their medical training, desire to undertake lay mission work among the heathen, and are willing to undergo at least one year's training with that object. (CA 3 [1885]: 141–42)

These additional, time-consuming conditions of recruitment to medical missionary service filtered out many doctors who were not ordained yet who may otherwise have gone to the mission field. This policy, which lasted until 1899 in Malawi, and the requirement that European staff members remain celibate certainly contributed to the chronic difficulties the UMCA had in finding doctors throughout the mission's entire existence. Only unusual individuals could be expected to forego a career and family life in Britain for the isolation and uncertainties of the mission field.

In Malawi the UMCA did not secure the full-time services of a doctor until 1899, fourteen years after the diocese's re-establishment. In the meantime, the missionaries often had no doctor at all due to illness or absence. For more than a decade they experienced notoriously high rates of mortality and morbidity that decimated their ranks. In 1894, Dr. Fred Robinson of Guys

Hospital, London, arrived to serve as the mission's Medical Officer (MO) with the primary charge of looking after the missionaries' health. Robinson had filled the post for only a few months when he became so ill that he was invalided to England. John Hine, Bishop of Likoma, and an Oxford graduate with a medical degree from London, stepped into the breach to serve as the mission's MO until 1899. Hine was personally more inclined to his pastoral work than to medicine, and was eager have another doctor take over the work.[25]

It was widely believed by the 1890s that missionary medicine in the British dominions offered unparalleled opportunities for proselytizing and discipleship. The key proviso was that medicine should not be allowed to take precedence over the doctor's fundamental charge of saving heathen souls. In his global review, *The Way of the Good Physician* (1915), Dr. Henry Hodgkin of the Church Missionary Society typified the outlook of many Protestant missions:

> The medical mission is, in both its aspects, a presentation of the Gospel, and no man can truly claim the title of medical missionary who does not believe that he is proclaiming his message in the acts of healing as truly as in the spoken sermon. To exalt either aspect of the work in antithesis to the other is to miss the inmost meaning of the medical missionary's vocation. (Balme 1921, 23–24)

By the mid-1890s, missionaries representing dozens of denominations were rapidly expanding their presence across eastern and southern Africa. Malaria and blackwater fever were rife and virulent among Europeans, yet tended not to be life threatening among adult Africans who experienced repeated exposure. Improved sanitary control and prevention and treatment of many microbial diseases now seemed within reach.

Ignorance of malaria transmission and the absence of professional medical care meant that missionary staffs had high levels of exposure and great risk of infection until the twentieth century. Death, especially from malaria, exacted a heavy toll among the UMCA's men and women in Nyasaland. Their mortality rate rose to a disastrous 120 per thousand in 1897–98.[26] Public alarm in England finally pressured the Foreign Office to support an on-site investigation. In 1899, about the time Ross presented his mosquito-malaria cycle, the Royal Society sent a Malaria Commission to Africa with instructions to visit Malawi first. Mortality from malaria (but not blackwater fever) began to ease dramatically the following year, dropping to 27 per thousand for the statistical year 1904–5 (Howard 1908, 3). Within a few more years malaria was seen as "the only disease with which European settlers in British Central Africa have to contend" (ibid.). Dr. Howard, who became the mission's first, full-time Medical Officer in 1899 and a vigorous campaigner for public health, attributed their local success against malaria to improved staff housing, expansion of the medical and nursing staff, and better medical screening of volunteers for mission prior to acceptance for an African assignment. However, few who qualified as doctors in Britain or elsewhere seemed prepared or willing to sacrifice their own careers and health for the sake of the UMCA's "received" mandate.

Almost as soon as he arrived in Malawi, Robert Howard began a comprehensive investigation of the human ecology of malaria up and down the UMCA's sphere on eastern side of the lake (Howard 1904, 1908). Decades later the improvements Howard had facilitated in the health of UMCA staff members continued to be described as "almost miraculous" (Wilson 1936, 110). He oversaw the destruction of mosquito breeding sites and widely promoted progressive forms of malarial prophylaxis, including adoption of the various barrier methods. Mission staffs were admonished to use mosquito nets, stay indoors from sunset onwards to avoid Anopheles bites, and practice "segregation from native children" in the evenings. Quinine was valued "as a subsidiary measure," although it was seen as "the least certain . . . [strategy] if employed alone" (Howard 1908, 16).

A Paramedical Strategy

In 1893, a conference of doctors sponsored by the Church Missionary Society established Livingstone College in London "for the instruction of foreign missionaries in the elements of practical medicine" (Hailey 1956, 1066). The nine-months' course at Livingstone was conceived as a way to enable missionary recruits and veterans to improve their chances of keeping themselves and their communities fit, and better able to survive the health insults they would inevitably encounter in the field. Lectures dealt with tropical diseases, hygiene, basic physiology, and surgery. Attendance at hospital clinics gave students practical exposure. It was emphasized, however, that graduates of the course could not expect to call themselves "medical missionaries" or to take over the positions of "qualified medical men" (ibid.). Given the growing prestige and gate-keeping capabilities of certified physicians and medical scientists, paramedical education was at best a stopgap measure, not a solution to the scarcity of real doctors.

Livingstone College remained a unique institution in Europe until 1906, when a German counterpart was established. By then this institution had already drawn members of mission societies from several countries for elementary medical training, and more were expected.[27] The college claimed that completion of the course gave a missionary sufficient training "to teach the hygiene required in tropical climates, and to deal scientifically with outbreaks of epidemics."[28] Such training promised to have "direct application to problems of defective sanitation in native tropical towns or districts," and it qualified the missionary "to instruct others, more especially children in native towns."[29] This loftier aim for graduates, to apply their practical training in public health matters to the benefit of the indigenous peoples, could not have had more than minimal influence on the well-being of Africans. After all, the college's primary purpose was still

> to safeguard the health and lives of missionaries, and whilst old students . . . were in many cases able to relieve much suffering among natives, and save many lives, yet they were not allowed to call themselves medical missionaries, nor could they do the work of such.[30]

Livingstone College attracted support from influential representatives of the Church of England, the medical community, and the universities. Sir Patrick Manson delivered the address on the college's Commemoration Day in 1908, by which time 299 students, including 56 associated with the Church of England, had finished the course. Anglican postings ranged across the entire realm of British imperialism, from Malawi and Uganda to Melanesia, mid-China, and the Falklands. This same year the UMCA's Medical Board in London approved a resolution requiring all its missionaries to obtain "at least" a certificate in first aid, sanitation, and hygiene, and urged that some should be required to attend Livingstone College.[31]

By 1910, ten British and six continental missionary societies had trainees at Livingstone. The institution had not become self-supporting, and its niche as a place that specialized in providing less than a full medical education was uncertain. In his annual review, the principal offered anxious commentary about the lower than expected enrollments, particularly from among "the great British Missionary Societies," and the decreasing subscriptions and donations.[32]

Medical Missions: Theory Revisited

The writings and firsthand reports of Livingstone, followed by other late-nineteenth-century explorers and travelers, dramatically strengthened the missionary movement. Livingstone had extensive direct experience with the slave trade, including that within the Lake Malawi region. His fervent messages to the outside world characterized East and Central Africa as "sick" and "wounded" places, afflicted by the depravity and humiliation of the slave trade, heathenism, and the spread of Islam. He was emphatic in his views that Africa's best hope lay in the abolition of slavery, its opening up to the civilizing influences of Christianity and legitimate trade, and ultimately the integration of its vast interior with Christian Europe (Kimambo 1989; Vaughan 1991, chap. 3).

Through most of the colonial period, certainly to World War II, medical and nonmedical missionaries generally perceived Africa as a danger to itself, a continent inhabited by backward, pagan peoples who suffered from inherent illness and a host of indigenous, pathological evils and defects. While important differences in concept and practice existed between Protestant and Roman Catholic missions, and respectively between their sects and orders, the general discourse of missionaries was steeped in the idea that "suffering and sin were inseparable" (Vaughan 1991, 66). Africans' sick bodies mirrored the sickness of their souls. If patients became well after treatment, "the physical transformation was taken as a direct sign" of their potential or actual spiritual transformation (64). Thus, according to some interpreters, it was just a short step for many missionaries (and mission-educated Africans) to the belief that disease, the African condition, was "the sweat of sin in Adam" (Beidelman 1982, 110). Health, on the other hand, was "an external sign of inner salvation" that could only be won through the mediation of the Good Physician (ibid.). The seeding of Christianity in African soil would be facilitated by missionaries' use of "medical tools" for the "introduction or restoration of health in a sick universe, the establishment of order in a world of disorder, madness, corruption, and diabolical illusions" (Mudimbe 1988, 52, cited in Olumwalla 2002, 113).

In 1912, Godfrey Dale, the UMCA's Canon of Zanzibar, felt compelled to contrast secular and missionary medicine as distinct planes. For government doctors, he said the primary business "is to look after Government servants, whether European or native, and the care of non-Government patients is added as a secondary consideration; whereas the Medical Mission exists to demonstrate practical Christianity, and makes its appeal to all who come to it" (Dale 1925, 240).

Alice Simpkin, a UMCA nurse in Malawi who had been "trained to full efficiency in a great London hospital [St. Bartholomew]," described a "lifeboat" concept of missionary medicine in her memoirs. Simpkin served the UMCA from 1914 to her death in 1935, during which time she became one of the mission's most effective nurses, managers, and benefactors. In her view:

> The astounding cures worked by the new injections, or the restoration to sight of a patient suffering from cataract, are even to the looker-on from a distance an obvious miracle, but what must they be to the sufferer? Imagine the power of the Gospel when preached to patients by the person who has saved them from a life of misery or dependence on grudging relatives. The bodily help is a guarantee of the reality of the spiritual blessing offered. (Simpkin 1926, 21)

As doctors gained in professional status their role in missions also acquired unprecedented influence within the worldwide missionary movement. Medical practice was increasingly viewed as a plane of Christian witness comparable to that of ordained ministers of the Word. Williams's position is that "medical missions, far from being subordinate to the spiritual, were rather its necessary expression" (Williams 1982, 282).

Most missionary doctors saw themselves as too occupied with their curative calling, their occasional preventive initiatives, and administrative responsibilities to take advantage of their singular opportunities for research and publication. Dr. Robert Howard's studies (e.g., Howard 1908) on malaria ecology rank as one of the important exceptions. However, by the mid-colonial period other missionary doctors had also begun to contribute to scientific medico-epidemiological studies. Specific examples include C. C. Chesterman (Congo) on drug therapy (tryparsamide) in connection with a rapidly expanding foci of Gambian sleeping sickness; and A. C. Fisher (Congo) on schistosomiasis (Browne 1979). While mission doctors did not in general take the lead role in medical science, many recognized that "the future of imperialism lay with the microscope" (Lyons 1988, 245).

TECHNOLOGY AND MEDICINE FACILITATE THE UMCA'S RISE IN MALAWI

Uses for a specific technology, the timing of its introduction, and its strategic value varied from one mission field to another. Where a mission society chose to locate its base and outstations, and how its underlying philosophy was understood, often proved decisive with respect to how much technology it could access and introduce.

Markedly different views of technology occurred among missions operating in essentially the same regional environment. For example, in late precolonial and early colonial Malawi, the Free Church of Scotland Mission (FCSM) headed by the powerful Dr. Robert Laws vigorously sought to stimulate a capitalist economic revolution that would benefit both Africans and European settlers. In the early days Laws collaborated closely with the privately operated African Lakes Corporation. Aided greatly by introduction of river and lake steamers, this Scottish trading firm proved successful at commercial penetration of the lake region and its northern hinterland. Beginning in the mid-1890s, Dr. Laws launched ambitious training programs for Africans in industrial trades, engineering, and entrepreneurship as well as in bookkeeping, teaching, and the ministry. Some 302 pupils were receiving instruction in 1897 (Laws 1898). Laws installed hydroelectric power to run machinery and provide lighting, and promoted agricultural experimentation and the training of medical orderlies (Gelfand 1964; McCracken 1977; Livingstone 1921).

As the twentieth century opened, Laws's economic philosophy and educational policy attracted thousands of Africans into the Livingstonia mission's sphere and the colonial labor system. Using rhetoric appropriate to the "globalizing" world of the twenty-first century, Laws (unwittingly echoing Marx's words) advised his peers in 1908 that the "annihilation of space" by electricity and improved surface communications had made it possible for even the most peripheral peoples to benefit from exchange with "complex civilizations." The world, he said, "has become one market, to which every nation may bring its own wares.... The world is rapidly becoming one workshop."[33]

Livingstonia's training programs did benefit the colonial economy. They also provided impressive opportunities for individual achievement and upward mobility among its graduates, who migrated by the hundreds to the Rhodesias and South Africa.[34]

In the neighboring UMCA domain, the mission philosophy strikingly contrasted with that of the Scottish Presbyterians. With their headquarters on Likoma Island some one hundred miles from Livingstonia across Lake Malawi, the UMCA's Anglicans stood resolutely opposed to colonial capitalism and commercial participation (Ranger 1981). Some African men did receive training in printing, carpentry, and building under UMCA auspices, but there was little inclination to systematically educate Africans to gain employable technological skills. While the UMCA's celibate missionaries often spoke of the Scots' programs at Livingstonia with frank admiration, the education they delivered to Africans had "a strong academic bias" in contrast to the Scots' vocational and technological orientation. Created to "civilize and Christianize" (Elston 1972, 357–58), the UMCA focused on promoting the domestic arts and family life modeled on ethnocentric European ideals.[35] That they did not actively try to advance African participation in the colonial economy was partly a reflection of their own class and university backgrounds. Quite a few UMCA missionaries were "ignorant of or repelled by the dynamic, self-assured world of Victorian industry" (McCracken 1977, 177). To them, limiting education to religious aims was a defensible means to avert the social upheaval that would occur if Africans turned themselves into what Bishop Smythies, who was consecrated Bishop of Likoma in 1884, called "bad caricatures of the Englishmen" (ibid.).

With the mission's rebirth in 1875, technology assumed a high profile in the UMCA's efforts to stake out its interests in Malawi. Steam power and Western medicine provided specific strategies designed to support the UMCA's goals of evangelization, the building up of a native ministry, and diluting the influence of Islam (Mills 1911; Roome 1926; Bone 1982). During its pioneering phase the mission saw "Mohammedanism" as the foremost, head-on threat in this vast frontier region.

In common with many mission societies around the world, the UMCA came to identify itself as a medical mission. Symptomatic of its difficulties with medical recruitment throughout its entire existence, the mission was unsuccessful in its efforts to commission a full-time European doctor for the Malawi field until 1899. In the UMCA's flagship journal, *Central Africa* (1883–1964), the inaugural issue publicized the mission's "very great need" for ordained "medical men." This plea was aimed at doctors who would care for Africans. On the other hand, medical help and public health measures were also sorely needed for the European staff in the mission's early decades. Terribly high mortality and an incidence of serious illness among the missionaries threatened their entire enterprise. Pleas for volunteer doctors continued in varying form throughout the colonial era. According to the UMCA's Bishop Smythies, the ideal medical man was one "who uses all his medical knowledge for a missionary end... [and] who longs not only for the healing of bodies but for the salvation of their souls" (*CA* 11 [1893]: 51). Smythies assured his readers in Britain and elsewhere that the UMCA's medical practices would be firmly grounded upon modern scientific principles, reflecting the "sympathetic and harmonious" relations that had recently developed between science and theology in the late Victorian era (*CA* 15 [1897]: 39).

At last, in 1899, Dr. Robert Howard arrived in Malawi as the UMCA's resident doctor. An exceptionally talented physician-epidemiologist, Howard proved a godsend for the mission. He quickly proceeded to make enormous contributions to African and missionary health, including an infrastructure of hospitals and dispensaries, during his ten years in Malawi. Howard's initiatives led the mission for the first time to effectively add basic elements of Western medicine and public health to its arsenal, including principles of hygiene, antiseptic treatment of ulcers and other lesions, operations with chloroform, and cataract surgery. Unfortunately for all concerned, Howard was forced to retire from both his medical work and residence in Malawi due to the UMCA's stubborn application of a self-defeating social policy.

Philosophy and good intentions aside, the reality for Africans was that even rudimentary Western medical services would not be available to them for many years. Furthermore, the UMCA never thought of itself as a development agency. Its own philosophy of minimal vocational training meant that few Africans connected to the UMCA through its schools, churches, and employment received training sufficient to help support the mission's espoused agenda for medical services. Possibly the UMCA's main claim, correctly so, was that until after World War I they far surpassed anything done by the Protectorate administration.

Chapter 2 examines the dynamic regional and historical settings in which the UMCA set about the task of shaping a physically vast mission field in the heart of Central Africa. I focus on the tumultuous changes that overturned and redistributed the balance of established indigenous power in the Lake Malawi region during the last quarter of the nineteenth century. In this drama the missionaries found themselves on the leading edges of imperialism's first and sometimes violent contact with African societies and slavers.

NOTES

1. The region along the western and southern shores of Lake Malawi (Lake Nyasa before 1964) was named the Nyasaland Districts Protectorate (1891), British Central Africa (1893), Nyasaland (1907), and Malawi (July 6, 1964). For simplicity, I write of Lake Malawi and Malawi throughout this book, except when context requires otherwise.

2. Although not concerned with medical care, an interesting and important analysis in this genre is by Nancy U. Murray (1986). She correctly portrays many of colonial Kenya's mission societies as extremely competitive and land hungry, so much so that they "dropped all pretense to amity" (187) in a rush for land that was reminiscent of the colonial powers' "scramble" for African territory following the Berlin Conference of 1884–85. Land has quite justifiably been the most central theme in studies of colonial Kenya. However, nowhere in this article is there a reference to any contribution the missions may have made to the African societies the missions invaded.

3. Rita Headrick (1994) points to the case of the (American) Brethern Missionary Society in interior Ubangi-Shari, who "devoted great amounts of time to caring for their own needs and suffering from bouts of fever. What was left went primarily to evangelical work. Very little time and resources were spent aiding sick Africans" (257–58). "On the other hand," says Headrick, "the French administrations attempted to barricade their French Equatorial Africa territories with regulations designed to keep out Protestant and non-French speaking missionaries. As a result, people were deprived of medical care from missionaries who might have come had they felt welcome" (256).

4. A Malawian social scientist (Msukwa 1987, 24) observes that, up to independence, the churches' concentration of resources in health and education meant little was left to apply to other fields such as agriculture, marketing, communications, water supply, and village sanitation.

5. World Council of Churches for Malawi Christian Council, Survey of Christian Medical Work in Malawi, Central Africa, July 31–August 15, 1965, 5 (mimeograph); and Msukwa 1987.

6. PHAM, Member Institutions 1987 (mimeograph).

7. *Impressions of South Africa* (New York: The Century Co., 1897), 240, quoted in Hammond and Jablow 1992, 79.

8. Peltzer 1987, 54–56. Faith healers use symbolic forms of healing such as prayers, holy water, laying on of hands, or Koranic scripts.

9. Customarily done without asking questions, in general contrast to biomedical procedure.

10. As many as one of each kind for every fifty to three hundred people (personal field estimates).

11. Cannibalism was greatly feared in the past. In his *Nyasa the Great Water* (1922) Archdeacon William Johnson, the person who lived more closely with Africans than any other UMCA missionary, wrote that "most, if not all natives are more or less obsessed with this fear of the dead being exhumed and devoured and with belief in cannibal wizards from which it springs. . . . I have often heard quite sensible natives mock at my unbelief in wizards" (120–21).

12. Usually plant poisons. See Munday 1941, 33.

13. I frame this discussion of witchcraft and traditional healing in the present tense because these institutions continue to operate, adapted to the practicalities of modern life. Witchcraft is widely invoked as a means of dealing with the stress that occurs in workplace relationships, competition in schools and business, love, kin group relations, politics, competitive sports, and major illness. It has grown along with forces that promote individualism, competition, and materialism. Bond and Ciekawy (2001) see no distinction between witchcraft and sorcery. They "use witchcraft as the general term for harm created through the manipulation of magic" (26, n. 1).

14. Schoffeleers 1976; Peltzer 1987, 52–53; Kaspin 1993. A European at the UMCA's Kota Kota station reported that local "heathen tribes" believe that *vinyao* "give pleasure to the departed spirits" (*Central Africa* 67 [1949]: 26); *Central Africa* is hereafter cited as *CA*.

15. Olumwalla's post-structural mode of analysis relies heavily on insights derived from Steven Feierman's work. See, e.g., Feierman 1990 and 1995.

16. London Missionary Society (c. 1900). I am indebted to Dr. Robert Stock of the University of Saskatchewan, Saskatoon, Canada, for his gift of "The Healer."

17. These ideas are further developed in Olumwullah 2002, chap. 1.

18. Personal observation. The practice of referring difficult-to-treat, or to save, patients from biomedical facilities to the indigenous healers apparently grew considerably in the post-colonial era of declining government health services and the rise of the HIV/AIDS pandemic.

19. On the main witch-eradication movements that spilled across Malawi and neighboring territories in colonial times, see Richards 1935, and Marwick 1950.

20. Often the first choice even in the post-independence period.

21. In 1963 a UMCA official described the the raison d'etre and challenge presented by the separatist churches: "The intimate connection between healing of the body and healing of the mind and soul is basic to Africa's life-view, and it is a connection the Christian Church neglects to its peril" (*UMCA Annual Review*, 1963, 34).

22. Lankester 1897, 246.

23. O. Tempkin, *The Double Face of Janus* (1977, 48), cited in Arnold 1988, 12.

24. Ross was the founding editor of the *Annals of Tropical Medicine and Parasitology*.

25. Hine also became Bishop of Zanzibar and Bishop of Northern Rhodesia.

26. Of the 423 staff who represented the UMCA between 1862 (the pioneer party) until 1905, 88 (21 percent) had died. This was despite efforts to recruit, "weed-out," and retain only the hardiest individuals. *CA* 24 (1905): 11–12.

27. "Livingstone College: Report for 1905–6," *Journal of Tropical Medicine and Hygiene* 10 (Jan. 15, 1907): 29.

28. "Livingstone College." *Journal of Tropical Medicine and Hygiene* 11 (March 2, 1908): 71–72.

29. Ibid., 72.

30. "Livingstone College Commemoration Day," *Journal of Tropical Medicine and Hygiene* 11 (July 15, 1908): 218.

31. UMCA Box List: A3 Medical History and Reports, 1882–1934. c. 1908. Rhodes House Library, Oxford (RHL).

32. "Livingstone College," *Journal of Tropical Medicine and Hygiene* 13 (Jan. 1, 1910): 11.

33. McCracken 1977, 196, ref. Livingstonia Papers, Box 3, Malawi National Archives (MNA).

34. Yet strong doubts have arisen about whether Livingstonia had a net positive influence on the development of African village economies in Malawi. See McCracken 1977, 209–10.

35. The Anglicans chose not to cooperate with the other Protestant missions to create a uniform system of education since their main goal was religious education not secular. See Pachai 1972.

CHAPTER TWO

The Lake Malawi Region: Forces of Change in the Late Nineteenth Century

'PLACES OF SKULLS' MARK THE VARIOUS ROADS ON WHICH
THE SLAVE TRAFFIC IS CARRIED ON; SKELETONS ARE STREWN
ON THE BEACH. THE COUNTRY BEHIND IS A DESERT FOR A
WEEK'S JOURNEY; AND AT EVERY STEP SOME NEW EXPERIENCE
OF THE DESOLATION OF THE SLAVE TRADE IS APPARENT.

J. F. Elton, *Travels and Researches among the Lakes and
Mountains of Eastern and Central Africa* (1879, 102)

EAST-CENTRAL AFRICA IN THE LATE PRECOLONIAL DECADES: SOCIAL, POLITICAL AND EPIDEMIOLOGICAL PERSPECTIVES

In the nineteenth century several overlapping forces powerfully affected the internal political order and trade relations of east-central Africa, including the Malawi area. They also dramatically helped to shape disease environments and health through unwitting human design. Several examples will provide context for the UMCA story.

First, whereas the Atlantic slave trade in West Africa was suppressed around 1840, such commerce continued to grow on the Indian Ocean side of the continent. Carried by wooden dhows powered by the seasonal monsoon, a centuries-old trade existed in slaves, ivory, copra, mangrove poles, and other items between the East African ports of Lamu, Mombasa, Zanzibar, and Kilwa, and Arabia, the Persian Gulf, India, and beyond. From about 1840, the islands of Zanzibar and Pemba, situated twenty miles off the mainland coast of Tanganyika and renowned for their clove plantations, came under the control of the Sultanate of Oman. As the Omanis also gained authority over the East African coastal strip, the hunt for slaves and ivory in the interior of east-central Africa greatly intensified—especially in Tanganyika, the eastern Congo, Uganda, Zambia, and Malawi.

Long-distance trade routes, all eventually connected with Zanzibar, fanned out from the coastal towns of Kilwa Kivinje, Bagamoyo, Pangani, Tanga, and Mombasa into the far reaches of the interior. These routes directed slaves and ivory to the coast for external markets, filled a demand for domestic slaves along the coast itself, and also served as cultural conduits for the spread of Swahili and Islam far inland. In response to demand at the coast, large areas inside east-central Africa thus became part of an international commercial system that was initiated and mainly controlled by Africans (Kimambo 1989). By one estimate the minimum number of people drained from the East African economies between 1830 and 1873 was 6,480,000, while the maximum was 21,160,000.[1] Regarding captured slaves, Burton said, "no man was foolish enough to spoil his own property" (1860, 1:51). Yet there can be no doubt that many captives who survived the journey to the coast also endured great hardship and suffering.

Second, in the southern interior, the "Kilwa routes" that linked the coast with Lake Malawi were "probably the oldest" in the entire East African system (Kimambo 1989, 238). These routes originated in response to the demand for slaves from French planters on the islands of Reunion, the Seychelles, the Mascarenes, and Madagascar (Issacman 1989, 185). The Yao in what are now Tanzania, Mozambique, and Malawi, and the Bisa, in Zambia, dominated this southern portion of the trade. By 1850 the mainland port of Kilwa Kivinji was the principal destination for slaves and ivory from the hinterlands of Lake Malawi, and it ranked as "the most important town on the coast between Mozambique and Zanzibar" (Kimambo 1989, 222). A trickle of slaves continued to be traded out of Malawi into the early years of the twentieth century (fig. 2.1).

Third, the demand for slave labor in Brazil persisted until 1878. In response, the middle and lower Zambezi valley, like the areas to its north, was integrated into the international capitalist system of production. It became a thriving focus for the capture of slaves purchased by Afro-Portuguese and Afro-Goan *prazeros* for shipment to sugar planters in Brazil, Cuba, and the West Indies. Places such as Quelimane and Ibo Island, on the coast of Mozambique, developed into major slave markets (Issacman 1989, 180–89). The growth of this trade also helped to weaken the the external political and trade ties of the Maravi Confederation, which had grown in the seventeenth and eighteeenth centuries from a focus near the southwest coast of Lake Malawi.

Fourth, aggressive Ngoni immigrants from southern Africa began arriving in pulses in Malawi and Tanzania, fighting their way along the western and eastern sides of the lake between 1840 and 1845 (Newman 1995,

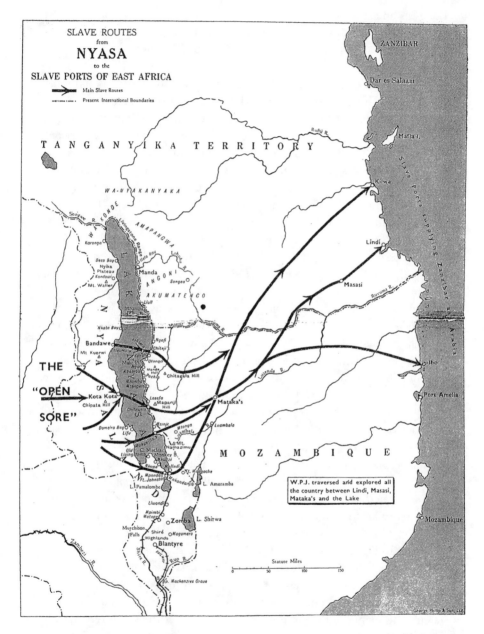

Figure 2.1. Slave routes from Malawi to the slave ports of East Africa.
(Source: Barnes (1933). From the archives of the USPG.)

174–75). Organized militarily, they brought terror and havoc to many indigenous populations into the 1880s, by which time UMCA missionaries had also seen and felt their presence. Yao immigrants, mostly farmers and traders, and primarily Muslims, also spilled over from Mozambique into the lands east and south of Lake Malawi, including the Shiré Highlands. Yao chiefs such as Makanjila and Mponda became heavily involved in the capture of slaves and their long-distance trade to the Indian Ocean ports. Ultimately, the Yao near the lake found themselves defending their interests against the UMCA's pioneer missionaries and British colonial power (Kimambo 1989). These developments, not excluding the growing European presence, exposed Malawians to social upheaval and new epidemiological pathways. Extensive violence and loss of life occurred as settlements broke up and people were forced to take refuge in new and often precarious places. The scenario compels attention to such consequences as hunger and disease, abandoned children, physical injury, death, and the breakdown of human community (see chapter 6).

In sum, slave trading was a terribly disruptive and debasing activity that brought drastic changes in the social organization, settlement patterns, ecology, and health of many peoples in this vast area (Pike and Rimmington 1965; Kimambo 1989). As seen through the eyes of James Stewart,[2] who explored Malawi east of the Shiré River, the area was

> "a lonely land of barbarism, of game and wild beasts, of timid and harried but not unkindly men, harassed by never-ending slave raids and intertribal wars. . . . We had passed through many villages burnt and deserted, just as their unhappy occupants had left them when they fled for life—that is those of them who were not speared or shot or captured. We saw in these villages heaps of ashes of charred poles in circles like the shape of the huts, broken pottery, a good many bones, but no bodies—the hyenas had attended to that. (Stewart 1903, 209, cited in Hanna 1956, 10–11)"

While reliable demographic records do not exist for this time, there is general agreement that many African societies lost large numbers of people to disease, gross mistreatment, and warfare. Patterson (1993), for one, views the years 1880–1920 as "the most deadly in history for much of the continent" (450). A most notorious example of social and economic destabilization (and extraordinary human resilience in response) is the genocide in King Leopold II's Congo Free State (CFS), where ten million Congolese—"a death toll of Holocaust dimensions"—are believed to have died from all causes, including murder, torture, starvation, exhaustion, exposure, and disease (Hochschild 1998, 4, and chap. 15). Leopold apparently sanctioned the "Swahili network," Tippu Tib's vast inland empire in the eastern CFS based on the collection of slaves and ivory. Trade routes linked it with Zanzibar, and it "became the first base for colonial penetration into the eastern part of Central Africa" (Vellut 1989, 306–7).

Epidemic Disease and Poverty in East-Central Africa and Malawi

Areas of Africa that experienced the most disruption and exposure to human and animal pathogens included central and southern Tanganyika, the Lake Malawi area, and the eastern Congo Basin. The terror tactics of slave raiders (burning villages and scattering remaining populations) and elephant-hunting groups, together with infected caravan members, served to introduce or re-introduce epidemic diseases. Smallpox, cholera, sleeping sickness, relapsing fever, and dysentery easily spread along trade routes or rivers into adjacent and then more distant settlements. For example, in East Africa, inhabited by scores of cattle-keeping cultures such as the Hima and Maasai, disastrous epidemics of rinderpest introduced to Ethiopia spread southward into vast swaths of territory in successive epidemics beginning in the 1890s and into the 1920s (Harlow et al. 1965). This lethal zoonosis, related to measles, killed thousands of cattle and also spread through many wild cud-chewing animals (Diamond 1999, 206–7). In Uganda, rinderpest reportedly moved twenty to thirty miles a day, "leaving a trail of carcasses in its wake" (Thomas and Scott 1935, 202). Having lost the core element of their subsistence, many thousands of people starved to death during such epizootics. Kjekshus argues that "the great Rinderpest of the 1890s . . . broke the economic backbone of many of the most prosperous and advanced communities, undermined established authority and status structures, and altered the political contacts between the peoples. It initiated the breakdown of a long-established ecological balance" (Kjekshus 1977, 126).

In Malawi, the pioneer missionaries who began to arrive in the mid-1870s (CSM, FCSM, UMCA, and later the White Fathers) witnessed the human consequences of slaving, the circulation and intensification of new infectious diseases, and deepening material poverty. For example, evidence that smallpox had become epidemic by 1890 comes from Mponda's, a place named for the Yao chief who controlled it. Strategically situated on the Shiré River near where it exits Lake Malawi, this Muslim town was about a mile wide, stockaded, and contained more than 5,000 inhabitants. Here, within the southern reaches of east-central Africa's slave and ivory domains, three French White Fathers had secured a tenuous welcome. They managed to hang on as tolerated and sometimes useful guests of Mponda for fifteen months in 1890–91 before Cardinal Lavigiere, their superior in France, ordered them to withdraw. While interest in learning about European Catholicism was minimal, the priests did make use of their modicum of basic medical skills and kept accounts of health conditions they encountered. They noted that it was customary to isolate people with serious illnesses in special huts located outside town. Treatment of smallpox sufferers relied on a form of quarantine, and members of slave caravans with smallpox had to remain outside the town until completely recovered. Nearly perennial food shortages meant that the population also experienced "the full gamut of vitamin deficiency diseases" (Linden 1974, 30–31). This undoubtedly compromised immune responses in many people, thus increasing their susceptibility to infection and disease.

Large crowds formed whenever the White Fathers ventured outside Mponda's on medical safaris. With their small stocks of Western medicines the priests reportedly managed to gain the upper hand in competition with Muslim *mwalimu* and their Swahili amulets (ibid., 30). In addition to epidemic smallpox, the priests recorded in the Mponda Diary that "scabies" was rife. Several years later D. Kerr Cross, the Nyasaland protectorate's Medical Officer, insisted that scabies was "the most common of all African skin diseases. Almost every native suffers in his wrists or hips or thighs. It is highly contagious" (Cross 1897, 18).

As for evidence of material poverty in Malawi, a study of the West Shiré District in 1893 recorded that families entered one-room houses at night that were furnished with a few mats, wooden basins, and clay pots (Iliffe 1984).[3] Owners of mortars and pestles lent them out to those without them for a handful of meal. Housing typically lacked windows. The political insecurity caused by the slave trade in Yaoland, on the southeast side of the lake, caused such fear that people moved into stockaded settlements, of which Mponda's was a prominent example. By the early 1890s the crowding of people inside these defenses had "produced an unprecedented level of squalor" (Linden 1974, 30). Decades later, UMCA nurse Alice Simpkin observed that "no sunlight enters the huts" (Simpkin 1926, 23).

ORIGINS OF THE UNIVERSITIES' MISSION TO CENTRAL AFRICA

Missionary penetration of Malawi in the interior of Central Africa is forever connected with the travels and profound public influence in Europe of David Livingstone. The Scottish medical missionary, explorer, and naturalist began his journeys (1841–73) in southern Africa at the age of twenty-seven.

At age forty-three he completed a remarkable three-year walk (1853–56) from the Atlantic in Portuguese Angola to the Indian Ocean in Portuguese Mozambique. He returned to Britain a national hero, resolved to see the African interior opened to European trade and Christianity.

In his famous speech to the students and faculty of Cambridge University on December 4, 1857, Livingstone, a member of the Free Church of Scotland, appealed to the English universities and the established Church of England to plant a mission among the peoples of the Lake Nyasa region (Bennett 1970; Hanna 1956). For decades, this vast area had been severely destabilized by the African, Arab, and Swahili slave trade. Intertribal conflicts fomented by the militant intrusions of the Nguni peoples from southern Africa had also taken a heavy toll on the region's habitability. "I go back to Africa," Livingstone told the assembly at Cambridge, "to try to make an open path for commerce and Christianity; do you carry out the work which I have begun? I leave it with you." His appeal catalyzed a movement to put down the notorious slave trade in east-central Africa, using to advantage England's guilt and consciousness about its role in the Atlantic slave trade (Latourette 1943, 348). Thus in addition to evangelization, there was a parallel motive for sending an English mission to Central Africa. Samuel Wilberforce, Bishop of Oxford, highlighted this sense of a national, collective culpability when he spoke to the Oxford and Cambridge Mission in November 1859. England, he said, "can never be clear from the guilt of her long continued slave trade till Africa is free, civilized, and Christian" (Anderson-Morshead 1955, 5; cited in Elston 1972, 345).

Within a few years of Livingstone's death in 1873, missionaries from the Church of Scotland and the Free Church of Scotland entered the Lake Nyasa region. The Free Church opened the first of several Livingstonia Mission stations at Cape Maclear near the southwestern end of the lake in 1875. Its development benefited from access to the trade and transportation services on Lake Malawi provided by the *Ilala,* a steamer operated by the Scottish-owned, Glasgow-based African Lakes Corporation.

The first attempt to establish a UMCA mission in Malawi was directly encouraged by David Livingstone, who accompanied the missionaries up the Zambezi in 1861. Led by Bishop Charles Mackenzie, a Cambridge mathematics don (Isichei 1995), work began among the Mang'anja peoples at Magomero, and later at Chibisa's village, in the Shiré Highlands (White 1987). From their arrival in Malawi the missionaries had to deal with rival chiefs and confronted persistent slave raiding. The party's decision to use guns in self-defense and free slaves created dissension among themselves and anxiety about the reaction of their Christian supporters in England. After a few months the mission settlement at Magomero reportedly resembled a "refugee camp," with some 160 liberated slaves (Elston 1972, 346). Evangelical work was severely hampered by the lack of a Mang'anja vocabulary and continued tribal warfare.

Bishop Mackenzie succumbed to malaria in 1862. Following this psychological blow, coupled with Magomero's general unhealthiness and isolation, the missionaries decided to relocate farther south at Chibisa's village. They remained there for fifteen months, again hampered by illness and local interference. Meanwhile, Bishop William Tozer, Mackenzie's successor, arrived on the scene in mid-1863. Tozer was keenly aware of the criticism many UMCA supporters in England had voiced regarding the mission's militant involvement in the slave trade and its lack of success with evangelism. He ordered the missionaries to withdraw and begin anew in the adjacent Portuguese territory. After brief but unsuccessful attempts in three sites, Tozer notified the UMCA's home committee that mission work in the region could no longer be sustained and must be withdrawn. Tozer then left for Zanzibar on his own authority, where he was to begin laying the groundwork for a future diocese and a base from which to reestablish evangelization on the mainland (Elston 1972; Rowley 1972).

By the early 1860s, Zanzibar had already been East Africa's greatest slave market for a half century. The UMCA authorities reckoned that after a few years in this heavily Muslim but less-risky location, they might be better positioned to renew their efforts to open the Lake Malawi region for evangelistic work. From its coastal base at Mkunazini on Zanzibar, the UMCA established new mission stations in the 1870s at Magila and Masasi on the mainland.[4] Representatives of the UMCA returned to Lake Malawi for reconnaissance in 1875. But it was not until 1886, when their first steamer was put into operation, that Likoma Island became the mission's staging point for expansion in the lake region.

Meanwhile, Zanzibar, on the route between the Cape of Good Hope and the Gulf of Suez, remained the de facto headquarters of UMCA's Africa operations and its main place of investment for several decades. When the Diocese of Nyasaland added the embryonic "Steamer Parish" to its accounts in the mid-1880s, the mission's London office was obliged to cast a larger net in search of increased private contributions and legacies to support its growing initiatives in east and central Africa. Northern Rhodesia, the third diocese, was added just before World War I. Territorial reorganization produced a separate Diocese of Masasi in southeast Tanganyika in 1928, while the Diocese of South West Tanganyika was cut from the Diocese of Nyasaland in 1952.

The Diocese of Nyasaland received on average about 30 percent of all operating funds distributed from London to UMCA missions from 1899 through 1961. During this time the number of dioceses grew from two to five, with a sixth added in 1961. Whereas all dioceses increased in number and responsibilities, relative support for the vast scope of education, evangelization, and medical work in Malawi varied little until 1952. Financially, this meant that the Malawi mission was deeply in the red most of the time. Then, in concert with the Central African Federation crisis and the creation of the South West Tanganyika Diocese, allocations to Malawi nose-dived more than 40 percent. Small declines continued into the 1960s when, with national independence imminent, most of the British staff and UMCA funding for the Diocese of Nyasaland basically faded away, along with the UMCA itself.[5] Ironically, support to carry on some services was successfully solicited from the American Episcopal Church.[6]

ENVIRONMENT AND COMMUNICATIONS IN THE LAKE MALAWI REGION

The elongated region that became the Nyasaland Districts Protectorate (1891), and thereafter British Central Africa (1893), Nyasaland (1907), and Malawi (July 6, 1964) covers some 46,000 square miles. This territory, entirely within the Southern Hemisphere, extends 560 miles from north to south and varies in width from 50 to 150 miles.

Lake Malawi, scene of the first naval engagement of World War I, dominates the country's physical environment (fig. 2.2). It is Africa's third largest body of fresh water after Lakes Victoria and Tanganyika, and its dramatic shifts in weather are legendary. Scenery in the basin is spectacular. Situated in the Great Rift Valley at 1,565 feet above sea level, Lake Malawi is a vast stretch of "astonishing lapis lazuli blue" water and supports over four hundred species of fish (*CA* 66 [1948]: 58). High mountains and plateaus rise several thousand feet above the lake and often descend steeply into it, particularly on the northern and eastern sides. Coastal access and settlement are often limited or prohibited. In the north the lake's depth reaches 2,300 feet, where the Rift Valley floor descends more than 700 feet below sea level. Forests and woodlands encroach on the lakeshore, although the human-modified ecology of the more accessible areas shows the effects of centuries of human influence, particularly in vegetation patterns. Some stretches of the western and southern coasts are characterized by grassy plains dotted with borassus (fan) palms and great stretches of the spectacular baobab tree, with its girth of up to eighty feet.

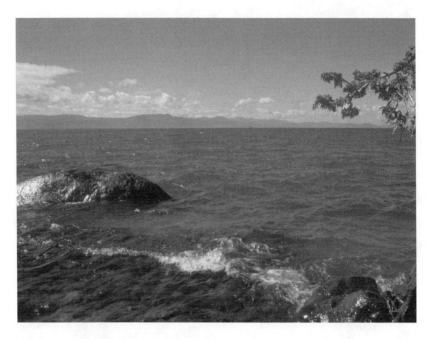

Figure 2.2. Lake Malawi, south end.
(Source: Author's photograph.)

Several small rivers drain into Lake Malawi (or Nyanja = "big water"), mostly along its western coast. The lake's size generates substantial local effects on surface winds, cloud cover, and rainfall. During the dry season (May–October), and occasionally throughout the year, powerful tradewinds from the south known as *Mwera* dominate the lake basin. An English observer in 1910 remarked that the winds caused "waves on the surface that would not discredit the Atlantic" (Mills 1911, 11). Severe southeasterly gales are a frequent seasonal phenomenon, producing rough seas and dangerous navigation.

The lake region also attracts great clouds of small midges called *kungu*. These insects mass and make a buzzing noise similar to a swarm of bees. They form columns of "smoke" that billow into clouds of "fantastic shape," forty to two hundred feet high. A six-inch deep, writhing mass of kungu could accumulate on the deck of a lake steamer in four hours. A protein delicacy, Africans captured them by the basketful, pounded them into "cakes," and ate them with delight. On November 28, 1886, UMCA layman and diarist William Bellingham sailed on the *S.S. Charles Janson*, the mission's new steamer. Just as his party sat down to their evening meal, a cloud of kungu descended on them: "they put out the candles, got into our food, and we could take them off the table by handfuls."[7]

Lake Malawi drains southward into the Shiré River (pronounced shee-ray), whose waters travel nearly three hundred miles to join the Zambesi in Mozambique. Beginning in the last quarter of the nineteenth century, the Shiré served as the major corridor into Malawi for European missionaries as well as for traders and administrators. Livingstone evaluated and encouraged the use of this river link to the Zambezi on his visit to Lake Malawi in 1859. It offered an important alternative to the overland slave caravan routes from the Indian Ocean coast that passed through Portuguese East Africa. However, a series of five cataracts that begin about midway between the Zambezi and the lake posed serious obstacles. These navigation barriers (the Kapichira, Hamilton, Tedzani, Nkula, and Kholombidzo Falls) forced a break-in-bulk, a shift to overland transport, and a heavy investment in human portage. European men and women generally traveled overland by *machila*, a canvas, covered hammock slung on two bamboo poles carried by four men at a jog trot. African relay teams of twelve to sixteen men carried loads of fifty to sixty pounds each, up to forty miles in a day (Winspear 1960). The extreme unhealthiness of the Elephant Marshes and adjacent malarial plains around the Shiré-Zambezi confluence was also a danger. Malaria and blackwater fever, its deadly sequel, proved all too common among the ever-increasing numbers of whites and African porters using the Shiré route (Gelfand 1964).

In March 1908, the Shiré Highlands Railway reached the town of Blantyre, providing a 112-mile link between the protectorate's center of white settlement and Port Herald in the extreme south. Certainly this development was a major improvement in transport, but the journey from the Indian Ocean still took seven days (ibid.). Travelers had to board a river steamer at Chinde on the Zambezi delta in Portuguese East Africa. They would then sail up-river for about one hundred miles to the confluence of the Zambezi and the southward-flowing Shiré River. The steamers could then navigate the Shiré northward for about seventy-five miles, crossing into southern Malawi.

THE SCOTS OF LIVINGSTONIA: FIRST STEAMER ON THE LAKE

Scottish missionaries and traders were the first Europeans to establish a permanent base of operations in the territory of the future Malawi. The advance party that arrived at Cape Maclear on Lake Malawi in

October 1875 included members of the Free Church of Scotland's Livingstonia Mission and representatives of the (established) Church of Scotland. Inspired by Livingstone and engineered through the dedicated efforts of James Stewart (see above), the mission organized for the purposes of evangelistic, medical, educational, and industrial work. The missionaries strongly believed that the ultimate success of their diverse enterprise depended on supplanting the Arab-African slave trade with "Commerce and Christianity." Livingstonia's missionaries had also been deeply influenced by the late explorer's insistence that trade should be based on steam navigation. They believed that use of steamers would divert trade southward, away from the notorious dhow ferries and overland routes to the Indian Ocean used by slavers and African traders. It would also stimulate agricultural exports and other legitimate commerce (Latourette 1943; Gelfand 1964; McCracken 1977). Within a short time the UMCA followed the example with its own steamer.

Livingstone's legacy virtually insured that the advance party of Scots who set up their temporary mission headquarters at Lake Malawi would arrive by steamer. Their vessel, the *Ilala*, was named for the village in modern Zambia where Livingstone died. Built in London by Alfred Yarrow for the Free Church of Scotland, the *Ilala* was forty-eight feet long with a beam of ten feet. It was constructed of a new lightweight metal known as "mild steel," at a cost of £1,600. This "mild steel" had exceptional strength, permitting hull plates to be made of metal only 1/16 inch thick. According to its template, the *Ilala* had to be assembled quickly, disassembled, and carried in pieces around the Shiré's many cataracts. Originally designed with three boilers, it was instead fitted with two, and bolt assembled, instead of riveted, in preparation for its successful trial run on the Thames (McKinnon 1977). Afterward the contractor disassembled her and packed the parts in three to four-hundred pound units, each containing several smaller parcels weighing fifty to one hundred pounds. In this condition the *Ilala* was loaded on the ocean-steamer *Walmer Castle* and shipped to the East African coast via Cape Town.

At the Kongoni mouth of the Zambezi, the *Ilala's* frames and steel hull plates were bolted together again for the river voyage to the Shiré River. When the party reached the Murchison cataracts on the Shiré, the craft required disassembly a second time. Some eight hundred to a thousand African porters (*tenga-tenga*) carried the pieces for about thirty miles around the falls to the upper Shiré at Matope. There it was reassembled a third time, apparently once again with bolts instead of rivets, and fitted out for lake duty (ibid.). This procedure of steamer disassembly, African overland portage, and final reassembly at locations above the Shiré's cataracts remained standard for the next twenty-five years.

Having left London on May 21, 1875, the *Ilala* steamed into Lake Malawi on October 12, 1875. On this accomplishment the *Ilala* rightly held the distinction as the first steamboat on the upper Shiré and Lake Malawi (McKinnon 1977), and possibly on any African lake. With its captain drawn from the Royal Navy, other members of the party on this first voyage included two engineers and a seaman as well as a medical doctor (the influential Reverend Dr. Robert Laws), a carpenter, and an agriculturalist (Gelfand 1964). Their first and primary destination was Cape Maclear, which became the first (and temporary due to malaria and slavers) Presbyterian mission site in what is today Malawi.

The missionaries dropped anchor at Cape Maclear, which offered shelter from wind and rough seas. This place was situated uncomfortably close to one of the half-dozen or so main routes across the lake used by slave traders operating from dhows (W. P. Livingstone 1921, map). Muslim Yao peoples controlled the sparsely inhabited hinterland of Cape Maclear. Recent arrivals from northern Mozambique, they had rapidly become the principal slavers in southern Malawi's notorious slave trade.

Remote from population clusters, hot, and unhealthy, Cape Maclear proved a poor setting for the Scots' Livingstonia Mission. After three years the missionaries abandoned the cape, leaving behind the graves of three comrades who had succumbed to disease.

A new coastal site for the mission was chosen among the Tonga people at Bandawe, some 125 miles farther north on Lake Malawi's western coast. Larger concentrations of population and local rivalries made it politically impossible for the Livingstonia missionaries to remain aloof from tribal affairs. The Tonga eagerly received mission schools and trade goods, and expected the missionaries to engage in their local politics.[8] By 1894, when the main base for Livingstonia moved north once again, the mission claimed thousands of adherents at and inland from Bandawe.

In 1878 the Livingstonia Mission acted to separate mission work from its transport and trading interests. That year the General Assembly of the Free Church of Scotland transferred ownership of the *Ilala* to the Glasgow-based Livingstonia Central Africa Company, founded in 1875 and shortly thereafter known as the African Lakes Corporation (ALC). Made up principally of entrepreneurs from Glasgow and Edinburgh, and managed by John and Fred Muir, the ALC aimed to profit by using armed force if necessary against Arab and African slavers and by encouraging Africans to redirect their trade in ivory and other goods to the Company. Ivory was its single most important item of trade and income during the 1880s. Although the ALC chose to establish its headquarters near the Church of Scotland's new (1876) mission station at Blantyre, south of Lake Malawi (McCracken, 1977), the northerly Livingstonia missionaries remained economically allied with and dependent on the company.

"Legitimate" trade on Lake Malawi, especially ivory, cloth, and food staples, was built on foundations created by the missionaries. It expanded despite the ALC's poor management and irregular delivery of goods in the lake basin. These circumstances reflected uncertain steamer maintenance and navigational difficulties on the Zambezi, as well as delays experienced when the steamers made stops to trade, mainly calico for ivory. By 1884 the ALC was carrying goods and people and providing services for the two Scottish missions (CSM and FCSM at Livingstonia), the London Missionary Society (LMS) at Lake Tanganyika, the UMCA on Likoma Island, and King Leopold's Belgian Association (McKinnon 1977). Some of the surplus revenues went into opening numerous small trading posts on the Zambezi and Shiré Rivers and on Lake Malawi as far north as Karonga. ALC stores and trading stations also spread into neighboring Northern Rhodesia. Described as the "economic arm of the Livingstonia mission," the ALC also set up the first labor bureau for the purpose of supplying African laborers to white planters in Malawi's Shiré Highlands (Tapela 1979, 71).

As part of their scheme for developing transport and commerce, in 1879 the ALC also placed the *Lady Nyasa II*, a sixty-foot paddle-wheel steamer, in service on the lower Shiré. This vessel operated on the Zambezi River, carrying passengers and mail bound for Blantyre. This town was then emerging as Malawi's commercial center for white planters and traders. In 1887 the *Lady Nyasa II* was complemented by a stern-wheel paddle-steamer, the *James Stevenson*, to expand services on the Zambezi and lower Shiré (Williams 1982).

In 1894 the Free Church of Scotland once again moved its headquarters farther north to a large tract of land known as Khondowe, situated among the Tonga and Ngoni peoples. Here the land rises steeply from the lakeshore to the beautiful, temperate Nyika Plateau over 7,000 feet above sea level. Some five miles inland, at 4,500 feet on the eastern side of this plateau overlooking the lake, Dr. Robert Laws established the Overtoun Institution (later renamed Livingstonia) and Gordon Memorial Hospital (Laws 1934).

TOWARD PAX BRITANNICA: BRITISH CENTRAL AFRICA
AND THE PROTECTORATE

After Cecil Rhodes's British South Africa Company (BSAC) was formed
in 1889, it quickly gained financial and administrative control over most of
Central Africa as well as the ALC's stock shares in 1890. A few other trading
companies also competed for profits on Lake Malawi in the 1890s and early
1900s, leading to mergers and buyouts that most benefited the ALC. The
ALC continued to operate under its original name throughout the colonial
era and was a key player in the extension of British rule (Latourette 1943).
Its monopolistic hold over river and lake transport and trade goods drew
criticism at least into the late 1890s. A UMCA missionary, Arthur Fraser
Sim, complained in 1895:

> "The Company has descended to being a kind of agency for European
> travelers and missionaries. Their prices are enormous, and everything
> brought out here is purchased at a premium of seventy-five percent. The
> route up the Zambesi and Shiré is practically in their hands, and here too
> they charge exorbitantly. . . . Fancy, [they] charge £15 passenger fare from
> Ft. Johnston to Kota Kota—two days' journey and no night traveling—
> cargo, £7 a ton the same distance. The charges on the [larger, faster]
> German steamer [*Hermann von Wissman*] are £8 per passenger and £5
> per ton cargo. What wonder that we try and escape these by using our
> own boats. (Sim 1897, 108, 270)"

In May 1891, following a period of tense competition with the Portuguese
over control of the lake region, and treaty signing with African chiefs, the
Foreign Office declared all of the territory that became Nyasaland a protectorate of Great Britain. This had been preceded a few months before
by the appointment of the experienced and capable Harry H. Johnston as
first Commissioner and Consul-General of British Central Africa (BCA).
Johnston had been the administrator for Central Africa in Rhodes's BSAC.
In this role he had been directly instrumental during 1889–90 in negotiating
"friendship" treaties with various African chiefs and Arab slavers whose collective interests ranged from the northern to the southern parts of the lake
region. In a classic example of European territorial competition, Johnston
had also managed to outmaneuver the strong Portuguese interests in the
region. This was ratified by the Anglo-Portuguese Convention in June 1891,
which followed by a year the Anglo-German Convention that recognized
what became the protectorate's boundaries with German East Africa.

The village of Zomba, situated in the Shiré Highlands about fifty miles from Blantyre and adjacent to clusters of European planters, was selected as the BCA government headquarters. Ft. Johnston (formerly and now Mangochi), on the banks of the Upper Shiré, was strategically chosen to serve Britain's imperial interests in the Lake Malawi region. Situated a few miles from the lake, astride a major route followed by slave caravans, Ft. Johnston became a staging point for punitive expeditions against the slave traders and powerful African leaders who continued to resist British domination. The government also located its Marine Transport Department at this site. Since the Upper Shiré was then navigable, the larger steamers on the lake could reach Ft. Johnston by sailing across the Bar and down-river for a few miles (Murray 1922).

Between 1891 and 1895 BCA Commissioner Johnston and his staff built up a territorial system of twelve districts together with their administrative headquarters, or *bomas*. Many of these *bomas* would serve as nuclei for Malawi's town development. In 1893 Johnston recruited Sikh soldiers from the Indian Army to help carry the fight to the slavers. Pacification was often violent and required several years to complete. The northern Ngoni region of Malawi did not come under British control until 1904.

In a space of six years Johnston's administration established policies for land and minerals exploitation and introduced a hut tax, superimposed on the indigenous exchange economy. English coin, placed in circulation in 1892, was quickly accepted. This action, and the hut tax, which was intended to get Africans to pay for government administration, helped to spread a money economy in the protectorate. It also provoked deep and lasting social and economic repercussions, discussed later in this study. Lack of work in the protectorate led thousands of "Nyasa men" to leave their homes and families in search of jobs in the mines and factories of Rhodesia and South Africa. It did not take long for long-distance labor migration to become institutionalized in colonial Malawi, with up to a quarter of adult males employed outside their homeland at some period in their lives.[9]

Before his tenure ended in 1897, Johnston had also overseen the construction of nearly four hundred miles of roads, and the introduction of public services including a postal system, customs, and police. Johnston's successor, Alfred Sharpe, established a new system of justice with a high court with lower traditional African and European courts. English law became paramount in the protectorate. The territory was renamed the Nyasaland Protectorate in 1907, and placed under a typical British Crown Colony constitution with a hierarchical form of administration consisting of a governor, executive council, legislative council, and provincial and district commissioners. With revenues just covering administrative costs, colonial law and order was now in effect. At the same time, "all questions of education, health and agriculture were left to the missionaries, and economic development was left in the hands of a few small [European] planters" (Pike 1968, 95). When Sharpe retired in 1910 Nyasaland was viewed in Britain as "a model colonial territory" (Tindall 1968, 187). Two years later the African population was organized under a system of indirect rule that replaced what remained of the traditional native authorities.

By the late 1890s the protectorate's population, while overwhelmingly African in composition, also included small numbers of European missionaries, civil servants, administrators, and traders. Clusters of European planters had established first coffee, and then tea, tobacco, and cotton estates, mainly in the Shiré Highlands and on the slopes of Mt. Mlanje and in the Thyolo Highlands. Also in the south, Blantyre developed as the territory's main commercial and transportation hub (fig. 1.2). However, the absence of a railway connection to the Indian Ocean greatly retarded economic progress in the protectorate. Conditions deteriorated further during the trade depression of the 1930s. When the rail link to Beira in Portuguese East Africa was finally completed in 1935, so few European settlers remained in the protectorate that "the British government began to exclude European development as a factor in the country's economic advancement" (Pike 1968, 96).

In 1945 the protectorate's estimated African population exceeded two million and was entering a period of rapid growth, balanced by very high infant and child mortality. Slightly over half the total lived in small villages on the plateaus and highlands south of Lake Malawi. In the same year less than two thousand Europeans, mostly farmers, civil servants, and missionaries, lived in the protectorate. By 1960, a few years before independence, the predominantly British European population had expanded to 9,500, nearly half of whom lived in Blantyre. About 1,600 Indians had settled in Malawi by the early 1930s. Sikhs, the earliest arrivals, had assisted in pacifying the territory. Most of those who followed played an influential middle role as shopkeepers, artisans, and professionals in the colonial economy. Others had created large commercial firms. When self-governance arrived 1964, Malawi's South Asian population exceeded 10,000 (Pike and Rimmington 1965, 143–44; Nelson et al. 1975, 64–85).

Before and after World War II, the structure of the colonial economy remained based on African subsistence agriculture with limited cash cropping. Migratory workers, mostly adult males, sent remittances home. South Asians provided traders, middlemen, craftsmen, and professionals; and Europeans managed plantation production of tea, tobacco, and other commodities, which depended on supplies of cheap African labor. South-central Malawi became the primary focus of infrastructure and of what little economic development was realized. Despite the movement south of some (largely Presbyterian-educated) Africans for employment, the north remained spatially and socially isolated from the south.

THE SLAVE TRADE AND PACIFICATION

Commissioner Johnston's accomplishments were such that he is credited as the individual "singularly responsible for creating the administrative machinery of the protectorate established in 1891" (Crosby 1980, 62). Suppression of the Lake Malawi slave trade proved to be a particularly significant accomplishment of Johnston's administration, as it both symbolized and concretized the arrival of the Pax Britannica. With the aid of Sikh, Tonga, and Makua mercenaries and three small gunboats, the *Adventure, Pioneer,* and *Dove,* stopping this rampant commerce finally became a reality in 1895.[10] Johnston went so far as to execute the Arab slave dealer, Mlozi. To the south, Mwinyi Kheiri, the fourth Jumbe of Kota Kota, who was eventually deported to Zanzibar, became the last coast Arab to serve as the Sultan's local representative (*wali*) in the Lake Malawi region.

Prior to 1895, Arab slavers had dominated the slave and ivory trades in the northern (Karonga) and central (Kota Kota) lake regions for fifty years (Shepperson 1958; Langworthy 1971; Wright and Lary 1971). Yao chieftans controlled the slave trade south and east of Lake Malawi. Kota-Kota, the Jumbes' headquarters beginning in the mid-1840s, was the principal assembly point on the western coast of the lake for slaves captured from as far away as the Congo basin. Each year, reportedly 10,000 to 30,000 slaves were transported across Lake Malawi in wooden dhows bound for Kilwa and Zanzibar. The primary overland route leaving the east coast of the lake passed through Mataka's village in what was nominally Portuguese territory (figs. 2.3 and 2.4).[11]

Five slave dhows apparently operated on the lake at the time the Livingstonia missionaries arrived (Young 1877). Arthur Sim, the first UMCA missionary based at Kota Kota, described a dhow as "about the size of a small fishing smack. It has one sail, and carries about 10 or 12 sailors and a passenger list of about 80" (Sim 1897, 176). If a dhow typically carried eighty slaves per run from Kota Kota, sailing roughly west to east across the lake to slave ports such as Losewa (or Lusefa), Makanjira's village, or Mponda's village, it would have required 125 trips, or one dhow load every three days,

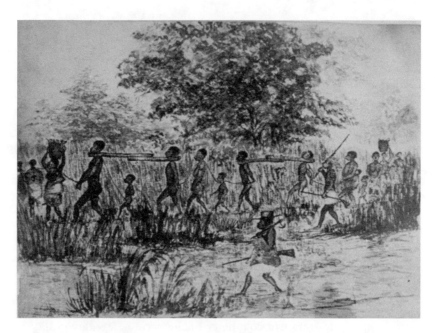

Figure 2.3. Slave caravan.
(Source: USPG.)

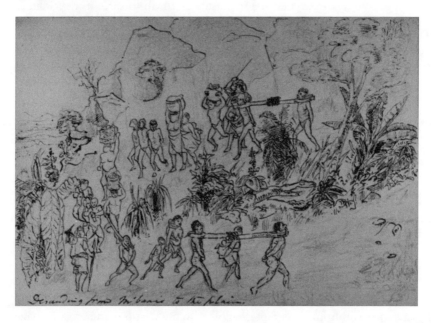

Figure 2.4. Slave caravan.
(Source: USPG.)

to transport 10,000 slaves in a year. Carrying this number of slaves with so few dhows meant almost continuous sailing. Also, the 10,000 slaves did not include the people captured and sold by Mlozi at the north end of Lake Malawi, nor those taken on its eastern side.[12] A later UMCA map of slave routes dramatically labels Kota Kota as the "Open Sore" of the lake region (see fig. 2.1).

Losewa, on one of several precolonial trade circuits in the lake region, became an Arab-controlled settlement[13] and the main east coast destination for slaves from the Kota Kota market prior to their transshipment to the slave markets of Kilwa and Zanzibar. Livingstone visited Losewa in August 1866, during his second journey to the lake, hoping to obtain transport to Kota Kota by dhow. Apparently fearing his intentions, the captains of two slave dhows slipped in and out of Losewa quietly enough to be unnoticed by Livingstone and his men. Consequently, to reach Kota Kota he was compelled to walk around the south end of the lake and then north along the west side. Shortly thereafter reports surfaced that Livingstone was "lost," or had been murdered by the Angoni. Edward Young, who headed the Royal Geographical Society's Livingstone Search Expedition, journeyed to Losewa in 1867 to seek clues about his disappearance and to gather more systematic information about the east coast of Lake Malawi. On arrival at Losewa he remarked on the settlement's great slave sheds and its considerable population of "half-caste" Arab-Africans (Young 1868).

In the years 1891 and 1892, the BSAC contributed about £10,000, and from 1893 to 1895, £17,500 per annum for the maintenance of the new protectorate's police force. The BSAC also allowed Johnston to have free use of the ALC's boats and steamers so long as he did not disrupt its commercial pursuits. Ivory, customarily transported to the coast by slaves, was the most important item of legitimate trade in the protectorate during the early 1890s. This commodity, so highly valued in many parts of the world, accounted for 79 percent of Nyasaland's exports (£5,530) in 1891, and rose to 42,495 pounds, or 82 percent of exports worth £18,252 in 1893 (Murray 1922, 169; Crosby 1980). In 1895 Arthur Sim recorded that "I have seen some tusks of ivory more than six feet high, weighing more than 100 pounds, and measuring round the curve more than seven feet" (Sim 1897, 108).

By 1895, Johnston's forces had conquered the powerful Yao territorial chiefs, including Mponda, Zarafi, Kawinga, and Matawiri. They had controlled the slave trade at the south end of the lake and in the upper Shiré region. By 1895–96 these chiefs had either surrendered or fled the protectorate. Only Makanjila continued the trade into the twentieth century, transporting slaves by dhow from a hideaway inside Portuguese East Africa (Murray 1922; Linden 1974).

Johnston's remarkable tenure as commissioner ended in 1895. The British Treasury officially stopped the BSAC's financial hold over the protectorate, although the company maintained its annual contribution until 1910–11 (Murray 1922; Crosby 1980). Most of Malawi's current Northern Region, originally acquired from African chiefs by the ALC, was transferred to and remained the property of the BSAC until 1936.

EXPANSION OF THE LAKE MALAWI STEAMER FLEET

The steamers on Lake Malawi served a variety of imperial, geopolitical, and missionary interests. Lakeside missions and trading firms virtually depended on the steamers for their existence. As dramatic symbols of European technological and military superiority, steamers had both tactical and strategic value in their ability to project the British presence and establish colonial law and order. As noted, the task of getting the vessels from England to Malawi was enormously difficult. Looking back, the protectorate's chief clerk would write: "In the face of almost insuperable transport difficulties, and in the absence of proper roads, the steamers were placed on the rivers and on Lake Nyasa" (Murray 1922, 23).

The pioneer era of steamers thus began with the Livingstonia missionaries and the ALC in 1875. Their vessel the *Ilala* remained the only steamer on the lake until 1885, when the Universities' Mission (UMCA) launched the *Charles Janson*. By the time of Harry Johnston's departure from the protectorate a decade later, five steamers plied the lake (Murray 1922; Williams 1958). Without the introduction of steamers it is unlikely that Johnston, in his dual role as British consul and BSAC representative, would have succeeded in his efforts to simultaneously make treaties with African chiefs, thwart Portuguese designs on the lake region, survive civil wars, and fight the slavers. Overland travel was still slow and dangerous. Given the great length of the lake and the elongated shape of the territory claimed by British interests, the ALC's *Ilala* and *Domira*, and the UMCA's *Charles Janson*, offered Johnston and his Indian and African mercenaries exceptional mobility within the lake basin. The little steamers projected imperial power and could move a sizable quantity of men and supplies at an average speed of about six to eight miles per hour (Murray 1922). Ultimately, the steamers proved a significant factor in Britain's ability to consolidate control over territories adjacent to the lake. Treaties with Germany (1890) and Portugal (1891) followed, establishing formal boundaries and paving the way for the proclamation of a British Protectorate in May 1891.

In 1891 the *Charles Janson* was the only missionary (UMCA) craft on the lake. The ALC had replaced the *Ilala* in 1887 with the *Domira*, a ship of one hundred tons and ninety feet in length. In 1892 the Admiralty placed two gunboats on the lake, the *Pioneer* and *Adventure*, as well as the *Dove* on the Upper Shiré. Also in 1892 the German (Berlin) Anti-Slavery Society launched the *Hermann von Wissmann*. Displacing ninety tons, this gunboat was intended to help suppress the regional slave trade and facilitate the establishment a coastal mission at Langenburg, some 130 miles north of Likoma. Unsuccessful in persuading the UMCA missionaries to abandon the work they had already started in what was in one sense a German sphere, the Germans eventually chose to cooperate with the British missionaries and even offered free transportation to places on the lake (*CA* 12 [1894]). In 1895, Arthur Sim, the lone UMCA missionary at Kota Kota described its functions as "half gunboat and half trader" (1897, 93). Eventually acquired by the German government, the *Wissmann* was in the first naval engagement of World War I. Captured by British forces, it was repaired and re-named the *King George* in 1919 (Murray 1922; Williams 1958; Hayes 1964).

Four additional steamers had been added to the combined lake fleet by the turn of the century. The *Queen Victoria*, 120 feet long, was built in Glasgow in 1898 to carry cargo and passengers for the African Lakes Corporation. The *H.M.S. Guendolen*, a gunship of 350 tons and 135 feet long, began service in 1899. Launched about 1900, the *Vera* was built to support the activities of the Berlin Missionary Society in Tanganyika at the far north end of the lake. A second UMCA steamer, the resilient *Chauncy Maples*, was built in 1899 and became operational in 1901 (Murray 1922; Williams 1958). Its arrival on the lake greatly helped to expand contact along the widening missionary-African frontier, enabling the continued growth and consolidation of the emerging "Steamer Parish."

NOTES

1. Kjekshus (1977, 14–16). Possibly only one-third of this number actually made it alive to the slave markets of Kilwa, Zanzibar, etc. Some authorities held that the survival rate was even smaller, with four or five slaves dead for each one who reached Zanzibar alive. Livingstone reckoned that ten slaves died for every one sold. See Elton 1879, 102, cited in Kjekshus 1977, 15.

2. Stewart was a theological student in Edinburgh who became a passionate lobbyist for a Presbyterian mission in Malawi.

3. I observed similar poverty among the elderly in the environs of Mua Mission (WF) in 1990.

4. Masasi station, opened by Bishop Steere in 1876 in the Yao country of southeast Tanzania, became a major staging point on the missionaries' route from Zanzibar to Lake Malawi.

5. This financial overview is based on an analysis of statements contained in a convenience sample of seventeen *UMCA Annual Reviews* from 1899 to 1961, kindly supplied by Catherine Wakeling, archivist, USPG, London. In 1899, the Likoma Diocese in Malawi assumed a debt of £9,715 when it purchased its second lake steamer. In 1910 the Nyasaland Fund was still overdrawn by £4,600. In the years surveyed, Nyasaland was funded at roughly 90 percent of the level of Zanzibar Diocese.

6. See, e.g., UMCA, S.F. Series, SF 29 XVI. General Secretary, UMCA, to Bishop of Nyasaland, Dec. 15, 1961.

7. *CA* 29 [1911]; Mills 1911, 263; Johnson 1926, 9; and Yarborough 1888, 116.

8. From 1875 to 1883 the Livingstonia Mission distributed at Cape Maclear, Bandawe, Ekwendeni, and other locations some "500,000 yards of calico [could be used as currency to purchase food supplies]; 25 tons of beads; [and] 7 tons of soap" (van Velsen 1960, 7).

9. The preceding and following sketch of colonial developments paralleling missionary activity is drawn from several of the numerous sources available. See., e.g., Pike and Rimmington 1965; Pike 1968; and Nelson et al. 1975.

10. The *Adventure* and *Pioneer* each had a naval doctor on board (Gelfand 1964, 270).

11. Mataka was a Yao chief whose importance grew with and through the expansion of coastal Arab-Swahili slaving interests in the region. At Mataka's (Mwembe) court, in the Lujenda River valley in extreme northern Mozambique (fig. 2.1), William Johnson was passed by a coast-bound caravan containing over five thousand slaves (Johnson 1926, 69). For a high-end estimate of the annual volume (30,000) of the slave traffic, see King and King 1991, 28.

12. W. G. Blaike, *Life of Livingstone*, 270, reported that a British Consul in Zanzibar in the 1860s told Livingstone that "19,000 slaves from this Nyasa region alone passed annually" through the town's custom house. Cited in Barnes 1933, 41.

13. By 1880, Arab-Swahili slavers and traders had established themselves at the headquarters of "every major Yao chief in Malawi" (Pike 1968, 69).

CHAPTER THREE

The Return of the UMCA to Malawi: Technology and Political Relations in the Quest for Permanent Influence

RETURN TO THE LAKE

Renewed efforts by the UMCA to establish a mission field in the Lake Malawi region got underway in 1875–76. From Zanzibar, Bishop Edward Steere, the mission's third bishop, envisioned a chain of stations along an overland route from the Indian Ocean to the lake. Positioned between two of East Africa's busiest slave-trade corridors that linked the coast and the interior, the proposed missionary road would have extended across southern Tanganyika and Portuguese East Africa (Mozambique) to Lake Malawi. Some in the UMCA believed that this route could ultimately open up a broad zone of Christian influence extending from Zanzibar to Lindi (a sea connection) and then inland some four hundred miles to the shores of Lake Malawi (fig. 1.1). The mission did establish several stations along this route. Most notable was Masasi, located some 130 miles inland and built up around a nucleus of Christianized former slaves of Nyasa origin. They had lived as free persons on Zanzibar for some time, and now the UMCA proposed to repatriate them. Many of these "Nyasalanders" chose instead to terminate their journey in southern Tanganyika and settle in the Ruvuma district. There they helped to found the first mission centers in the region (UMCA 1903).

In 1881–82 the Reverend William Percival Johnson and the Reverend Charles Janson, his ill-fated older colleague, became the first UMCA pioneers to reach Lake Malawi. They had selected an overland route across southern Tanganyika and Mozambique. Johnson's experiences at the lake and his imagination and moral authority would soon carry the day in favor of the UMCA implementing a technological approach to building up the Nyasa mission field. What better method, given the lake's expanse and the spheres of influence already staked out by the Church of Scotland and Livingstonia Missions, than to exploit the advantages of steam-driven water transport. The emergence of the lake steamer as a central feature of UMCA strategy in Malawi would render the overland route through southern Tanganyika and Portuguese East Africa (P.E.A.) obsolete almost overnight (Elston 1972).

William P. Johnson's pioneering role in planting the UMCA in Malawi was extraordinary and unparalleled by any other member of the mission. An Oxford scholar-athlete (stroke of his college eight) possessed of remarkable linguistic skills and boundless energy, Johnson surrendered a prestigious appointment in the Indian Civil Service to become a UMCA missionary. He and Chauncy Maples, his life-long friend and fellow Oxonian who was later briefly the Bishop of Nyasaland, joined the mission in 1876 during their early twenties (fig. 3.1). A staunch Anglo-Catholic evangelist and in lifestyle an unyielding ascetic, Johnson was unforgettable both to his colleagues and to the Africans with whom he identified more than any other missionary. A paradoxical man, he was both deeply caring and, at times, stubbornly difficult. Thoreau would have said that Johnson listened to a different drummer.

The young Johnson had blonde hair, high cheekbones, and an angular face. His colleagues knew he had an uncommonly genuine and deep love for Africans. Johnson also had an uncompromising need to minimize contact with worldly possessions and even simple comforts. At the time of his death he had spent fifty-two years in the service of the UMCA, including the years 1896 to 1926 as Archdeacon of Nyasa (*CA* 46 [1928]; 47 [1929]; and 72 [1954]). Blinded in one eye and two-thirds so in the other in 1885, from 1886 Johnson made his home base aboard the UMCA's cramped lake steamers. Bishop J. E. Hine remarked that "personal comfort was the last thing W. P. Johnson ever thought about" (Hine 1924, 78). When Bishop Fisher (1911–29) arrived in Malawi, he found Johnson living on the UMCA's steamer, "but he refused to have an ordinary cabin and had a corner of the native dormitory boarded off—a horrible little hole dark and unventilated in which he lived and worked."[1]

In a retrospective after Johnson's death in 1928, his superior wrote that he had been disorganized and unwilling to adopt a rational, prudent

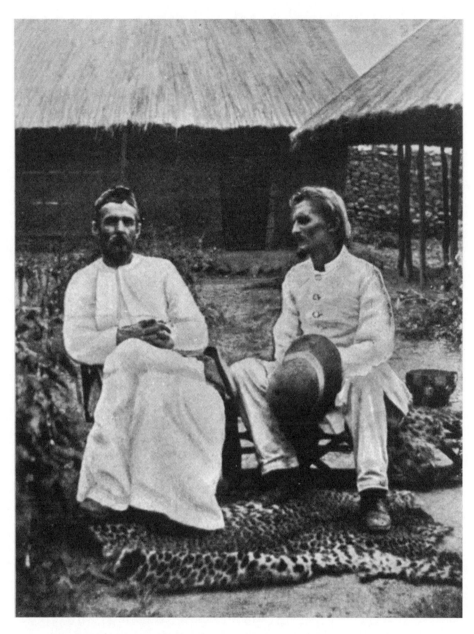

Figure 3.1. Archdeacon Chauncy Maples (left), and Rev. W. P. Johnson at Likoma.
(Source: The National Archives of Zimbabwe.)

approach to managing resources such as money and food supplies. Johnson was perceived as unwilling to live according to any formula or timetable except his own, a condition that caused terrible frustration all around.[2] In missionary circles he became known as the "Apostle of the Lake" because of his constant preaching, teaching, and pastoral work among the dozens of villages scattered along two hundred miles of Lake Malawi's eastern shoreline (*CA* 72 [1954]). Johnson shouldered the brunt of work done by the UMCA's "steamer clergy."

Despite the many aggravations of trying to work with him, even Johnson's critics such as Bishop Fisher saw him as "ready to do anything, bear anything or learn anything; he seems salted to any vagaries of climate or exposure, able to pick up any language in a month or two and to get through work or distances which would be astonishing in a man half his age" (Blood 1957, 58).

Despite his severe vision impairment, Johnson learned to read Arabic and frequently carried both the Bible and the Koran (Barnes 1933). He single-handedly translated the complete Bible into Chinyanja (*CA* 37 [1919]: 131). Oxford University awarded Johnson the degree of Doctor of Divinity, *honoris causa*, in 1911 (Winspear 1956). Reflecting on his Nyasa career, particularly the lonely and difficult first decades, one obituary observed that only "a new Johnson" could fill the gap left by his death. But the new man "will never be called upon to go through what Johnson did—there is no slave trade now, no starvation, no danger of being lost, no impossible distance from doctor or nurse, no murderously inclined chiefs nor fighting among tribes—government sees to that" (*CA* 46 [1928]: 204).

Few if any Africans with memories of Johnson are still living. The man is now largely lost to time, folklore, and whatever Europeans chose to write about him. While Johnson's alleged "nativism" tended to distance him from some of his European colleagues, most of them stood in awe of his achievements, humility, and desire and ability to identify with Africans. Writing twenty-five years after the archdeacon's death, a UMCA priest seemed to reflect an appraisal of the man that was widely if not universally shared among Europeans both within and outside the missionary enterprise. Johnson, he said, "will always rank as one of the great heroes of the century, a man of the same stature as Livingstone" (*CA* 72 [1954]: 58). Wrote Bishop John Hine, "Johnson was always reticent about himself; his letters and speeches were obscurely expressed . . . he seemed one apart, different from all others, a solitary soul called to do a great work and doing it with all his might . . . he had no great gifts of utterance, he was no pulpit orator; there was nothing of the popular missionary preacher about him. At a public meeting his words were often vague and hard to follow. Yet there was something so arresting about this man; it was he himself who impressed others and who appealed to them. There was a distinction and a sense of power in reserve which made him a notable figure in any company and marked him out as one who was cast in the mould of the saints. We might compare him with Ramon Lull in the thirteenth century, or still more with Francis Xavier in the sixteenth: men who mostly lived alone and worked alone and whose life was hid in God."[3] In 1953, the bishop of the new Diocese of South West Tanganyika (formerly part of the Diocese of Nyasaland) observed that "very large numbers of Africans who live here are convinced that William Percival Johnson is a saint. They observe the day of his death as if he were already canonized; . . . his tomb in Liuli pro-Cathedral is an object of pilgrimage from time to time" (*CA* 72 [1954]: 64).

Johnson first reached Lake Malawi in 1881 via an overland route from Masasi in southern Tanganyika. His first attempt to establish a route to the lake through the Yao country in 1879 had been unsuccessful. On the second exploratory expedition he was accompanied by his Zanzibari attendant and apparently had no intention to visit the lake. By the time he reached Mataka, the powerful Yao slave-dealer at Mwembe in P.E.A., Johnson had run out of European provisions and was sick with fever and ulcers. At Mataka's village he experienced "a rough reception" (Laws 1934, 205), but did learn that the Scottish Mission's steamer *Ilala* made occasional visits to the Yao slave-dealer Makanjila on the eastern side of Lake Malawi. Johnson believed that "the way ahead [via Mtonya] had been made clear by the war parties and plenty of Indian corn had been left to eat along the track" (Johnson 1926, 66). With Mataka's consent he changed his original plan and set off for the lake. Once at the lake he hoped to find a way to cross it to secure medical help from Dr. Robert Laws of the Scottish Livingstonia Mission at Cape Maclear.

Johnson received a friendly welcome at Makanjila's, but was chagrined to learn the *Ilala* last visited about two years' earlier! In increasingly poor physical condition, and relying again on his ingenuity and gritty determination, Johnson used one of his two "precious" Maria Theresa dollars to hire canoe-men to paddle him across twenty-five miles of treacherous open water to the east side of Cape Maclear. On landing, Johnson sent a messenger to Laws, who quickly came around at night in the steamer to rescue him. His meager possessions consisted of "a reed mat, a small bundle and a little earthenware pot"; and the boils on the patient's head and hands were so severe that "he could not put on his coat or use a knife and fork" (Laws 1934, 206).

After a "delightful month" in the care of Dr. and Mrs. Laws, Johnson pronounced himself well. The doctor provided him with a supply of trade goods so that he could negotiate the return journey to Zanzibar via Mataka's territory. Laws later recalled that it was "characteristic of Mr. Johnson that, as soon as his health improved, he must needs be off to his work again" (ibid.). Years later, after several medical-social visits to Livingstonia, Johnson remained deeply impressed by the Laws's hospitality, remarking "Oh the Paradise to me in my weakness of a well-organized station with a lady in charge!" (Johnson 1926, 67).

Johnson and the Reverend Charles Janson began walking west from Masasi in December 1881, with the goal of setting up a mission station on Lake Malawi. To avoid Ngoni warbands they used a more southerly route than followed in previous attempts to reach the lake from the east, traveling through Unangu (later a UMCA station) in Yaoland, P.E.A. They reached the lake shore at Mtengula in mid-February 1882. It had been an arduous trek, undertaken during the rainy season. Janson, feverish and weakened by dysentery towards the end of the journey, struggled against his health to walk north along the coast with Johnson. He died for his effort a week after their arrival at the lake. Johnson buried him in the lakeside village of Chia, about twenty miles from Mtengula (UMCA 1903; A. E. Anderson-Morshead 1955). With his companion now gone, Johnson was suddenly the only European on the eastern coast of Lake Malawi.

For nearly two years, Johnson wandered alone up and down the coast of Lake Malawi and in the adjacent Ruvuma and Lujenda river basins. He wanted to "observe the habits of the people, to learn their language, and, lastly, to form a plan for mission work amongst them" (UMCA 1903, 33). The village of Chigoma on the lakeshore became his base. He began proselytizing there under the authority of Chiteji, a hospitable Nyanja chief who also controlled about half of nearby Likoma Island. Situated just four miles offshore on a slave route, Likoma was destined to become the UMCA's first station and its headquarters in Malawi.

The UMCA missionaries viewed the local Nyanja peoples of the immediate coastal zone as "peaceable" fishers and cultivators. In contrast, militant African tribes including the Gwangwara Ngoni (recent invaders of Zulu origin) and the Yao inhabited the interior country east of the Lake. The Yao had long raided the Nyanja and sold them to Arab-Swahili slavers from the East African coast. At the time of Johnson's arrival the countryside was plagued by extreme insecurity,[4] and the "continual fear of Ngoni raids unsettled everything" (Winspear 1956, 21–22). Chiteji had built a stockade about two miles away from his village. The chief's people slept there every night, and Johnson found safety among them (ibid.).

Europeans recorded that fear and vulnerability pervaded the existence of African communities in the greater lake region. How people adapted their settlement patterns to survive the depredations of hostile neighbors provide striking illustrations of their response to the terror. In some localities people had clustered their conical-roofed grass huts into large villages surrounded by "impenetrable stockades, or perched on rocky peaks or headlands" (UMCA 1903). In other places, particularly on the coast north of Likoma, people built villages on piles on low-lying rocks and reefs in the lake just a few feet above the water, accessible only by canoe.

Some pile-villages achieved considerable scale, "with platforms four to five hundred feet long and possibly thirty broad. Some were two stories high; a lower story for cattle and goats, while the men lived above." The life in the pile house was hard, and they have been abandoned since more settled times (Johnson 1926, 105). Small islands might also be crowded with refugees. People on Papai Island would "swim their cattle across to the mainland in the morning and back again in the evening" (106). Johnson saw pile-villages off-shore around Manda in 1883 (*CA* 55 [1937]: 209). They had disappeared by the end of the century, when he could find "no trace of the people I had found living in the cities of refuge from the enemy" (Johnson 1926, 104–5). Africans reported that the dreaded Ngoni, whom Johnson called the "Philistines," had killed all of the former inhabitants of the pile-villages and nearby slopes above them. The Ngoni and Yao from the hills apparently had a superstitious dread of water; hence the perceived security of pile-villages for people near the lake. Only a few feet of water proved an effective deterrent against these marauders. As late as 1899, when raids were no longer common, lakeside villages on the east coast continued to be either stockaded or defensively sited on the water (Winspear 1956; Elston 1972).

Territories on the western side of Lake Malawi remained a Scottish Presbyterian sphere, excepting the heavily Muslim area of Kota Kota. Tonga and other African peoples subjected to the Ngoni raids and reign of terror responded by building settlements of remarkable ingenuity. An important eyewitness account in the 1880s records caves and holes dug into the ground; and huts placed on ledges ten feet wide on cliffs two-hundred-fifty feet high, partly shielded by dense vegetation and accessed by fissures in the rock. In other places people converted sheer mountain walls into terraces for huts, sought security in river gorges and behind waterfalls, or built flimsy shelters and perched like sea birds on piles of boulders out in the lake (Elmslie 1899, 83–89).

Travel on the eastern side of the lake was also slow and dangerous in 1882. Narrow, winding footpaths connected the coastal villages, but the primary African means of travel was on water in dugout canoes (UMCA 1903). Word of Johnson's existence traveled quickly across the lake to the western side. The *Ilala* stopped occasionally near Chiteji's village. Johnson and the *Ilala's* captain became friends and the latter brought his boat and occasional European visitors "to and fro [Chiteji's] at long intervals" (Johnson 1926, 91–92). Johnson sailed on the *Ilala* to Karonga at the north end of the lake with five of his future catechumens, seeking friendly contact and potential opportunities for evangelism among other African peoples. The return leg was a long overland journey, through the Livingstone Mountains and along the east side of the lake. Johnson became quite ill and disabled by "an ulcer with two openings in his thigh" (Winspear 1956, 22). It was May 1883, and his African companions carried him back to Chiteji's. There, he had the good fortune of an offer of transport on the *Ilala* to Dr. Laws's Scottish mission, which had been relocated on the western coast at Bandawe. Once again Johnson recuperated for several weeks under the care of Dr. and Mrs. Laws.

On recovering his health, Johnson sailed on the *Ilala* to the south end of the lake and then walked into the Shiré Highlands to collect his mail and visit the Church of Scotland Mission at Blantyre. With his letters he found a months-old cable from the UMCA's Home Committee, requesting that he return to England for consultations. Johnson departed Blantyre shortly thereafter, uncharacteristically armed with a revolver (Johnson 1926, 112). He had decided to explore the hill country on the southeast side of the lake in order to "be able to report to the new Bishop [Smythies] on the state of the whole country" (110). In his memoirs he observed that he wasted no opportunities to proselytize on his journey back to the lake: "As usual I preached at places on the way, showing the people my credentials, as it were" (109–10; Elston 1972, 349). He descended to the lake at Losefa, where he met a slave caravan and talked with its leaders. The party included "two Mohammedan teachers . . . a good one and a bad one ; the bad one begged for revolver bullets and immoral French medicines" (Johnson 1926, 111).

Upon reaching Chigoma[5] Johnson reaffirmed his cordial and strategic ties with Chiteji before leaving the lake region for Zanzibar. He had already settled upon a plan and strategy for missionizing the lake region and would soon present his proposal to the UMCA authorities. He sailed from Zanzibar to England, arriving in the summer of 1884.

During Johnson's initial investigations, and for several years following, geopolitical claims by a rival colonial power, in this instance Portugal's claim to Mozambique, restricted the UMCA's freedom of action on the eastern side of the lake. The UMCA grudgingly accepted that the middle third of the coast and all of the adjacent interior to the Indian Ocean was Portuguese territory, although the final agreement on jurisdiction among Britain, Portugal, and Germany was delayed until the end of the century.

Stimulated by the Arab-African slave trade, extensive areas around the lake had become part of a vigorous frontier of Islamic expansion in the nineteenth century. The arrival of Christian missionaries promoted mutual hostility and a heightened sense of competition between crescent and cross. In addition, several powerful African chiefs competed for territorial influence and control of the slave trade in this region until the late 1890s, thereby slowing European penetration for more than a decade. Describing the lake coast in the 1880s, William Bellingham observed:

> There is not a village but what has its dealings in slaves and its slaves. . . . Passing through Mponda's country coming home, we saw several places where Mponda's caravan of slaves encamped. There were hundreds of places where fires had been, and at each fire there would have been four or five people. (Yarborough 1888, 139)

S.S. CHARLES JANSON: THE UMCA'S FIRST STEAMER

Johnson's extensive itinerations around the Lake Malawi basin persuaded him that the mission could probably realize its goals sooner and more efficiently with the assistance of a small lake steamer. Twenty years earlier Bishop Mackenzie, writing in 1861 shortly before he died on the Lower Shiré, had requested "a University boat" for the Nyasa mission field. Bishop Steere had advanced the idea of purchasing a native dhow "to carry missionaries up and down Lake Nyasa" (*CA* 43 [1925]: 87). While the two bishops seem to have been the earliest proponents of a nautical strategy for the UMCA in Malawi, as a practical matter it was Johnson who fleshed out the idea and brought it to reality. He certainly gained the reputation as "the main promoter of the steamer enterprise" (Buchanan 1885, 256). Johnson briefly considered the possibility of recommending that the UMCA adopt the use of a large canoe, a steel boat, or a dhow to launch its mission activities. He rejected each of these options because none of these craft offered realistic or safe choices (given the frequent violent storms on the lake) for a mobile, floating school and missionary residence (Barnes 1933; Winspear 1956). During his solo, pioneering work in 1882–83, Johnson had acquired extensive first-hand knowledge of the coastal zone and parts of the interior uplands situated on the eastern side of Lake Malawi. In writing up his travels for the *Proceedings of the Royal Geographical Society* he also described several transverse water routes across the lake used by slavers and others, as well as a number of shorter ferry routes (Johnson 1884). Johnson had sailed on the *Ilala* several times during this period, and benefited from its being used as an ambulance, courtesy of Dr. Laws, during a debilitating illness.

With his detailed expertise of the lake region Johnson seems to have had no difficulty convincing the UMCA leadership and his fellow missionaries of a steamer's several advantages. He emphasized that they could rapidly establish and maintain contact with different African peoples settled along the lake shore and in the adjacent interior in far less time, in greater safety, and more cheaply than overland routes permitted. European missionaries and African teachers could work on land during the day and return to the steamer at night, avoiding contact as much as possible with "fatal mias-mas" in the low-lying, often swampy, coastal areas (another fifteen years would pass before malaria was linked to its mosquito vector). And there would be a greater possibility of avoiding or undercutting the influence of hostile African groups such as the Gwangwara and the slave-raiders. The missionaries clearly recognized the advantages of a steamer in light of the lakeside environment they wanted to "open up." A steamer's range and great relative speed would facilitate the UMCA's strategy of working among different tribes and polities. The vessel would serve as "the centre of work" and through its mobility enable the mission to "avoid the jealousy caused by residence under one particular chief" (*CA* 3 [1885]: 172). The UMCA wanted to believe that it could maximize the geographical scope of their re-ligious agenda while minimizing "disturbance" to African social conditions (Barnes 1933, 69). Such compartmentalized and contradictory thinking ev-idently meant that the missionaries hoped to revolutionize and "manage" the spiritual life of Africans without having to confront directly the enor-mous implications of the other social and cultural changes that followed as the frontier unfolded. By all means, the UMCA should avoid creating black Africans who behaved like Englishmen.

The steamer was to move north and south on the lake, serving as a float-ing headquarters, a "Training Home for African Teachers," and a catalyst for an expanding chain of mission stations and schools on land (*CA* 2 [1884]: 55; Buchanan 1885). Trained African teachers would be placed among the villages on land. European priests, transported by the steamer that served them as a dormitory and a church, would make regular visits to the villages.

The missionaries reasoned that African social life was less likely to be disrupted if they restricted their activities to visiting as opposed to living in the villages. A mission steamer would also encourage efficiencies in the use of personnel, and offer more independent and direct lines of supply among the stations and with routes to the outside world. Not least important, steamer transport could exploit a local fuel source.

But was this list of anticipated advantages too sanguine? John Buchanan, a Church of Scotland Mission staff member, coffee planter at Zomba, and later the British Consul, thought so. Considering the *Ilala's* experience, he warned that the lake was subject to severe storms that would render the steamer not "permanently reliable." Furthermore, the lake and its coastline as well as the connecting Shiré and Zambezi valleys remained "inimical to European health." Should the UMCA avoid these serious threats, "then the vessel may become a precious auxiliary to the Mission, like the famous Southern Cross yacht of Bishop Patteson of Melanesia" (Buchanan 1885, 256). What Buchanan did not directly mention was how much time the steamer might be hors de combat because of mechanical problems, repairs, and shortages of spare parts involving engines, boilers, and plates, particularly under the conditions of a tropical climate (Sim 1897).

In England the UMCA Home Committee and Bishop Charles Smythies, who himself had carried out a reconnaissance of the region between the Indian Ocean and Lake Malawi in 1875, approved Johnson's steamer plan for Malawi. Johnson spent six months of 1884 in Britain successfully raising money for the steamer. He evidently had little difficulty soliciting the necessary £2,312 needed for its construction (*CA* 3 [1885]: 5). Moreover, Charles Janson had written into his will a specified sum of money for building a UMCA steamer for use on Lake Malawi (Johnston 1897). Upon launching there seemed little doubt that the vessel would immediately be named the *S.S. Charles Janson*, in memory of Johnson's colleague.

Messrs. Yarrow and Headley of London, a firm specializing in building small craft such as fast river and cross-channel ships, built the *Charles Janson* at a cost of about £5,000 (Buchanan 1885). It was sixty-two feet long, twelve feet wide, and displaced twenty-five tons (the ALC's *Ilala* was only forty-eight feet long). The *Charles Janson* had a single screw propeller, auxiliary sails (two masts), a speed of eight knots, and a draft of five feet (Williams 1958). Friends of the mission donated its anchor, compass, canteen, and other fittings (Yarborough 1888). Immediately after its construction, the steamer was disassembled into about eight hundred pieces. These parts were then packed into headloads of sixty pounds each and fitted in turn into about

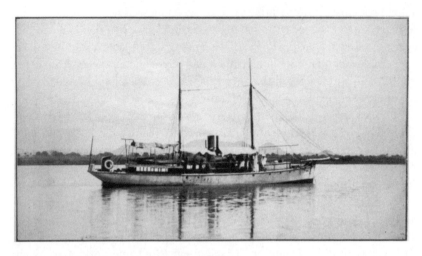

Figure 3.2. The Mission Steamer *Charles Janson*.
(Source: Johnson (1926), facing p. 138. From the archives of the USPG.)

three hundred eighty cases. The entire cargo, including stores for the party's first six months' existence on the Upper Shiré and Lake Malawi, was then shipped in the hold of the *Hawarden Castle* to Cape Town, from which the *Florence* carried it to the mouth of the Zambezi.

W. P. Johnson, assisted by a naval officer and five laymen, had charge of the expedition transporting the *Charles Janson* to Lake Malawi. On arrival at the mouth of the Zambezi, Johnson was stricken by virulent ophthalmia that blinded him and forced his evacuation to England for surgery. His illness prevented his presence on September 6, 1885, when the reassembled *Charles Janson* was dedicated and floated out of its dry dock at Matope above the Murchison Falls into the Shiré.[6] The UMCA rented a crude dock and sheds at Matope from the African Lakes Company, which originally built them for the construction of the *Ilala* a decade earlier. It was dedicated in an English-Swahili service by Charles A. Smythies, the newly appointed first Bishop of Likoma (Yarborough 1888, 51, 65). The *C. J.*, as the steamer became known, remained in the UMCA's service for fifty years (fig. 3.2).

William Johnson came back to the Lake Malawi region in November 1886, several months later than planned. Following his eye surgery in England, and while en route to the embryonic mission at the lake, he became seriously ill and went to South Africa for medical care and recuperation. When he finally reached Malawi he was permanently blind in one eye and nearly so in the other. He found it difficult to focus the eye that gave him partial sight, and in bright light he typically peered between two fingers (Winspear 1956). Handicapped but unwilling to be "disabled," he continued his career at the lake for another forty-two years.

LIKOMA ISLAND HEADQUARTERS: CENTRALITY OR ISOLATION?

For reasons related to the decision to adopt the steamer strategy, and to security, the UMCA authorities acquired rights in Likoma Island and made it the mission's Nyasaland headquarters. While Johnson was recuperating in England, Bishop Smythies in Zanzibar made one of his five visits to Lake Malawi, where he visited Likoma and negotiated an agreement with Chiteji that allowed the UMCA to set up a station on the island. Situated approximately midway between the north and south ends of the lake, Likoma ("desirable," "pleasant," or "beautiful") is roughly four miles from the eastern coast. It is about four and one-half miles long and two and one-half miles wide (figs. 3.3 and 3.4). Likoma and neighboring Chizumulu, seven miles farther west, are the only important islands in Lake Malawi.

UMCA missionaries thought of Likoma first and foremost as a haven of safety against attacks by slavers and hostile Africans, even though it lay astride a main slave-transport route. It was also seen as a healthier place for Europeans. Bishop Smythies mandated that the east coast of the lake was malarious and "so unhealthy that no mission stations were to be built there" (Howard 1904, 45). Some in the mission wanted to believe that Likoma was merely a few hours away from Dr. Laws and medical help at the Scottish mission at Bandawe. In fact, canoeing time across the widest part of the lake ranged from twelve to twenty-four hours in fair weather, with passengers and craft exposed to strong winds. The journey was "always long, difficult, and exceedingly dangerous," making dependable connections between the east and west coasts difficult (*CA* 34 [1916]: 33). On the other hand, Likoma residents could reach the Portuguese-administered east coast in about an hour. Over time, intermarriage and social relations forged strong ties between the islanders and the east mainlanders (ibid.).

While the lake offers essentially unimpeded navigation, there are few good harbors, and sand banks and bars often limit anchorage. Likoma was an attractive place because it has the excellent, well-protected harbor of Mbamba, which could be easily reached at night or in bad weather (Howard 1904). William Bellingham, a UMCA engineer, established the station during the four months that followed the dedication of the *Charles Janson* and its first sailing on the lake (Yarborough 1888, 20–26, 61–62, 105-6; *CA* 2 [1884]: 188).

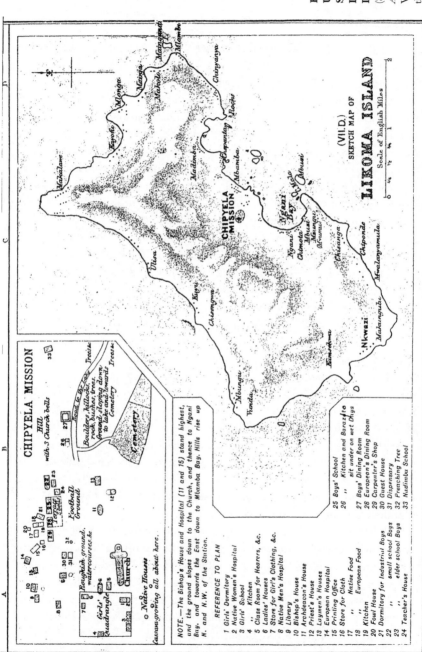

Figure 3.3. UMCA Head Station, Likoma Island. (Source: *UMCA Atlas* (1903), pl. VII.D. From the archives of the USPG.)

CHIPYELA MISSION

HILL
with 3 Church bells

Road to Ba-Fort

Bouldlers, hillocks, rock, bushes, trees. Ground sloping down to lake and towards Cemetery.

Cemetery

Treess

Treess

Football Ground

Roughish ground, watercourses.&c.

Girls' Quadrangle

Church

o *Native House*

casava growing all about here.

NOTE.—The Bishop's House and Hospital (11 and 15) stand highest, and the ground slopes down to the Church, and thence to Ngani Bay, and towards the East down to Mbamba Bay. Hills rise up N. and N.W. of the Station.

REFERENCE TO PLAN

1 Girls' Dormitory
2 Native Women's Hospital
3 Girls' School
4 " Kitchen
5 Class Room for Hearers, &c.
6 Ladies' Houses
7 Store for Girl's Clothing, &c.
8 Native Men's Hospital
9 Library
10 Bishop's House
11 Archdeacon's House
12 Priest's House
13 Laymen's Houses
14 European Hospital
15 Printing Office
16 Store for Cloth
17 " Native Food
18 " European Food
19 Kitchen
20 Foul House
21 Dormitory for Industrial Boys
22 " small school Boys
23 " elder school Boys
24 Teacher's House
25 Boys' School
26 " Kitchen and Baraza to sit under on wet Days
27 Boys' Dining Room
28 European's Dining Room
29 Carpenter's Shop
30 Guest House
31 Dispensary
32 Preaching Tree
33 Nutimba School

SKETCH MAP OF

LIKOMA ISLAND

(VII.D.)

Scale of English Miles

CHIPYELA MISSION

Makasilawe
Kayoko
Mlonga
Msinga
Mwalo
Mwalo
Manganja
Mkombo

Chanyanya

Chapankay Mlochis

Madimoto

Mbamba

Ulisa

Kuyu

Chirenyuva

Mbungu

Wanda

Ngani Bay
Chimoto
Mbwasi
Msungu
Mvunwi
Chisanga

Ngani Bay
Pt-Msala
Mbwasi

Chiponde

Mwalanyamula
Makanguiu

Nkwazi

Kanselema

John Bartholomew & Co

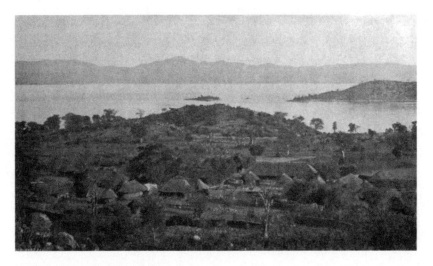

Figure 3.4. Likoma Mission Station, 1890s.
(Source: Anderson-Morshead (1903). From the archives of the USPG.)

The *C.J.* made its first call at Likoma on January 22, 1886, just fourteen months after it was shipped from London in small parcels.

Until August 24, 1885, Likoma remained jointly under the authority of Chiteji, Johnson's former host on the mainland, and his neighbor, Mataka of Kobwe. The arrival of the first UMCA missionaries was unannounced. Yohanna Tawe, one of the very few African witnesses of record during the UMCA's century in Malawi, recalled that he saw "a white boat coming from the south of the Island." After they anchored the boat inside the bay, two Europeans (the Reverend George Swinny and William Bellingham) came ashore and pitched their tent. Four foreign Africans accompanied them: "SoSongolo the teacher, Augustine Ambali, Nicholas Faraji, and Frank the Zuluman" (*CA* 53 [1935]: 254). The island's chiefs responded by sending a messenger by canoe over to the mainland to inform Chiteji, their patron and Johnson's benefactor, of the strangers' arrival. While we can only speculate on his motives, Chiteji's response indicates that he had calculated it would be advantageous to permit the missionaries to settle on Likoma. He decided to enter into an agreement with the UMCA that called for him to transfer land to the mission and promise other considerations in exchange for various "articles of barter" (Barnes 1933, 75).

The site chosen for the station on Likoma was immediately adjacent to the *chipyela,* or "place of burning," the ground where witches are burned alive.

Elston (1972) asserts that the mission site was "purchased according to native law." A formal agreement regarding Likoma did not, however, materialize until 1890. At the urging of John Buchanan, the British vice-consul, the UMCA negotiated written agreements with many of the African chiefs on the adjacent coast in order to establish rights to anchorage, landing places, fuel wood, and building sites. In exchange the chiefs received quantities of white and sometimes blue calico (e.g., thirty to sixty fathoms), blankets, beads, and bars of soap.[7] Such transactions generally took place through "friends" in a village who acted as go-betweens for the two parties. Barter with trade goods remained the sole medium of exchange at Likoma until 1892, when the first coin was introduced (Johnson 1926). As late as 1905, soap, cloth, salt, and beads remained interchangeable with cash at Likoma and some of the mainland villages.[8] The Likoma agreement with Chiteji established the boundaries of the mission area; it accorded the UMCA full jurisdiction over the adjacent harbor, including the slope leading to it; and it abolished witch burning on Likoma.

Likoma Island sat in splendid, nearly unimaginable, isolation from the early centers of commercial and administrative activity in colonial Malawi (cf. Elston 1972). The UMCA's initial location decision strongly emphasized security concerns, and physical accommodation of their adopted technology in the form of a good harbor for the *Charles Janson*. At the time it was known that other suitable harbors existed along the east coast at Mtengula and Mluluka, forty to fifty miles south of Likoma (Johnson 1926, 139, 148, 161–62, 183–84, 207). Yet effective control over either of these places would have required difficult if not impossible negotiations for territory on which to establish a mainland station.

In the 1880s, the locations of these other harbors would not have offered the missionaries "safe asylum . . . from the incursions of marauding tribes" (Maples 1899, 308). Monkey Bay, near Cape Maclear at the southwest end of the lake, was also well sheltered with good anchorage. Since it was under the control of Mponda, the prominent Muslim slave-dealer, and also within the Scots' Livingstonia sphere, Monkey Bay was not a reasonable choice for a head station in 1885. The UMCA had started evangelical work in this district (at Mkope) by 1889, but it was done from the safety of the steamer (Johnson 1926, 139, 185). Thus, for the UMCA to do what it did in the lake region in the 1880s, both the steamer and Likoma Island proved necessary elements of strategy. The key players believed that the absence of a suitable base on the mainland was an insufficient excuse to ignore Livingstone's charge.

The friendly reception and willingness of the people to provide firewood for the steamer cheered a traveler arriving at Likoma on the *Ilala* in 1885. He remarked that "nothing can exceed the beauty of this spot" with its "capital anchorage" and "picturesque park-like glades with numerous villages" (*CA* 3 [1885]: 171). A generation later another observer noted:

> Every bay round the island has its village, and apart from the Mission stations no house on the island is built more than fifty yards from the shore . . . because of the carrying of water and . . . the white ants. This is a country where, when white ants are to be considered, the gospel has to be reversed. It is the wise man who builds on the sand and the foolish who builds on the rock. (*CA* 42 [1924]: 220)

On a visit to Likoma in 1888, John Buchanan, the Acting British Vice-Consul on Lake Malawi, remarked on the large bay that lay below the station, and the "simply charming" view of the mountainous mainland claimed by Portugal. The landscape was not a place one would select for agriculture, and was densely studded with gigantic baobab trees that formed "a magnificent cordon all around the island, close to the water's edge." A "wonderful variety of trees," especially the fig, grew on the island, although the baobab was the commonest species. For the consul, an experienced man in such matters, the place had a romantic aura: "a picture of quiet rural life." Men guarded herds of twenty to thirty cattle. Large herds of goats with sleek, colorful hides roamed the island. Strolling along the shore in the late afternoon, Buchanan was captivated by the scene. Lake Malawi's deep blue coloring was accentuated by the white waves that washed onto the sandy beaches. Children dug holes in the sand, amusing each other, or wove nets or carved miniature canoes while their mothers prepared the evening meal. Returning fishermen beached their canoes (*bwato*) and spread their nets out, mending some in preparation for the next day's return to the water. Overhead an occasional fish eagle sailed toward its roost in a tree (*CA* 6 [1888]: 125). The lake's spectacular environs invited spiritual feelings regardless of one's religious persuasion. Decades later a UMCA official from England undoubtedly spoke for many when he wrote that "the beauty of the whole place [Likoma] really lies in its tiny bays, with their rocks and their islets and deep blue water swarming with fish, and so clear that one can easily count the stones on the bottom" (*CA* 42 [1924]: 218).

John Buchanan also observed in 1888 that "a stranger visiting Lukoma [*sic*] is at once struck by the utter want of display of riches" (*CA* 6 [1888]: 153). Its people inhabited numerous small villages scattered on plains between the hills and the shoreline. In other places the hills dropped sharply to the lake. Fish and fishing played a central role in the life of the settlements all around the lakeshore, as is true today. Cassava flour and fish (fresh, smoked and sun-dried) formed the basic dietary staples.

Because granite is Likoma's defining geological feature, the island is covered by poor, sandy soils that do not hold water, and there are no permanent rivers or springs. Drinking water is obtained from the lake. Within an hour after a rain, the ground surface is dry. Likoma's hilly central spine rises over five hundred feet above the lake, and granite boulders punctuate the terrain. Most of the rain (c. 35 inches) falls from December to April, followed by generally cooler and pleasant months during a long dry season that culminates in a period of hot, oppressive weather. From October to December shade temperatures along the lakeshore often reach 120°F. Sensible nighttime temperatures can be extremely high and bothersome during this season owing to the island's dense covering of rocky boulders that absorb heat during the day and re-radiate it at night (Howard 1904).

Dr. Robert Howard, the diocesan medical officer from 1899 to 1909, believed that the island's barrenness was a great liability because it limited the production of fresh vegetables, fruit, and milk.[9] Maize would not grow due to the thin soils (Howard 1904). Dr. (later Bishop) Hine also emphasized that building material was extremely scarce. The bamboos, poles, reeds, and grass used in local house construction all had to be procured from the mainland. One had to travel twenty to thirty miles inland from the lake in order to find limestone. Sometimes the men sent to bring back these materials would be intercepted and held or attacked by the Ngoni, causing a delay in building plans (CA 12 [1894]: 169).

For the resident missionaries there was another, much harsher side to this setting—whose appearances and symbols they interpreted freely, if not always accurately, and had committed themselves to change. Day in and day out the islanders lived in and with the "horrors of heathenism," and the "terror of the Gwangwara" (Ngoni) on the adjacent mainland. While the countenance of the Africans was "outwardly fair and pleasant," even "lovely," the missionaries thought they could sense that "a feeling of intense sadness lurked on the inside"—and over-stretching poetic license—where "all is foul and dark" (CA 6 [1888]: 125).

Likoma's population in 1885 was estimated at 2,600, approximately two-thirds Nyanja speakers and the rest people from the west coast, mainly Tonga (CA 34 [1916]: 33). In common with the Nyanja (closely related to the Chewa of southern Malawi and southwest of the lake) and Yao peoples on the adjacent coast and in the interior behind, Likoma's populations had a matrilineal social structure. Rights, obligations, and duties pass through the female line, while authority over a man's children is strongly vested in their maternal uncle (mother's brother), and marriages tend to be unstable. Many Likomans had sought refuge there from the insecurity of their original homes on the mainland. By the early 1900s, with the evolution of more settled conditions under British colonial rule, perhaps a quarter of the population had returned home (Howard 1904). In 1914 Likoma's population was expanding through natural increase, and the island was reportedly already overcrowded and chronically short of foodstuffs.

The existence of the mission with its amenities also stimulated a flow of African immigrants from the adjacent Portuguese territory. As an island, Likoma was portrayed as the perfect dodge for mainland peoples who came only to "evade taxation." Yet many people had family members in both places. Since the mission had established Likoma as its headquarters, the need to transact domestic and economic business produced a regular movement of people back and forth across the water. By 1919, tensions with the Portuguese authorities on the mainland had grown over the issue of food exports from Kobwe to Likoma. A long-standing source of friction centered on the loss of customs duties on cassava and other foodstuffs. The Nyasaland government claimed that "the island had ten times as many natives as it can support," and the Resident argued that in the absence of a permanent agreement Africans should adhere to Portuguese regulations.[10] Resolution of this quandary was no further along three years later. Portuguese authorities had resorted to seizing Likoma canoes and allowing unsupervised police to engage in brutality toward both Likoma and Portuguese Africans. Bishop Cathrew Fisher hoped that the Portuguese would face the reality of an essentially harmless but relentless flow of people:

> Likoma and the coast opposite are one show and no regulations that can be made will ever make the natives regard them as anything else. The people are all related, the distance is trifling, and they simply will not recognize the political boundary. They go to and from all the time and without the most elaborate police system nothing will stop them doing so.[11]

The Original Mission Station on Likoma Island

Occupied continuously from 1885, the original site selected for the mission's head station was a plot of ground one hundred yards square. It lay on a sloping piece of land about six hundred yards from the lake and one hundred feet above the water level at Mbamba Bay, called "the place of crocodiles" by local Africans (CA 53 [1935]: 254). Two African villages lay a half-mile apart on the lakeshore, roughly equidistant from the mission. The missionaries' food was poor, luxuries were very few, and there was much exposure to malaria and its sequelae. They generally disregarded hygienic principles. Based on their perceived local experience, the missionaries' lay health practices often proved unreliable if not fallacious. There was "almost complete ignorance of the special precautions necessary in a tropical and malarial climate" (Howard 1904, 16). Greatly complicating matters was the fact that until the close of the century malaria was still attributed to "miasmas."[12] Thus a practical scientific understanding of its causes and transmission would not be available for another fifteen years.

All African huts were round (straight lines were little used in local cultures) and windowless, featuring one room and one door. Their poor quality and modest size was thought partly to reflect the operation of a social leveling mechanism. A man who built a house larger than those of his peers surely invited them to tear it down and deflate his ego (Yarborough 1888, 138). In the early days the UMCA missionaries used wattle (reeds) for their own houses and other necessary structures, which they built (without daub) in semi-African style. These structures lacked windows, but a space was left between the walls and roof so that air and light could enter. Archdeacon Chauncy Maples believed that reed houses were both healthier and "more native!" (Howard 1904, 16). The early UMCA missionaries lived in "rude houses" (excepting the ladies quarters) that were "unfit even for a native's occupation." They subsisted on an African diet of "bad food, badly cooked." Commissioner Harry Johnston believed their strategy was a futile, self-defeating exercise. At Likoma it was "pathetic to see highly educated men from Oxford and Cambridge hollow-eyed and fever-stricken, crouching in little huts which no native chief would deign to occupy" (*CA* 14 [1896]: 179). For nearly ten years the missionaries led an ascetic, primitive lifestyle of self-sacrifice, believing that Africans would identify with their example and show a greater openness to their ministry.

Even after the UMCA had abandoned its strategy of shared poverty with Africans, ideas of simple living and sacrifice remained philosophical cornerstones of mission life. In contrast, according to a disenchanted English visitor, Church of Scotland missionaries in the "little Arcadia" at Blantyre opted for an alternate position on the hardship spectrum. They were carried around in machilas [hammocks], "with troops of native savages dangling behind them"; moreover, "they have the best houses, stores, workshops, gardens and anything else worth having, all paid for by their friends at home" (Colville and Colville 1911, 47).

Likoma, however, "provided nothing but granite rock" and this produced "a constant sending backwards and forwards of the mission boats"

(Hine 1924, 153). Nearly two decades after the mission opened "all firewood, timber, and most of the food for native schoolboys" still had to be brought from the mainland by boat (Howard 1904, 14). But the island supplied "very good stone," and "excellent mortar" was made from white anthills. The first stone and brick buildings went up in 1889, and others followed by 1892. These structures included a hospital, schools, a building for a printing press, and stores, but no European-style dwellings. Late in 1892, two disastrous fires at Likoma destroyed nineteen of thirty reed houses, including the ladies' quarters as well as the library and book collection. Nonetheless, by mid-1894, the Likoma station had grown to "thirty-nine roofs," including a European Hospital, Industrial School, both with stone walls and grass roofs, and the first house built of stone with glass windows. Twelve African builders and up to 160 day laborers contributed to the construction of the tiny but essential hospital (*CA* 12 [1894]: 169). Between 1897 and 1900, all Europeans on the station received houses built with permanent materials, and also glass windows.

By 1896 these events, together with high levels of illness and mortality in the ranks, and the arrival of new members and ideas, helped to sway the UMCA's Home Committee against the ascetic principles of Johnson, Maples, and the other pioneers. A decade of harsh experience had turned up little evidence that their evangelism had been enhanced because they maintained a more or less "African" material existence.

Twenty years after Likoma's founding a great cathedral was put up and dedicated a few yards from the *chipyela*, the burning-place of witches.[13] Preceded by two temporary churches, Likoma Cathedral is a massive, cruciform structure constructed of local granite and bricks (fig. 1.3). Some of this stone was "imported" on the *Charles Janson* from Amelia Bay (Manda) in Tanganyika, about one hundred miles northeast of Likoma. Here, the Livingstone Mountains rise to ten thousand feet, and dip precipitously into the lake. Set with "mortar" prepared from the compacted soil of termite mounds, the cathedral measures 320 feet long, 85 feet wide from transept to transept, and 45 feet along the ridge (*CA* 78 [1960]). Together with its chapel, library, chapter house, and cloisters, the building's area exceeded 37,000 square feet. It was at once a stunningly powerful symbol of European culture and dominance, and an exotic and romantic (respectively for Africans and missionaries) place in and from which to stimulate the spread of a new faith. Its construction was overseen by a qualified architect who was also a missionary. The Africans he recruited as masons and other workers came from the ranks of either "Christians or catechumens," and each day's work began with prayers.[14] Even in the 1920s the cathedral was believed to be "the largest single building in Central Africa" (Dale 1925, 195). It remains a truly remarkable edifice, symbolizing ecclesiastical and imperial aspirations in one of tropical Africa's most isolated areas.

Reverend Chauncy Maples

In mid-1886, the Reverend Chauncy Maples moved from the UMCA's pioneer station at Masasi, in southern Tanganyika, to bolster the staff at Likoma. Within three months, Bishop Smythies of Zanzibar appointed him Archdeacon of Nyasa. Maples supervised the expansion of the work at Likoma for nearly a decade. Overall responsibility for policy and personnel in the Nyasa mission field continued, as always, in the hands of the bishop in Zanzibar, situated over one thousand (route) miles away. In 1892, the UMCA, its work growing steadily, decided to subdivide this huge area by forming the new Diocese of Nyasaland and appointing a bishop to supervise it.

Maples also provided significant and sustained support for the efforts of William P. Johnson, his close college friend from Oxford, to build up his ministry among the lakeshore villages (fig. 3.1). In many ways there could hardly be more contrast between two men. Maples was socially at ease and highly articulate, even eloquent; whereas Johnson lacked polish and often had difficulty expressing himself. Nevertheless, their friendship and liking for each other remained strong. It was bolstered by a shared belief that mission work should focus almost exclusively on evangelism, primarily based on itineration rather than on the expansion of stations and substations. Johnson held a much more radical version of this position than Maples. He had a strong aversion to encouraging large mission stations such as Likoma because in the process of becoming large, well ordered, and prosperous, their spiritual influence on the local Africans might ultimately be weakened (Barnes 1933, 146–47). Yet Johnson sometimes failed to appreciate the inconsistencies in some of the positions he so staunchly defended. One key mission member observed that "the steamer *Chauncy Maples* was as alien as Likoma Cathedral and probably as costly—but while the Cathedral was pegged down solidly to one place, the steamer was at least floating hither and thither and justifying its existence in many places" (144).

Johnson often visited more than two settlements daily from his base on the *Charles Janson.*[15] Recalling the early years, he wrote:

By December, 1886, Archdeacon Maples had fairly started me in regular visiting and preaching on the east side of the Lake, as far south as ... Chikole [fifty miles from Likoma]. The *Charles Janson,* which had the reputation in after years of being the swiftest steamer on the Lake, was about the length of a college eight. How we slept, had our meals, often had a school on board, and always had a chapel, and all this in a cabin which is now a baggage-room, is a thing to remember. "The world was young," says Dr. Smith, in describing Rebecca's gladsome drawing of water, and so it was with us. . . . The skipper and the engineer came in for the rough-and-tumble work when the natives were hostile. Often we had to run the gauntlet from Monkey Bay to Mtengula or Msumba, without landing and with the knowledge that if we ran ashore we should fall into enemy hands. (1926, 138–39)

Maples, whose name became virtually synonymous (posthumously) with the "Steamer Parish," was a man of penetrating intellect and legendary social gifts. Charismatic, musical, and humorous, he was, said Bishop Hine, "at home in any company and everyone made him welcome wherever he went." His attractive personality "made him popular with all and loved by many." People often remarked that "he is so unlike a missionary," and "steamers called at Likoma and visitors came up just to have a chat with Maples" (Hine 1924, 103). Among the "eminent visitors" was the British Commissioner, Harry Johnston, as well as "missionaries of all sorts, Presbyterians, White Fathers, [and] members of the Dutch Reformed Church" (ibid.). Johnson recalled that "our very good friend Captain Berndt," in command of the German steamer *Hermann von Wissmann*, "was a very frequent visitor in Maples' time" (Johnson 1926, 211; cf. *CA* 12 [1894]: 71).

Maples drowned in Lake Malawi on September 2, 1895, when the *Sherriff*, the mission's tiny steel sailing boat named after the late captain of the *Charles Janson*, ran into a violent storm at night and capsized. He was en route from England to take up his new appointment as bishop of Likoma Diocese. At forty-four years of age he had already given the UMCA twenty years of service, and except for Johnson was the mission's senior cleric. Maples was anxious to reach Likoma as quickly as possible. Accompanied by Joseph Williams, a devoted layman with long service to the mission, Maples had his crew follow a course that took them up the western side of the lake toward Kota Kota. This decision was ill advised and inappropriate, and the men's deaths ultimately avoidable. Both missionaries perished two and one-half miles from shore despite rescue efforts by the African crew. All eighteen African men and boys swam safely ashore (*CA* 19 [1901]: 124). Maples tried swimming to save himself but was dragged down by his wet cassock. His death was a tragedy for the UMCA, and the diocese remained without effective leadership for almost three years (Elston 1972).

COLLABORATION BETWEEN THE MISSION
AND THE COLONIAL GOVERNMENT

Events surrounding the evolution of the UMCA's headquarters offer a clear illustration of how the actions of the colonial administration could directly serve the mission's objectives, and vice versa. The mutual advantages of such collaboration served merely to reinforce the imperious manner in which Africans would be denied a voice in decisions that affected them. During a visit to Likoma in July 1895, Commissioner Harry Johnston, with the complicity of the missionaries, awarded by fiat and in fee simple all of Likoma and neighboring Chizumulu Island to the UMCA in perpetuity.[16] Arriving on a Sunday on the British gunboat *Adventure,* Johnston summoned the headmen and mainland chiefs to meet with him immediately. After church people assembled under the station's large "preaching tree" (also used for trials of serious cases) where Johnston told them how their islands would henceforth be governed. The Reverend W. P. Johnson served as the commissioner's interpreter. According to an eyewitness, Johnston entered the scene

> under a white umbrella, dressed in gray, and his hat adorned with the Administration colours, white, black, and yellow. After shaking hands with the Europeans he sat down, and business began at once. Sir Harry Johnston spoke very clearly and distinctly, so that every word was heard [!], and at the end of a sentence or two Mr. Johnston interpreted them to the people. He explained that the islands were under the British flag, and he left control of them to the paternal care of the Mission, except in cases of murder. He said that as long as the people gave no trouble, and did not make it necessary for the Administrator to visit the islands, he should not tax the inhabitants of either of them. (Mills 1911, 17)

Protests raised at this meeting by African chiefs such as Mataka, against the British presence in general and their arbitrary and confiscatory actions in particular, proved futile. Johnston set out their options, and pointedly warned them that if the English withdrew from Likoma the Portuguese or Germans would surely take them over. A quarter century later the UMCA's Johnson readily rationalized the protectorate administration's theft of African land in the mission's favor, saying that "we [missionaries] should have remonstrated but we thought it wise on the whole to accept the deed in the spirit in which [Commissioner] Johnston meant it: as a means of protecting the natives" (Johnson 1926, 126). In his memoirs Dr. J. E. Hine

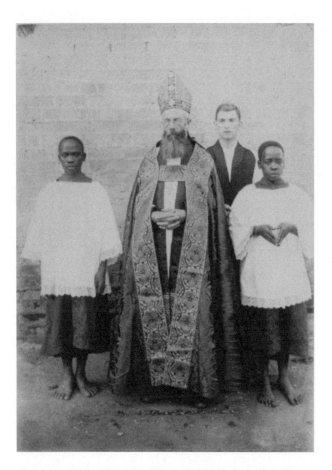

Figure 3.5. Bishop J. E. Hine, Rev. J. G. Philipps, and African Anglicans.
(Source: USPG.)

(Bishop of Nyasaland, 1896–1901) (fig. 3.5) rather less circumspectly praised "Sir Harry's wise foresight" in ensuring that the "'Nyasa archipelago' (all the islands in the Lake), were put under the English flag." In his opinion this act yielded "an inestimable benefit" to the UMCA, other missions, and to Malawi's African residents because "Likoma might have become the centre of an unfriendly German government or of Portuguese misrule." The conditions under which the island was "made over" to the UMCA included responsibility for its civil administration. According to Bishop Hine, "we undertook to be responsible for its order, though not to have any jurisdiction over criminal cases. We constantly acted as judges in what the natives call 'Milandu,' and kept up a fatherly oversight of all the people living on the island" (Hine 1924, 99).

The missionaries could hardly mistake the fact that they would advance their own goals if they obligated themselves to act on behalf of the fledgling British administration. In pursuing their own spiritual and secular aims they also directly served as reliable agents of low-cost "Indirect Rule" for the colonial state. The UMCA's colonialist alliance and "portfolio" of activities ran the gamut, particularly in the pioneer days. Early in 1888, for instance, foreshadowing its conscription for military purposes during World War I, the mission's *Charles Janson* was pressed ("lent," in mission idiom) into the service of the ALC and government. This particular activity was part of a long-term, unsuccessful effort to impress upon Mlozi, the powerful Arab slave-dealer at the north end of the lake, the idea that he should acquiesce and accept British "protection." Mlozi then commanded the trade in a large region around Karonga, and had also built a series of stockades to gain control of routes into Tanganyika. In a move that was surely a breach of the UMCA's own policy of noninterference in the slave trade, Johnson accompanied the British vice-consul and an emissary of the Sultan of Zanzibar on this expedition to Mlozi (Johnson 1926, 150–51). In addition to the steamer the UMCA was asked for, and Archdeacon Maples supplied, "a large quantity of native food, some powder, caps, bullets, my Martini-Henry rifle and 280 cartridges" (Elston 1972, 352). The men went ashore unarmed and were not attacked, but their brief negotiations failed to change the status quo. On the return voyage south the *Charles Janson*, only sixty-five feet long, was packed with seventy people—the crew as well as "Europeans who had gone up as volunteers [against Mlozi] and natives." After landing passengers at Likoma, the *C.J.* continued on a southerly course to Matope on the Shiré River (Johnson 1926, 151). Johnson, whose home was, in fact, the steamer, remained on board.

Meanwhile, a decision had been made by John Buchanan, at the time the British Acting Vice-Consul on Lake Nyasa, in collaboration with Johnson, that on the voyage south out of Likoma they would visit Makanjila at his large village on the east coast. A slave-dealer of great notoriety, Makanjila controlled commerce in Muslim-dominated Yao country at the southeast end of the lake. Johnson later admitted that he had been "trying pretty steadily" for a considerable time to establish a foothold for evangelism in Makanjila's village—"in a more hopeful way than by politics" (i.e. via the flag and a show of force). Yet in the end Johnson gave in to expediency. He concluded that he could win more immediate access to Makanjila's people by being part of an display of imperial power. Moreover, he "felt it right on this occasion to support Mr. Buchanan since it would produce a 'show' of the [British] flag and arms." From the Africans it "would mean a large present, for a flag was a luxury to be paid for" (Johnson 1924, 152–53).

When put to the test, Johnson's strategy of collusion with the British administration quickly backfired. Shortly after they had arrived on the *C.J.* and rowed ashore at Makanjila's, an angry crowd numbering in the hundreds took Johnson and Buchanan hostage. They were stripped and subjected to other indignities. Johnson would later recall with some amusement that this prompted Buchanan, the more roughly treated of the two men, to cry out—"And this to an Englishman!" (154). Kept hostage overnight, the two men were released the next day for a ransom of kegs of paint carried aboard the steamer. Makanjila evidently desired the paint for his slaving dhows. However, he was "shot by his own people" not long after this incident (156).

In explaining the mission's self-image and its strategy to supporters in England, Johnson adopted the familiar language of the Berlin Conference strategists in an effort to impress benefactors with the geopolitical scale and complexities of the mission's task at hand. He instructed that

> people who meddle without taking a party side, or enriching a chief, need a strong support and meet with continual rebuffs, and this why we are continually asking for funds, etc. *We have on the water a grand sphere of independent influence,* helping chiefs and their people; slavers and the oppressed all need help alike, none can be lopped off by us, while none welcome us wholly. . . . [I] feel a sympathy for Mlozi, even. . . . We don't want to be petty chiefs at Lukoma [*sic*], nor to flatter the people who oppress them. The people are nowhere enthusiastic for us, because all are concerned in the evils we have come to struggle against. But if we have fair scope, we do find what we have come to seek and to save. (*CA* 6 [1888]: 127, emphasis added)

Three other examples suffice to illustrate the early, often close interdependence of the UMCA and the government. In 1890 Commissioner Johnston borrowed the *Charles Janson* to transport his expeditionary force on visits to various African chiefs and Arabs in different localities around the lake, seeking to show the flag and sign treaties with them (Murray 1922). In 1892, British forces attempting to capture the Yao chief Zarafi encountered severe resistance. Commander Keane, R. N., came to the rescue and enabled the contingent to save its position on Zarafi's mountain. The UMCA, hearing that there was little native food available to these men, stepped into the breech and sent provisions to them on the *Charles Janson*. The favor was soon reciprocated. In May 1892, the government sent the first coinage, "about £100," for use at Likoma, signaling the beginning of the end of barter exchange. "In return for our help in bringing food" to Commander Keane, the government forgave the duty the UMCA owed on the coin (Johnson 1926, 204–5).

While formal collaboration between the mission and government was never implemented on a large scale, a distinct pattern of mutual assistance is evident throughout the colonial era. In 1920 the British Resident at Kota Kota indicated that he had succeeded in convincing the UMCA's Archdeacon Arthur Glossop to represent the government with "the powers of a Principal Headman on Likoma and neighboring Chisumulu Island." Glossop had offered "to keep and check the money received for hut tax till it can be conveniently taken to Kota Kota. He does not wish to receive any payment or to have a Magistrate's warrant."[17]

Archdeacon Glossop resigned his colonial office in 1937, "no longer a young man." He had remained tax collector and honorary agent for the District Commissioner on the two islands for seventeen years. He was appointed Justice of the Peace in 1926, arranged for cases to be brought before African courts, and oversaw the choosing of chiefs who tried them. In 1931, Glossop appeared on King George V's Birthday Honours List, the recipient of an O.B.E. At the end of Glossop's tenure Likoma had nine villages and six hundred taxpayers, while Chisumulu ("three hours sail from Likoma") had two villages and one hundred fifty taxpayers. The UMCA remained the unrestricted freehold owners of Likoma.[18]

The UMCA's presence in Central Africa by 1885 ensured that it would play a significant role in imperial geopolitics and territorial conquest. Advanced European technology, such as the Gatling gun and steamboats, gave the Europeans a huge advantage. Steamers operated by merchants and European navy units on Lake Malawi and on the Senegal and Congo Rivers opened routes and markets in formerly inaccessible interior regions. These assets were widely deployed to encourage the native populations into swift submission. Africans often responded with defiance and brave resistance, and sometimes used rifles they had acquired through trade or capture against the invaders. But in the end, faced with great firepower and the Europeans' clever divide and rule tactics, the native peoples could not prevail. In other cases African communities knew how to recognize a fait accompli, or they perceived advantages for themselves in coming to terms peacefully.

Few missionaries resorted to guns to acquire land for stations, schools, and dispensaries, or to maintain the "order" they hoped to produce. To achieve their objectives they found it necessary to systematically devalue and dismiss, overtly and subconsciously, many African social mores and culture norms. Despite sincere motivations underlying the desire to spread their own perceptions of civilized behavior, and the Gospel, years of cultural contact passed before some missionaries would stand back to observe and reflect on the fact that their own rules for living did not automatically serve African interests.

Clearly there was a fine and often blurred line between the missionaries' impassioned desire to expand Christ's kingdom on earth and their own imperialist instincts. Representing the established Church of England, and the middle and upper classes, it did not come naturally for the high-church Anglicans of the UMCA to try to distance themselves from the colonial administration. Archdeacon Johnson expressed this complementary relationship well:

> I can never be thankful enough to have been trained in a school where the duty of serving God both in Church and State was steadily put before us. The presence of any Government steamer calls for other steamers to trade, and for yet others to do the work of the Church specifically, and in the same way the Mission steamer calls for the government boat and the trading vessel. (Johnson 1922, 200)

Johnson's conscience evidently troubled him from time to time about such matters, even when he was not personally in a position to act differently. For instance, in connection with land acquisitions in the Portuguese sphere on the eastern side the lake, he remarked that among the Africans "one piece of paper was considered as good as another." This showed "how little the natives understood the meaning of the agreements" (Johnson 1926, 195).

The missionaries exposed their human natures whenever they pursued opportunities to acquire territorial influence and worldly dominion over the life of African peoples. Writing towards the end of his long career, Johnson, who had always been the UMCA's baffling eccentric, played the role of historian and philosopher and capably distanced himself from the drama in which he had been so prominent an actor. He observed that "when Europe turned her eyes acquisitively on Central Africa, details of the division were worked out comically or tragically as God saw fit" (ibid.).

GENDER, SOCIAL FORCES, AND SELECTION
FOR MISSION SERVICE

Health and disease invariably occur within specific cultural, social, and political contexts. In Malawi some of the UMCA's policies concerning the missionary lifestyle may over time have run counter to the missionaries' well being. For example, understandings today about the generally positive relationship of marriage to adult health and longevity suggest that the UMCA's dogmatic insistence on celibacy for its members may have been counterproductive to the quality of individual and collective mission life.

Celibacy in the UMCA's high-church subculture may also have indirectly affected the outcome of efforts to support the health of both Africans and Europeans. A case in point is Dr. Robert Howard, the energetic and highly respected medical officer of the diocese from 1899 to 1909. He was forced to leave the UMCA because he married Kay Minter, an English nurse who worked in the mission's hospital at Kota Kota. The Howards' "indiscretion" and the mission's marriage policy proved costly to the medical work. It would not be easy to secure another highly qualified, committed doctor, or nurses. Their departure left the entire Diocese of Nyasaland—already a vast and cumbersome project—without a doctor for about one and a half years. The loss of Mrs. Howard deprived the UMCA of a highly capable nurse with first-rate British qualifications.

For Africans, the UMCA strongly encouraged marriage but applied strict rules of entry into Christian matrimony (Africans would have interpreted any move to discourage marriage as unnatural and absurd; cf. Beidelman 1982, 69–71). While not entirely unsuccessful in its endeavor to impart a monogamous ideal, the mission discovered it was impossible to monitor all African behavior it sought to control. In contrast, among the European missionaries it was a simpler matter to enforce a standard of celibacy for all and an age barrier for women without regard to personal qualities or other circumstances. Along with sanctions against missionary nuptials, the UMCA's policy held that no female under age thirty, or (initially) over forty years of age, with or without a nursing qualification, was acceptable for mission work (*CA* 17 [1899]: 8). (This issue is revisited in chapter 8.) Presumably, the exclusion of younger white women from the field would eliminate the need to "protect" them from the possible advances of African men and the rigors of station life. Older women would be less inclined to marry, whereas younger ones might become a source of distraction and friction among both men and women. Married missionaries would also produce children!

Harry Johnston, the chief government official in Nyasaland from 1888 to 1895, was a keen and not uncritical observer of missionaries. In his view, women generally made better and "more lovable" missionaries than men, and with each passing year the rapid increase of civilization and growing European population made it easier for married women to share missionary work with their husbands. However, he advised against young unmarried women coming out to Africa as missionaries unless they were married. Even then, it was generally considered necessary to shield women of decency and "English prudery" from the inevitable shock of exposure to what was seen as a barbarous and sexually depraved culture. There was enough to worry about in the challenges of a sickly and enervating tropical climate. The commissioner offered a solidly Victorian appraisal of the challenge and risks confronting a young British woman upon her taking up mission work in Africa. She would face an "ordeal" of crudity, nudity, and indecent manners. Her own values and behavior would be susceptible to "moral deterioration" and a "certain loss of delicacy." Resorting to a Spencerian idiom, Johnston warned of a need to protect against degeneracy in the European. Thus "rude contact with [Africans'] coarse animal natures and their unrestrained display of animal instincts tends imperceptibly to blunt a modest woman's susceptibilities, and even, in time, to tinge her own thoughts and language with unintentional coarseness" (Johnston 1897, 200).

As a condition of acceptance into the UMCA, both women and men had to agree to undertake missionary work without a stipend. It is thus not surprising that missionary recruitment targeted those with private incomes who could be financially independent of the UMCA. "Sons of country parsons and small-town solicitors," they came from public school backgrounds and most had attended Oxford or Cambridge (McCracken 1977, 177). Passage out to Malawi or Zanzibar, and furlough or retirement back to England, was paid for them. However, lack of personal means was not considered a barrier to joining the mission. A woman could "live without expense to herself or friends as long as she remains in it" (CA 17 [1899]: 7). Support upon retirement was another matter, particularly for women lacking financial independence. In 1888 each missionary could draw £20 annually for clothing. For a woman this amount was judged "sufficient allowance for dressing plainly in the Mission style." A printed document describing a woman's outfit and dress code, "carefully considered by persons out in Africa," was available from the UMCA office in London (ibid.).

Many of the men who joined the mission came from middle- or upper-class backgrounds in Britain, with Oxbridge or somewhat similar

educational and social pedigrees. Archives contain little material on members' individual or collective wealth. Given the social status of so many of
the men, in particular, there is little doubt that a majority remained on
a financially sound footing during the course of their careers in Central
Africa. Opting for missionary work was nonetheless surely a matter of faith
and conscience. Religious commitments aside, for many if not most of these
men (and women) the decision to join the UMCA also involved (at least
in theory) a greater or lesser degree financial and professional sacrifice. As
one observer put it, in the UMCA "we find men of high endowments, and
many of them of fair University attainments, sacrificing a career at home,
and giving themselves with high minded devotedness to the work. Hence
we get real results" (*CA* 6 [1888]: 155).

Men and women could choose the diocese they wanted, but not the
specific work they would do after arrival in the mission field. Women needed
to understand and accept the reality that their "assigned places" would be
essentially limited to teaching, nursing, and midwifery, or housekeeping and
"industrial" work (laundry, ironing, supervision of gardening, etc.). Typically,
a nurse also had responsibility for housekeeping and basic supervision. All
work was to be undertaken "as a religious act, as an offering to God, as a way
of helping the whole work of the Mission." The missionary's purpose was

> not *merely* be useful, not *merely* to do good to others. It is not enough to
> come out with the idea of doing conscientiously a certain amount of work,
> what *you* conceive to be strictly your duty, and then of claiming the right
> of going your own way and seeking your pleasure outside the Mission for
> the other hours of the day. (*CA* 17 [1899]: 9)

An advice-giver urged women think and pray about whether they should
enter the mission field. Hasty action, "in some fit of enthusiasm," could
lead to great disappointment all around. It was "far better [to] discover
before you go out that you have made a mistake, than that you should find it
out six months after you have reached Africa" (ibid.). As spinsters all, their
paramount mission work was to win African women and girls to the Lord.
Through teaching and example, they would lead them to adopt a Christian
lifestyle, and presumably help them to raise their social status among men to
the standard suggested in the New Testament. Within the UMCA there was
a clear expectation that women missionaries would carry out an important
task in cross-cultural social and theological engineering: it was their job to
teach both African men and women "how the Incarnation has sanctified
and put honour on womanhood" (ibid.).

NOTES

1. Bishop Cathrew Fisher to Long, Nov. 12, 1928. UMCA 1/1/2. MNA.

2. Ibid.

3. Preface to Barnes 1933, 9.

4. Wilson (1936, 132) states that the last such raid within territory worked by the UMCA occurred in 1909. A raid on coastal villages staged from the hills on the *east* side of the lake was recorded in 1911 (see *CA* 34 [1916]: 30).

5. "Chigoma was home, but there are no creature comforts," as Johnson could not even obtain a native bedstead (Johnson 1926, 108).

6. The steamer idea was now gaining in popularity in east-central Africa. In the same year the ALC, under contract with the London Missionary Society (LMS), conveyed the sections of the steamer *Good News* up the Zambezi, across Lake Malawi, and then overland to Lake Tanganyika via the partly-completed "Stevenson Road" (Johnston 1897).

7. In exchange for lands deeded to the UMCA agents by African chiefs. Original handwritten stamped and sealed MSS: August 16, September 13, November 5 (six chiefs), and November 18, 1890. A letter dated Jan. 17, 1893 from H. M. Commissioner Johnston to the UMCA's W. P. Johnson criticizes the manner in which the UMCA agents obtained the land from Africans. UMCA, Misc. Pieces, Ux. No, 94. Rhodes House Library, Oxford (RHL).

8. Stores, *Likoma Diocesan Quarterly Paper* 8 (July 1905): 208. Cited in McKinnon 1977, 183, n. 59.

9. This problem was partly solved by Archdeacon Johnson's establishment of two gardens on the mainland opposite Likoma (Howard 1904).

10. Archdeacon Glossop, Likoma to Resident, Kota Kota, May 12, 1914, UMCA 1/2/20/5, MNA; and Resident, Kota Kota to Chief Secretary, March 7, 1919, S1/576/19, MNA.

11. Bishop Cathrew Fisher to Sir George [?], Aug. 18, 1922, S1-2006-22, UMCA Relations with Portuguese, MNA.

12. Miasmatic theories proved resilient through the end of the century. In 1881 mission houses (presumably the CSM) "were built to face inland to avoid 'miasmata' being blown in over the water, while double story buildings were favored since it was believed that the miasmata did not rise far above ground level" (Ransford 1983, 59).

13. The UMCA built their cathedral at Zanzibar on the site of the old slave market at Mkunazini.

14. The UMCA claimed 690 Communants at Likoma Cathedral by 1907 (Anderson-Morshead 1955, xxvii).

15. Maples "did not like the steamer but would go across to Bandawe, whatever the weather, if the need occurred" (Johnson 1926, 136).

16. An earlier Certificate of Claim to Likoma, not including Chizumulu, had been drawn up and signed by Commissioner Johnston and the UMCA representatives (Archdeacon C. Maples and the Rev. W. P. Johnson) in January and March 1893. No African participation in this process is acknowledged. UMCA Misc. Pieces, UX No. 94, Jan. 18, 1893, Registered no. 15. Copy. RHL.

Fifty-four years later an agreement was reached that transferred all of Likoma Island back to the colonial government. Lands Officer to Vicar-General, Aug. 23, 1949. UMCA 1/2/20/5. Malawi National Archives (MNA).

17. Resident, Kota Kota, to Chief Secretary, Zomba, July 8, 1920. Administration of Likoma and Chisumulu Islands. S1/311/19. MNA.

18. Glossop to Bishop Frank Thorne, May 29, 1934, UMCA/1/2/20/5. MNA; and Provincial Commissioner, Northern Province, to Chief Secretary, Zomba, Dec. 18, 1937. MNA.

{ CHAPTER FOUR }

Expanding the Steamer Parish:
Ten Thousand Square Miles for Mission

Consider again the extraordinary nature of the physical environment in which the UMCA chose to develop its mission work. During the mission's first decades its territorial focus grew into a greatly elongated region based on steamer transport and communication. Breathtakingly beautiful, this lacustrine region of blue water was hemmed in by mountains on every horizon. It stretched more than four hundred and fifty miles north and south in the Rift Valley, extending from the Livingstone Mountains of southwest Tanganyika to the Upper Shiré River in southern Nyasaland. Precolonial Africans relied primarily on water transport to get from one coastal village or fishing grounds to the next, while dhows carried the bulk of the nineteenth century slave-traffic to the lake's east coast. Winding paths connected villages near the lake, and roads were unknown (UMCA 1903).

Despite the indigenous systems of lake transport carried on primarily by dugout canoes, the UMCA's evolving regional structure had no precedent. Its organization and scope was qualified from the start by the mission's strategic choice in 1884 of Likoma Island as its diocesan headquarters and by the early importation of the *Charles Janson* to work Lake Malawi's east coast. Thereafter, the expanding regional definition of UMCA activity was manifestly a creation of the missionaries' appetite and energy for evangelism, and an increased frequency of steamer visits to coastal villages. Eventually the steamers acquired a more or less regular schedule and routes (*CA* 48 [1930]: 189). These developments helped to increase African mobility within and beyond the lake basin. They also contributed to some expansion of marine trade and a build-up of connections with other water and land communications at Ft. Johnston (Mangochi) and Matope on the Shiré River, and at Kota Kota.

For many Africans, the steamers eventually influenced fundamental elements of their everyday economic and social lives. Africans traveling by steamer carried and spread news and gossip, and acquired novel secular and religious ideas from throughout and beyond the UMCA's sphere. Paradoxically, the new mission region, which encompassed parts of the homelands of the Mpoto and Manda (in southwest Tanzania),[1] Nyanja (central), and Yao (south) peoples, also remained relatively remote, isolated, and materially poor during the colonial era. Such conditions partly reflected the UMCA's philosophy and decisions regarding the application of its resources. The mission viewed evangelism as its primary and, if necessary, its only calling. While a small number of Africans were systematically taught practical skills essential to the mission's operations, such as teaching, nursing and dispensary work, and construction techniques, the UMCA did not view itself as an institution responsible for economic development. Its stand was self-serving of its religious and spiritual aims. Yet the mission's position was on some level also arguably defensible. The mission's bishops and staff correctly foresaw that colonial labor policies and direct African participation in the colonial economy would bring a harvest of social dislocation and secularism inimical to evangelism and their interpretation of the Christian lifestyle and ideals.

CREATING THE MISSION'S SPHERE OF INFLUENCE

Two points bear reemphasis. First, without the steamers it would have been impossible for the UMCA to reach as many places and peoples as it did. Second, even with the steamers, and with grander and more reliable operating funds, the mission's strategic aspirations would have been checked by their physical scale and by the difficulty of securing and keeping the services of doctors, nurses, and trained African staff.

To found and sustain services to their their coastal and interior head stations, including the associated schools, church congregations, hospitals, and out-clinics, for decades the UMCA missionaries depended extensively upon the steamers to get them directly to their destinations. These vessels transported European and African mission workers, food, and supplies to coastal bays and settlements such as Mtengula. From this place one could go on foot to one of the UMCA's few inland stations such as Unangu (fifty miles) and Mtonya, the Yao towns in Portuguese territory (*CA* 16 [1898]).

Technology and Paradox

In the Lake Malawi region, it is a truism that mission work at a new site in the interior was likely to be more successful when a steamer could position missionaries and their baggage on the coast and within reasonable walking range of their desired destination. A great premium was placed on the steamers' advantages of speed and security relative to the perils of walking overland. This method served both the UMCA and the Scottish missionaries on the opposite side of the lake. However, since the mission had only one steamer until 1901, and thereafter never more than two operating at a given time, weeks often elapsed between return visits to a particular village or port. Certainly the pace of travel by steamer could be slow by modern standards. Mechanical breakdowns brought anguish and upset the most important plans (see chap. 5). Yet the UMCA had no practical alternative to lake transport once it had selected Likoma Island and the lakeside villages relatively nearby as the initial focus of its evangelistic efforts. In this part of Central Africa lake steamers offered great advantages, but also posed distinct liabilities. Once the decision was made to structure the mission field and related teaching, medical, and evangelistic activities around steamers, the missionaries did not have to wait long to experience the meaning of technological dependency. A commitment to the vessels encouraged high expectations, together with patterns and rhythms of movement from which it was hard to disengage. Disappointments and hardships followed, leading to greater realism about the ways technology could not always provide for the timely transfer of people, ideas, and goods. All things considered, however, there really was no satisfactory alternative to the steamers.

William Percival Johnson (1854–1928)

The combination of the arrival of the first steamer in 1885, followed at the end of 1886 by the return of the Reverend William Percival Johnson from medical leaves in England and South Africa, provided the specific form of technology and human energy and ingenuity the UMCA needed to proceed with its plans for evangelization in Central Africa. There is little doubt that the presence of this particular man, Johnson, and the availability of the *Charles Janson* were crucial factors in the relative successes the mission counted in its pioneer era. This convergence of time, place, person, and machine at Lake Malawi was a signal moment. No missionaries alive at the time would have disputed the claim made much later that "the importance of the *Charles Janson* in the overall strategy cannot be over-estimated" (Elston 1972, 350).

While Livingstone became the best-known European missionary in nineteenth-century Africa, Johnson's life story of persistence and accomplishment in adversity ranks him among the continent's true heroes of Christian endeavor. In the pioneer era of African missions it is not uncommon to be able to single out an individual who, whether humble or brash, by peculiar genius and force of personality had an extraordinary impact upon the entire enterprise. Steamer or no steamer, it is tempting to speculate about what the consequences for the embryonic Diocese of Nyasaland would have been had the brilliant Johnson's health, in particular his near-blindness, convinced him to retire from the mission in 1886. There is little doubt that the absence of this incredibly odd man, this so-called "Apostle of the Lake" who "won back the lost past of our first venture" (*CA* 46 [1928]: 208), would have left a wide if not unbridgeable chasm in the UMCA's accomplishment in Malawi. Johnson's truly heroic persistence over a half century under every manner of adversity, and his unstoppable drive to preach, teach, and minister in the villages scattered along two hundred miles of coast and the mountains behind, became legendary beginning with the early years of his long career. His legacy remained vivid while his witnesses still lived, and thereafter in the UMCA's published records. Few other outsiders could or would have dared to walk in his shoes or assume the risks he took. His early departure would almost certainly have diminished if not crippled the UMCA's second effort in Malawi.[2]

The Steamer Parish

More water than land, the UMCA missionaries called their region the "steamer parish." For all practical purposes the *Charles Janson* quickly became "a second head station," operating alongside and in support of the headquarters on Likoma Island. It served as Johnson's "floating home" and later that also of the Reverend Christopher B. Eyre (Wilson 1936, 109; Winspear 1960).

A widely traveled master seaman in the British Mercantile Marine, Eyre came out to Malawi in 1896. He worked on the *Charles Janson* until the *Chauncy Maples* came along in 1901, when he shifted to the larger steamer for the next five years. Although the two priests could have hardly differed more in their personalities—Johnson was the demanding ascetic and "one of the

hardest taskmasters imaginable" while Eyre was the genial yarn spinner—
they evidently enjoyed a long and happy association (Barnes 1933, 93). Eyre
excelled as the *C.J.*'s "husband." His responsibilities included "looking after
its stores, its provisions, its supply of firewood . . . [and] engaging the steamer
hands and paying them" (95). He was also the paymaster for the mission's
African teachers in the mainland villages. That job was complicated by
the fact that wages had to be in money equivalencies, yet paid out fairly in
corresponding quantities of goods such as cloth, soap, salt, beads, or perhaps
books for a teacher's personal use. Cash did not become the rule of exchange
until after 1910. By then the number of traders opening shops in settlements
along the coast had expanded, enabling teachers to choose how they wished
to spend their money (ibid.).

In 1888 the British Consul observed that "the *Charles Janson* is almost always under steam" in the hands of Captain Sherriff and Mills, his engineer
(*CA* 6 [1888]: 153–54). Its African crew of seventeen was "rather large for
such a small steamer," partly because the ship lacked room for a windlass
and required at least a half dozen men to haul up the anchor. Wood fuel
for the ship's engine also had to be brought on board and stowed. African
crewmembers included six sailors and a *capitao* (Portuguese for "head-boy"
or quartermaster in charge), five stoker-engineers and their *capitao*, a cook,
butcher boy, the captain's personal servant, and a night watchman. In addition to wages, crew members received a *posho* (maize flour) allowance in
the form of trade-calico or soap (Mills 1911, 62).

Initially, recruitment of the *C.J.*'s crew was difficult and dependent upon
locating men who could be enticed to sign on. Men able and keen to leave
home and to work far away with Europeans were scarce, and few of the
steamer's first crewmembers became Christians. Over time, however, and
reportedly before the pressure of compulsory taxes and competition for
industrial work took general effect, the recruitment process became more
discriminating. As training expanded after 1886, the coastal villages developed a good supply of men who were "extremely capable, both as sailors
with the boats and in the management and steering of the steamer, and also
with firemen and engine-drivers" (Barnes 1933, 93). It thus became easier
to locate men who could reliably fill either temporary or permanent vacancies on the steamer. Soon men who had become Christian converts on land
eagerly applied to join the *C.J.*'s crew (fig. 4.1).[3]

Throughout the pioneer period, the UMCA encouraged village Africans
to travel on the *Charles Janson* and, from 1901, on the *Chauncy Maples*. In 1893,
for instance, sixty Christians drawn from the villages of Chisanga, Pachia,
and Msumba on the central east coast traveled on an overloaded *C.J.* to

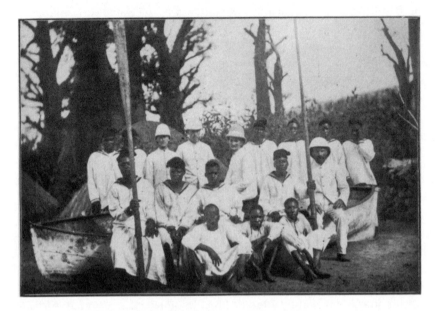

Figure 4.1. Crew of *S.S. Charles Janson* (W. P. Johnson, center rear).
(Source: Johnson (1926) facing p. 198. From the archives of the USPG.)

Likoma for the Easter holy days (*CA* 11 [1893]). In 1906, when the public found out that the *C.J.* was making one of its occasional trips to Nkamanga on the west coast, the mission was overwhelmed with requests for tickets. Severe space limitations meant that many with good reasons for going had to be refused.[4]

A few African sailors who served on the *C.J.* had training and skills almost from the start. Anticipating such a need, Johnson had recruited three Africans to accompany him to England in 1884. Hamisi (Yao), Manweri (Nyanja), and Tumani (Nyanja) had previously worked for Johnson. On arrival Johnson left these men under the wing of the Reverend A. G. Stallard of St. Peter's in Brixham, on the south Devon coast (Johnson 1926, 114). According to Barnes, Johnson's biographer, Stallard had long shown enthusiasm for the UMCA's work. He housed the three Malawian men (or Nyasalanders as they were then known) in his home, introduced them to local fishermen, and found opportunities for them to go out with the fishing fleet. The three "Blackmen" stayed in Brixham for seven months of seamanship training, supervised by local trawler captains. Before they returned to central Africa the Malawians had provoked considerable curiosity and respect among the English fishermen for the UMCA's work (Barnes 1933, 66).

Hamisi and Tumani, two of the three Malawians who apprenticed at Brixham, joined the *C.J.*'s crew and accompanied the steamer on its first voyage into Lake Malawi in September 1885. A rough sea had been stirred up by strong *mvera* winds from the south. Bellingham recorded that all on board became seasick except Hamisi and Tumani, who "enjoyed" the voyage (Yarborough 1888, 77).

Several of the Brixham fishermen eventually made their way south of the Equator to work with the UMCA in Malawi. The first was George Sherriff in 1886, who remained as skipper of the *C.J.* until he died in 1891. He was followed by at least three other Englishmen from Brixham who came out as mission workers. They had joined "as a direct result of the work of Mr. Stallard and the impulse given to their interest in Africa by these three 'boys' from Nyasa in 1884, and by Johnson, whom they held in veneration" (Barnes 1933, 66). Over the years, UMCA publications and the private letters of missionaries frequently remarked on the contributions of the "Brixham trawlers." Even fifty years later, the interest created by the Malawians was still in the air in Devon (ibid.).

In 1902, following the mission's deployment of a second steamer, the *C.J.* was assigned to the bishop and assumed a much-expanded responsibility for mission transport. In addition to its standard activities on behalf of the bishop and mission transport generally, the *C.J.* was assigned to operate at night in case of emergencies.[5] Edwin Ayers, the *C.J.*'s captain, observed:

> Each trip of the steamer is on a different errand, so life aboard is never monotonous. Sometimes it is a voyage to take the Bishop about for Confirmations, or the doctor in answer to an urgent call, or to pay one of his periodical visits to the stations, a trip to Malindi for mails and stores, or to some native village to buy food to supply Likoma's large demands for her hospitals and native boarders. . . . Once a quarter we take one of the Likoma clergy across the lake to Nkamanga, and there, running along the coast, pick up any scattered Christians from Likoma who have settled there, and take them to Nkata Bay for a Celebration of the Holy Communion. . . . We take our folks back to their village, and then return, laden with fruit and flour and a full passenger list, as there are a great many families from this district related to others at Likoma. (Mills 1911, 63)

The presence of the second steamer did not decrease the demand for the *C.J.*'s services; rather, the new mandate to facilitate the bishop's agenda meant that the *C.J.* was sailing more than ever. Within a few years, its previously stable running expenses rose 26 percent.[6]

Johnson remained set on training African teachers and starting schools in all the important villages along the east coast. He also believed that vigorous efforts to proselytize among Africans brought aboard the steamer would yield tactical and strategic benefits in carrying out the UMCA's mandate. Revealing a bit of social engineering, a contemporary recorded:

> Mr. Johnson endeavours to draw children from the various villages along the Lake-shore, into the steamer, and then bring together children of different tribes and peoples, laying what may be the foundation of friendships amongst those who hitherto have been at deadly enmity with one another. A school is kept on board, and the teacher does not spare himself. (CA 6 [1888]: 154)

In this early period the first African teachers were not local, but rather came from the UMCA's college on Zanzibar or the Masasi Diocese in southern Tanganyika. Several among them had been Nyanja slaves whom the UMCA had rescued and trained for evangelical work. They returned to Nyasaland to volunteer their services among their own people (UMCA 1903; Johnson 1926, 173). With a steamer on the lake the missionaries rapidly gained the confidence they needed to expand the territorial scope of their evangelistic activities. Depending on rainfall in a given year, they could also sail south on the Shiré River to Matope to collect stores. This perceived security of communications was also interpreted as the condition that enabled the mission to open the door for the recruitment of women.

In 1886, Johnson embarked on a new evangelistic campaign on the *C.J.* He was joined by the Reverend George Swinny, the new priest-in-charge at Likoma, together with his young wife, Mary, their infant daughter, and several African mission trainees.[7] They started to preach and teach at Chiteji's and other lakeside villages opposite Likoma Island. Johnson's method of choosing where and when to work was essentially "freelance" (Wilson 1936, 73). Backed by his close friend Maples at Likoma, he charted his own course in searching for places where people were willing to hear him preach. This process was gradual and risky for both the Europeans and mission Africans. It required steadfast persistence, acceptance of personal hardship, and an ability to confront sudden, militant reactions when their intrusion was undesired. The missionaries' propaganda frequently encountered frank disinterest among Africans, and outright hostility from the Muslims at the south end of the Lake. Johnson keenly understood that "the people are nowhere enthusiastic for us" (CA 6 [1888]: 127).

The UMCA followed a fairly consistent approach to securing a toehold among the coastal settlements. Initially, gifts would be presented to the local chief or headman. This was followed up with an attempt to negotiate what the missionaries interpreted as a tacit agreement for them to enter the area to establish schools. If this procedure went smoothly, transport was arranged to enable married African teachers and their wives (to teach women and girls) to be posted in or near a village to begin their work. Teachers' wives were assigned to teach village women and girls the alphabet and domestic tasks such as childcare, hygiene, and cooking (*CA* 6 [1888]: 127). The first school in a location was generally an alfresco arrangement with little more than a blackboard, slates, and chalk, a printed alphabet sheet, and a Hearer's Catechism (a handbook of questions and answers for teaching Christian principles and comportment to those considering church membership). Later, if conditions seemed promising, a more permanent school was built in the locality. Conversely, teachers would be pulled out and reassigned to another place if the response to the religious instruction was weak. The function of these schools was decidedly religious rather than educational (Elston 1972, 351).

In the 1880s, the missionaries' odds for success in promoting European-style Christianity in Malawi could not have appeared robust. Slaving activities and raids by the Tanganyika Gwangwara (Ngoni) persisted until the mid-1890s: "Anywhere one might see a band of Gwangwara, from five to thirty men in number, coming briskly along with their shields and spears, and sometimes one's heart would beat a little faster, but very seldom were they insolent or quarrelsome" (Johnson 1926, 147). Johnson's composure and taste for understating danger is evident in this remark.

In 1886, the Swinny family undertook what Johnson called "one of the most chivalrous efforts of our Mission by moving [from Likoma] to Chingomanji's village of Chikole, where they hired one of the very small native huts" (141). Depending on one's ideological outlook concerning missionaries as frontier agents, the Swinnys' leap-frog move of some sixty miles south to Chikole, into hostile territory occupied by the Muslim Yao, was an act of faith that is startling in its courage, or utterly foolhardy and offensive. We have only Johnson's word on this. He described the Swinnys' host Chigomanji as "nothing if not the head of a Yao slaving outpost... [and] a clever man [who] knew how to speak and act with strangers." Johnson preferred to sleep on the *C.J.* when the steamer visited Chikole rather than in the village, which was subject to raids and also used as a resting place by slavers and their human cargo. Upon going ashore to visit the Swinnys,

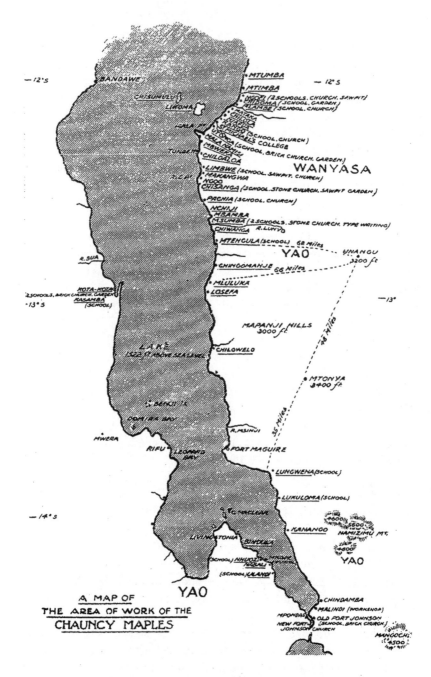

Figure 4.2. Area of work of the *Chauncy Maples:* Central Nyasaland, 1885–1908.
(Source: Howard (1908), 8.)

Johnson discovered that they had created "an English home in a village which was completely pagan with a veneer of cosmopolitan brigandage" (ibid.).

However, after eighteen months the UMCA had lost the entire Swinny family. George succumbed to fever and died while in the care of Dr. Laws of the Scottish mission at Bandawe, forty-five miles across the water from Likoma. His infant daughter had preceded him in death. Mary, his widow, started a school on Likoma and continued to teach girls and women. She, too, became ill and died in 1888 aboard ship while being invalided home to England.

Many months passed until the UMCA finally found a "suitable native" teacher to pick up the work the Swinnys left behind at Chikole. After a strong start, this individual reportedly fell from grace through "gross immorality." According to Johnson, the contradiction had been "too palpable" for the local people, and so they rebelled against efforts to teach Christianity (147).

In the first year and a half after Likoma's founding the *Charles Janson* sailed to the southern end of the lake "at more or less regular intervals." En route, the steamer visited the settlements of Makanjila (later Ft. Maguire) and Monkey Bay, and then sailed to Matope on the Shiré River.[8] The UMCA's political relations with the mainly Muslim Yao on the southeastern side of the lake region remained weak during the late 1880s, and for some time it proved impossible to plant a mission representative at any village south of Chikole (148). While a mission school was eventually organized at Liwonde on the banks of the Shiré in 1888, this was soon undone when "Mohammedan and partly slaving" influences forced the work to end (159).

Through Johnson's dogged perseverance, a chain of schools and groups of "hearers" slowly but steadily formed along the lake coast, initially in the villages of Ngofi, Chitesi, Chisanga, Pachia, and Msumba (figs. 4.2 and 4.3).[9] The last three places had become the largest of the Nyanja settlements on the eastern side of the lake, doubtless due, at least in part, to a greater sense of security in numbers. In time, after a small group of converts had been made in a place, a reed church was built to serve members and anchor a potentially growing number of new converts.

Johnson's persistence at forming alliances and playing one Nyanja or Yao chief, big and small, against another paid the UMCA dividends because the strategy ultimately succeeded in bringing down many of the barriers to missionary penetration. All the while the countryside remained unstable and often violent, and the boundaries of a chief's territory fluctuated "with the fortunes of war" (162). When the steamer carried the missionaries from one village to another they had no assurance of a cordial reception.

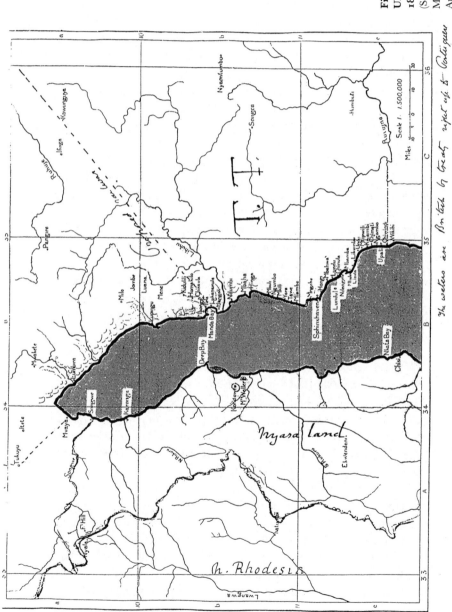

Figure 4.3. Northern UMCA Sphere, 1885–1900. (Source: Child (1924). Malawi National Archives.)

What Chauncy Maples called Johnson's "adventures" often referred to his colleague's difficult and sometimes life-threatening experiences with African protests against encroachment by the UMCA and other Europeans. Those actions included being pelted with garbage, attacked by spearmen, and seized, stripped, and held for ransom. There is no doubt that many Nyanja and, especially, Yao chiefs and their followers did not appreciate and did not at all welcome the missionaries' intrusions into their world. This was particularly true of those who benefited in one way or another from the slave trade.

Despite numerous obstacles, the UMCA's influence among new groups of Africans continued to grow in the late 1880s. Johnson would not be deterred from his goal of opening schools at every village of importance, and the *Charles Janson* was "almost always under steam" (*CA 6* [1888]: 153). At Mtengula, tougher African resistance meant a longer wait before the Bible was carried ashore. This village was situated on an excellent harbor midway between Msumba, with "its fish and its fertile meadows," and Chikole. One of Mtengula's chiefs appeared open to Johnson's overtures (Johnson 1922, 11). However, Makanjila, a more dominant regional authority on the southeast coast, was clearly hostile. In his memoirs, Johnson recalled that "the negotiations for landing [at Mtengula] fell through till after Makanjila's village had been conquered" (Johnson 1926, 184). Effective access by the UMCA was delayed until several years later, following a British punitive force (chap. 2) that had moved decisively against Makanjila and other Yao slavers. This action permanently altered the balance of power in favor of colonial and missionary interests.

In his penetration of the Muslim realm in the south, Johnson made good use of the hospitality and "civility" of Makandanji. He was a rival of Mponda, a powerful Muslim Yao chief and slaver whose headquarters was at the southeastern end of the lake (fig. 4.2). Mponda controlled much of the territory and commerce in this area. Johnson walked the eight miles from Makandanji's village to Mponda's and succeeded in striking up friendly and useful relations with him (ibid.).

By 1889 the UMCA had also carried its work to the settlement of Mkope in the Monkey Bay district. Located on the baobab-studded floor of the Rift Valley, Mkope is about one hundred fifty miles south across the lake from Likoma (fig. 4.2). In this area the population was mostly Nyanja, although Mponda was their paramount chief. Johnson recalled that upon their arrival at Mkope in the *Charles Janson*, Mponda had "sent up a spoilt young favourite, aged about fifteen" as his emissary and broker. This boy "was armed with a revolver, and it is a mercy he did not shoot any of us or even any of the people" (185).

Progress in building up a community of believers at Mkope was slow. In the missionary mind both the physical and cultural environment of Mkope slowed progress. Johnson observed that the morale of the population remained low. He attributed this to Mponda's frequent tendency to treat the Nyanja as slaves, and that the people were "obsessed" with witchcraft. Marauding hyenas also harassed the population, and for many years there was a "generally fatal" disease, said to be beriberi, that affected both the local population and the UMCA teachers who settled there. Later reports emphasized frequent failure of the rains and famine (*CA* 67 [1949]).

For an (always) married African teacher, the UMCA used a posting to Mkope as a kind of litmus test of the individual's "earnestness" and commitment to Christianity and the mission. The place was generally unattractive and far away from one's home and kin group. Considering these factors, Johnson said he was "not afraid to trust several young teachers who showed willingness to go to Nkope" (Johnson 1926, 186; Nkope or Mkope). The mission's persistence was not without reward, although another thirty years passed before Mkope became a principal station with a resident European staff.

From 1889 to 1894 the *Charles Janson* was deployed on a more or less regular pattern of itineration among the growing number of the lakeside villages where the UMCA gained permission to teach Christianity. The steamer traveled as far north as Mbamba Bay in German East Africa (Tanganyika) (fig. 4.3), and then to the far south and across as far as Matope on the Shiré River, a distance of over three hundred miles (fig. 1.2). Life was hazardous and tenuous for most of the lakeside African populations, and large and small tyrannies abounded. Missionary work was punctuated by Ngoni and Yao raids on local settlements. Johnson was convinced that his decision to make regular visits to villages in the *C.J.* had the effect of discouraging raids. Even though missionaries said they carried no arms on board, the little steamer nevertheless represented a superior and rather awesome technology in the eyes of local populations dependent upon dugout canoes. Said Johnson: "Our coming was one of the things that kept the weaker villages from isolation, and we brought them news of the outside world. It was a revelation to see strangers who did not trade, did not bully, kidnap, and murder, and yet did not fawn" (1926, 174). These interpretations may have been self-serving. Yet the archdeacon was certainly on the mark in his assessment of the steamer's symbolic and practical capabilities.

Beginning with Likoma, the UMCA established fifteen principal stations on land in Malawi and the adjacent territories of Portuguese East Africa (Mozambique) and Tanganyika between 1885 and 1925. Six stations opened before 1900. Likoma was followed by a smaller mission on Chizumulu, the neighboring island, in 1889. A third station was opened in 1893 by Archdeacon Chauncy Maples of Likoma and Dr. John E. Hine, some fifty miles inland from the lake at Unangu in the adjacent Yao country on the high plateau (over 3,000 feet) of Mozambique.[10]

At Unangu, a large Yao town said to contain "thousands of houses," Chief Kalanje permitted Maples and Hine to build a station there so long as they did not interfere with his slave trade and restricted themselves to religious matters (Anderson-Morshead 1955). In 1898 Yohana Abdallah, the son of a Yao chief, was appointed priest-in-charge at Unangu. It thus became one of two UMCA stations placed under the supervision of an African clergyman (fig. 4.4). The mission's ultimate objective in planting this inland station was to create a base to facilitate eastward expansion to link with the outlying district of Masasi (Zanzibar Diocese) in Tanganyika (Mills 1911).

A fourth UMCA station was opened in 1894 at Kota Kota, a place that was closed to Europeans until 1892 (Howard 1908). A village of some five

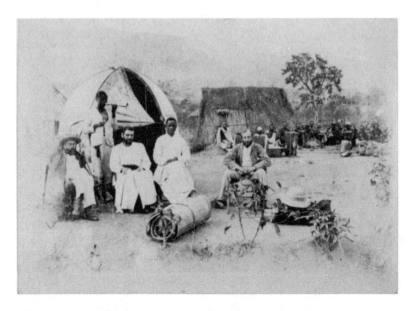

Figure 4.4. UMCA Camp in Portuguese East Africa (Bishop Hine, Rev. Margesson, Rev. Y. Abdulla).
(Source: USPG.)

thousand people and a major center of Islamic influence, Kota Kota had been for several decades the headquarters of several Jumbe and the major slave port on Lake Malawi's west coast. Mponda's (1896) and Malindi (1898) complete the roster of principal stations founded by the pioneer missionaries before the twentieth century.

TRANSITION FROM PIONEER DAYS: THE FRONTIER CHANGES

Excepting Unangu on the Mozambique plateau (and later Mtonya and Likwenu), each UMCA station was directly accessible by the steamer and had at least one permanent European staff member by the turn of the century. Mponda's village and the contiguous UMCA Mponda's mission station (from 1896) were situated on the right bank of the Shiré River where it emerged from Lake Malawi at the Bar. They lay astride a major slave route, with caravans moving overland around the south end of the lake, to and through Mponda's, and then continuing across the Shiré to Makandanji's village north to Mataka's (fig. 2.1). Mponda's was also only seventy miles north of the protectorate government's headquarters at Zomba and only six miles by land or ferry from Malindi station. This section of the river was infested with crocodiles, and thus a dangerous place for the adults and children who had no alternative but to go there to get water, wash clothing, bathe, or swim. Attacks on humans were frequent, resulting in loss of life and limbs, drownings, and other trauma. In response the mission built two semicircular stockades in the water so that people could bathe in safety (Dale 1925).

Around 1910, following old Chief Mponda's death and the emergence of his successor, Che Mambo, the government merged the two villages to gain more administrative control. The new Mponda's was relocated just outside Ft. Johnston, and Che Mambo proceeded to build his main residence about a hundred yards from the UMCA station. Under the scrutiny of the colonial administration, Mambo ruled this Muslim town and its surrounding district for the next quarter century (*CA* 53 [1935]: 247).

Mponda's became the UMCA's main stores center and treasury office. It proved difficult to conduct Christian proselytization because the local Yao population had strong ties to Islam. The Reverend John G. Phipps, the first UMCA priest-in-charge at Mponda's (1896–1902), developed gardens and established a local herd of cattle. Phipps succeeded in building up an early core of Africans adherents, and is credited with having laid the groundwork for a chain of schools on the banks of the Upper Shiré.[11]

Malindi station, seven miles northeast of the Shiré's mouth and with good anchorage, was carved out of fourteen acres of bushland the mission had purchased from the British government in 1897 (*CA* 17 [1899]: 180). Its first function was an engineering station for outfitting and repairing the mission steamers. Fitters and engineers from Glasgow came out to work and live at Malindi. Only intermittent missionary work was done before 1902. Soon thereafter, it grew into a "full-service" mission offering evangelical, educational, and medical services to the predominantly Muslim and rarely enthusiastic Yao. It was not long before the mission had extended its work from Malindi about thirty miles inland, encompassing villages in the hilly district of Mangoche (Dale 1925). During the 1890s the UMCA's goals surely were advanced as a result of the gradual reduction of the slave trade and the development of more settled if still harsh conditions (e.g., forced labor) that accompanied the establishment of British overrule in the protectorate. By the late 1890s the need for protection and security from slavers and the Ngoni that had earlier stimulated a defensive clustering of peoples into exceptionally large villages along the lakeshore had eased considerably. More peaceful conditions brought a fissioning of many of these larger settlements into smaller villages. People dispersed in small matrilineal groups along the coast and into the hills above the lake. These new patterns made villages more difficult to reach from the steamer, reducing it effectiveness. Some mission villages nearly emptied, causing a drop in attendance at local schools and churches (McKinnon 1977). From the UMCA's perspective this process of decentralization and dispersal expanded the need for new schools and teachers, and increased the pressure of the missionaries' workload.[12]

Despite the missionaries' best efforts, apparently there was always to be a gap between what they sought to achieve and how they comprehended the results. Understanding what was transpiring in the lives and souls of "their" Africans was not a linear process. Progress was never a straight line. Africans who in one way or another adopted Christianity and attempted to live according to Christian principles (quite apart from any sectarian ritualism or dogmas) experienced conflicts and contradictions on their journey to the Christian faith. These African experiences paralleled and surely often exceeded the kind of challenges faced by Christians born into a Western culture, not least the missionaries. Certainly, this quality of shared struggle with Africans regarding beliefs and ideas about sinfulness, sacrificial living, and forgiveness must have been apparent to the UMCA priests and teachers, even though it is difficult to recognize it as such in the mission's written records.

For the European missionaries, genuine conversions among Africans proved hard to certify and monitor. While many Africans sought to live as communicants and full members within the strict bureaucratic standards of behavior the missionaries set out, they were under constant surveillance and subject to church discipline. Fornication, marriage to non-Christians, and insistence on monogamy as the foundation of Christian marriage and family were among the missionaries' foremost concerns. Yet African custom, which had long accommodated broader concepts of family and appropriate sexual (and economic) relationships, including multiple wives and certain allowances for situational sharing of women, provided endless frustrations. Such departures from the European Christian ideal were also complicated on both sides by the fact that African societies, too, recognized adultery in their own terms and had customary remedies that dealt with it. Not least, Africans deeply feared and were motivated by the web of supernatural forces that pervaded many aspects of their daily lives. They also venerated and placated the spirits of their ancestors. From a missionary perspective, then, many African beliefs and practices proved nettlesome if not outrageous and unyielding. As for pioneer Malawian Christians, their full standing and degree of participation in church life was largely determined according to a rolling report card kept by the missionaries.

An effort to rehabilitate "lapsed" Christians was a regular feature of missionary work throughout the UMCA's tenure in colonial Malawi. In 1948, for instance, the parish priest at Mkope Hill near Monkey Bay compiled a census "of interest to fellow priests" on "600 cases of Christians under censure or discipline." He identified and ranked eight categories of serious breach of Church rules:

1. village (as opposed to "church") marriage with another Christian, or "trial marriage" (39 percent);
2. village marriage with heathen (28 percent);
3. bigamy (11 percent);
4. being second wife of bigamist (10 percent);
5. divorce and remarriage (9 percent);
6. marrying a divorcee (1 percent);
7. slackness (1 percent); and
8. "various" (1 percent) such as interest in Watch Tower [i.e., the Jehovah's Witnesses], "version to Islam," and complicity in indigenous dances.

This same priest also observed that more than half of the communicants who lived in the parish failed to make communion in the three months around Easter. Their laxity could be explained only by their "indifference to and ignorance of" the basic tenets of the faith (*CA* 67 [1949]: 75).

Other cultural and psychic barriers also slowed the rate of missionary acceptance among Africans, especially where more than one ethnic group inhabited an area. The Lake Malawi region was not simply a single African-missionary frontier. Numerous African peoples and languages co-existed there, and diverse cultural forces and political crosscurrents confronted each other (cf. Winspear 1960). In the Muslim-influenced locality of Ft. Johnston-Mponda's, at the south end of the lake, the presence of two languages and peoples, Yao and Nyanja, as well as the preexisting "other" universalizing religion, confounded the UMCA's efforts to "get any definite hold on the people."[13]

A parallel confrontation with Islam, which had entered via the slave trade, marked the UMCA's efforts to build up a viable center of Christian influence in the Islamic stronghold of Kota Kota. Muslim opposition to the spread of Christian influences would remain a perennial complaint among the UMCA missionaries (Blood 1957).

During the 1890s mission activity in the diocese had evolved geographically into four more or less distinct zones. Likoma, the diocesan headquarters, was the mission's policy and ecclesiastical center. Two women, a nurse and a teacher, who followed Mary Swinny arrived at Likoma in 1888 to work with women and girls (Elston 1972). Work on neighboring Chizumulu Island was administered from Likoma. In 1898 another sub-station was opened at Nkwazi at the south end of Likoma Island, followed soon by St. Andrew's training college. St. Michael's teacher training college was opened in 1900 near Utonga on the mainland opposite Likoma.

The *Charles Janson* carried on its steamer work in the mainland villages. This crucial activity stretched along the coast opposite Likoma for 150 miles, from the village of Ngofi in the north to Ft. Maguire and Makanjila's in the south. From Makanjila's the *C.J.* would steam to the southern tip of the lake, crossing into British territory and finally making a loop up to Monkey Bay. This southern leg had a fishhook contour and added another 125 miles to the steamer route. Outbound from Likoma this route covered a distance of about 275 miles and facilitated contact with villages in both Portuguese- and British-claimed territory. Stations at Kota Kota, on the west coast, and Unangu, over fifty miles inland from Likoma in Portuguese territory, formed the UMCA's other primary places of interest until the late 1890s.

Including its five main stations, the UMCA reported in its Easter Census of 1897 that it had established 28 schools in 18 localities in Nyasaland— more than a threefold increase in pupils in five years. Published maps of the period indicate an expansion to 31 schools and classes between 1897 and 1902 (UMCA 1903, plate 8). Total enrollment in 1892 was 508 pupils, with a boy-girl ratio of 3:1 in schools in the lake villages. By 1897 enrollment had grown to 1,270 pupils. All books needed for teaching in the schools and churches were printed in several vernacular languages by the Printing Office at Likoma.[14]

By 1897 a "typical" mission school had about 45 pupils, and a boy-girl ratio of 3:1. Likoma (5), Monkey Bay (6), and Kota Kota (2) accounted for almost half the total number of schools, but only 30 per cent of the pupils. In the "steamer district" the schools with the largest enrollment were located in the coastal villages of Pachia, Chisanga, Kango, and Ngofi in Portuguese East Africa.[15] By 1900 the mission's sphere of influence included 33 lakeside villages, worked by 33 African teachers who went about their duties with little supervision due to the "extreme shortage of priests." During 1900 several African teachers had been dismissed for "grave faults," while others had had been sent up to the training college.[16]

The UMCA recognized several categories of persons in transition to full membership in the church, including Hearers, Catechumens, Baptized, Communicants, and Adherents. By Easter 1892 the UMCA claimed over 860 adherents in Nyasaland, and more than 1,400 people had been baptized. Five years later the mission had fourteen European workers and twenty-two churches. Adherents numbered 6,705, an eightfold increase in five years or an average of 305 Adherents per church. In 1897 some 850 men and 478 women were confirmed in the church, which suggests that the annual rate of growth at the time was above 10 percent (*CA* 10 [1892]: 148, and 15 [1897]: 176).

At the turn of the century the UMCA could thus point to substantial, even remarkable, progress during fifteen years of voluntary hard labor and sacrifice on the part of its European missionaries and their African believers. They could legitimately claim to have "planted the flag" and to have secured a substantial presence, with a school, or school and church, in over thirty-three African settlements. All but one location was coastal. The identity of these settlements began to change when they became stops on the steamer route. Populations grew increasingly less isolated than ever before. Expectations and desires changed with greater access to material goods, new ideas, and travel.

Tenuously at first, and unevenly, the steamer acquired more influence as both message and messenger. It stimulated and represented processes that linked the lakeside peoples to new forces of commercial and social change occurring elsewhere on the lake and beyond. The *Charles Janson* had begun to enmesh Africans in a changing geography of communications that lessened isolation and enabled the outside world to penetrate the lake region. Slowly, new ideas, goods for personal and domestic use, and access to increasingly distant places became possibilities for greater numbers of people. Counterbalancing this opening-up was the fact that at least half of the territory the UMCA had chosen to evangelize was at least nominally Muslim and thus already a contentious religious frontier. It was unrealistic to expect a large number of conversions to Christianity, and likewise to readily draw many Muslim children away from their Koranic training and into mission schools. Furthermore, the Scottish Presbyterians had created a viable sphere of influence among the peoples on the plateau and highlands on the west side the lake. Geographically, then, the UMCA had little real choice but to occupy a kind of vacuum that had formed in the lakeshore zone (Elston 1972).

In 1899–1900 the mission's freedom of action in the lakeside villages was altered, technically, by the final geopolitical settlement involving British and Portuguese jurisdictions in the Lake Malawi basin. The highlands and west side of the lake remained British. Lands on the eastern side of the lake were roughly divided into five sections. Germany received two northern sections (in Tanganyika). The two middle sections stayed under Portuguese control (part of Mozambique), while Britain secured the southernmost section. Likoma and Chizumulu Islands, already occupied by the UMCA, remained British. Lake Malawi was designated international water. This configuration of territories reportedly came as "a great blow to the Mission in general and specially to Archdeacon Johnson, that almost all the villages in which his work lay were put under the Portuguese flag" (Wilson 1936, 114). However, in a practical sense Portuguese colonial control over the lakeside villages in the UMCA's sphere caused little interference in the day-to-day conduct of affairs.

In reality, sorting out the imperial domains, especially with the Portuguese, was probably more of an affront to the British missionaries' nationalistic pride than a loss of their capacity to influence people through mission work. Their reaction may also be seen as a Victorian expression of British intolerance of the general lifestyle and attitudes of the colonial Portuguese. In the British view, the Portuguese did not keep the proper social and sexual distance from African women and did not conduct themselves as gentlemen. Britons believed that the Portuguese set a poor example for European colonizers. A form of racism may also have been a factor. Some critics of the period assert that in the British mentality, "niggers began at Calais" and included all non-Anglo-Saxons (Hammond and Jablow 1992, 110).

In contrast to the founding of schools and churches, the UMCA's medical work during the 1890s was miniscule. A temporary dispensary for Africans opened at Likoma in 1890. It also accommodated a few hospital patients (*CA* 8 [1890]: 5), and gradually built up to an average of 900 attendances monthly.[17] A dispensary was opened in 1893 at Unangu, in Portuguese territory, and it soon became a busy and noisy enterprise (*CA* 11 [1893]: 60). In 1894, the mission constructed two permanent hospitals on Likoma, one for Africans and one, the first stone building with glass windows, for European staff (*CA* 12–14 [1894]: 71). The only other facility put up in the 1890s was a second native hospital at Likoma in 1899. Designed to accommodate six male patients, it either replaced or augmented the older hospital.[18]

This comparatively underdeveloped state of the UMCA's medical care facilities reflected its great difficulty in finding and keeping a qualified doctor, and also a lingering ambivalence shared in common by many Christian missions about the relative importance of healing and evangelism (Good 1991). Before the twentieth century, some foreign mission boards opposed the very idea of a medical missionary, arguing that "faith and prayer were sufficient to ensure native health" (Gelfand 1988, 14). There was also only a small pool of medical doctors who also qualified as clergy, the strongly preferred dual credential, and competition among missions for them was keen. For some it was more appropriate to press on with preaching than to encourage the recruitment of doctors who were not first and foremost trained clergymen.

Yet as the mission expanded and more Europeans came out to Malawi, the high levels of morbidity and mortality they experienced made it painfully obvious that if the work was to go forward some minimal infrastructure was needed to support their own health, at least. In a retrospective account, the UMCA's first full-time medical officer referred to the 1890s as "a period of remarkably bad health." The European death rate in Nyasaland rose from 97 per thousand in 1895–86 to 120 per thousand in 1897–98, "in a population where the great majority were young men in the prime of life" (Howard 1908, 2). For example, chronic ulcers forced Dr. John E. Hine, D.D., M.D., the mission's first doctor (and later a bishop) to leave Malawi within two years of his arrival in 1889. Treatment he had received from Dr. Laws of the Scottish mission at Bandawe produced little relief (*CA* 8 [1890]: 4). Hine recuperated and eventually returned, but the mission lost his services for two years. Dr. Frederick Robinson of Guy's Hospital in London succeeded Hine in 1894. He too suffered from poor health and within six months was invalided to England "partly paralyzed by fever" (Gelfand 1964, 10).

Malaria and blackwater fever posed the greatest threat to the missionaries. Of the twenty-eight missionaries who died in the 1890s, "twenty were due to malarial fevers, and of these sixteen to blackwater fever" (Howard 1908, 2). Fortunately, scientific knowledge of the cause of malaria, and improved means of prevention and treatment, emerged by the beginning of the twentieth century. Meanwhile, from 1894 to 1899, following Robinson's departure, the formidable task of diocesan medical officer fell once more on Dr. Hine's shoulders. After the turn of the century the UMCA missionaries' health status underwent distinct improvement. This change was facilitated in 1899 by the arrival of Dr. Robert Howard as the full-time medical officer for the Diocese of Nyasaland. Howard, who stayed on the job for ten years, showed keen interest in promoting practical public health among both missionaries and Africans. His insistence that the missionaries use prophylactic quinine on a daily basis appears to have contributed to a gradual decline in the frequency of virulent malaria episodes.[19]

By the end of the 1890s and the pioneer phase of mission, the *Charles Janson* had been in more or less constant service for nearly fifteen years. It had played a crucial role in opening the lake basin to mission influences, and it was heavily depended on for regular visits to more than twenty stations and sub-stations. By now this vessel had taken a beating in the line of duty and was judged as "aged and infirm." As a home for Rev. Johnson and temporary shelter for others, the *C.J.* was also small, cramped, and uncomfortable. She was said to be unable "to get along the Lake from village to village so quickly as formerly, while the time for her repair becomes greater, and so hinders the work which otherwise might be accomplished."[20] Thus it was realized that mission's work had expanded beyond the small steamer's capacity to cope with it alone. The European clergy increasingly felt responsibility to provide more counsel, support, and priestly services to African deacons and teachers in the lakeside villages. Mission supplies, mail, and passengers also had to be carried. Sentiment for a second steamer was building. The UMCA's pioneer phase was ending.

THE *CHAUNCY MAPLES:* FLOATING HEAD-STATION

By 1898, the UMCA's dependence on lake transport was firmly established. In fact, there was increasing pressure for the mission to acquire a new and larger steamer to help cover existing commitments, as well as to facilitate the further build-up of the mission field.[21] The Central African territorial and social frontier had been crossed and commitments had been made, with significant and permanent consequences. At this time the mission had to confront two interrelated challenges. First, it was essential to nurture the roots of the Christian faith among the early converts. Second, it had accepted a mandate to spread the Gospel to the many African communities in the lake region whose physical location, political ties, or religion placed them outside the UMCA's sphere of influence. To help meet these goals the mission placed an order in 1899 for a new and larger steamer that would take over a substantial burden of the work that had been carried on from the aging *Charles Janson*. There was no intention to retire the *C.J.*, which provided essential but more limited services until the 1930s.

As in the case of the *C.J.*, William Percival Johnson played a key role in the UMCA's decision to invest in a larger vessel. The new bishop, Dr. Hine (1896–1901), appointed Johnson Archdeacon of Nyasa in 1897 and supported his reasoning to acquire a new floating station. With Hine's support Johnson returned to England and led another successful campaign to collect most of the funds needed for the new steamer's construction and transport out to Malawi. John Crouch, an engineer and a former captain of the *C.J.*, drew up the technical specifications for the ship, incorporating ideas from Johnson and Bishop Hine. Its construction was supervised by two prominent engineers, Sir John Wolfe Barry, builder of London's Tower Bridge, and Henry Brunel (*CA* 17 [1899]; Barnes 1933).

Built in the yard of Messrs. Alley and MacLellan in Glasgow, the new steamer had a single screw propeller and displaced 250 tons. It was 127 feet long with a beam of twenty feet, and moved at a speed of nine knots (fig. 4.5). On its completion in October 1899, the vessel was disassembled and its parts, all galvanized, packed into approximately four thousand parcels. These items and the steamer's nine-ton boiler were shipped to Malawi on the steamer *Hollinside*, owned by the African Lakes Corporation (*CA* 17 [1899]: 199). Upon reaching the Zambezi's mouth the steamer parts were sent up-river to the Shiré confluence. From the Shiré, the packages were headloaded around a series of cataracts to Mponda's village. There, near the entrance to Lake Malawi, the components were handed over to five European technicians who had come out from Britain to supervise the work of reassembly. This process was to consume more than a year. The boiler, which could not be dismantled, was wheeled overland. Dozens of Ngoni porters pushed and pulled the huge cast iron boiler across steep hills and rocky river beds for sixty-four tortuous miles to the shoreline at Malindi.

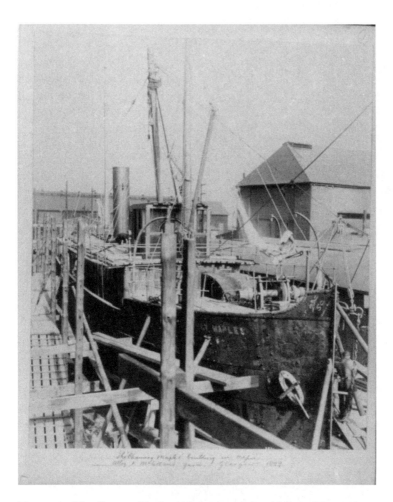

Figure 4.5. The *Chauncy Maples* under construction, Messrs. Alley and MacLellan Yard, Glasgow, 1899.
(Source: USPG.)

The boiler was subsequently installed there because of shallow water at Mponda's (figs. 4.6, 4.7, and 4.8) (Winspear 1956).

Total cost of the new steamer project was estimated at £16,500, including £9,000 for the original construction, £5,500 for transport to Malawi, and another £2,000 for reassembly at Lake Malawi (*CA* 22 [1904]: 190). Launched in June 1901, the steamer made a brief trial run on the lake in October 1901. In the early years it sported sails (Williams 1958), and was compared in size to "a Thames up-river steamer from Windsor to Oxford"

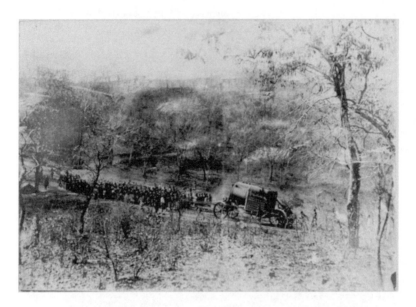

Figure 4.6. Overland hauling of the boiler of the *Chauncy Maples* to Malindi, Lake Malawi.
(Source: USPG.)

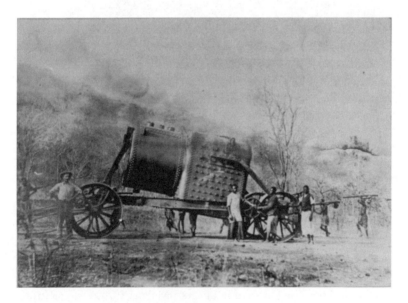

Figure 4.7. The boiler of the *Chauncy Maples*.
(Source: USPG.)

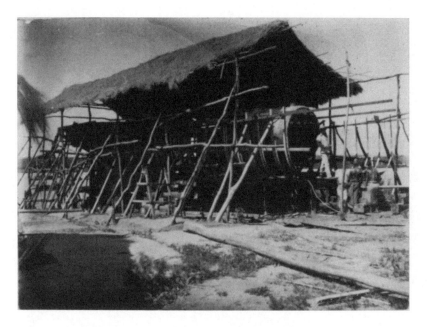

Figure 4.8. Fitting of boiler into the *Chauncy Maples* at Malindi.
(Source: USPG.)

(*CA* 54 [1936]: 207). At the time, it was the tenth steamer operating on Lake Malawi (fig. 4.9). This total included a much smaller vessel built around" 1900 for a German mission society working at the extreme north end of the lake (Williams 1958). Otherwise, only the UMCA's steamers functioned primarily for missionary purposes.

The remainder of the larger vessels on Lake Malawi included several gunboats under the control of the Royal Navy, plus a few steamers that carried cargo and passengers for the African Lakes Corporation (see chap. 2). At the turn of the century the mission also had its "Likoma Fleet," consisting of three small sailing boats (the *Charlotte*, *Mary*, and *Patience*) with an African crew of a *capitao* and two sailors. These craft ferried passengers to and from the mainland. Other boats included a dhow and three dugout canoes (*CA* 19 [1901]). The *Mary* was a small "little sharpie" (crew of two) used to transport Likoma priests to the villages around the island's harbor and neighboring bays (Mills 1911). By 1911, the *Mary* and *Patience* had been withdrawn from service. Taking their places alongside the *Charlotte* were the *Ousel*, a thirty-two foot, two-masted iron ship with an eight-man crew, and the *Chikulupi*, or *Hope*, a yacht-type metal boat. Both came as gifts to the mission. In addition, the

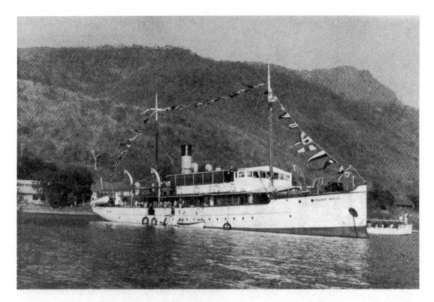

THE CHAUNCY MAPLES AT MALINDI READY FOR HER JUBILEE VOYAGE.
(Photo: Society of Malawi)

Figure 4.9. The *Chauncy Maples* at Malindi, Jubilee Voyage.
(Source: USPG.)

mission placed several old and dilapidated steel boats at Likoma, Kota Kota, Malindi, and Mponda's to assist in off-loading cargo from the steamers, and to carry clergy on short trips (ibid.).

The UMCA's new steamer made its first official voyage over Christmas 1901. Departing from Malindi, the vessel headed north to Likoma, stopping en route at Monkey Bay, Kota Kota, and several stations on the east coast. A large contingent of African passengers accompanied the captain and seven other Europeans. In April 1902 the steamer was consecrated by Bishop Trower (1902–10) and named the *S.S. Chauncy Maples,* memorializing the late archdeacon and bishop (1895) who drowned in Lake Malawi en route to assume his new duties at Likoma.

While the *Chauncy Maples,* or *C.M.,* was undergoing reassembly and outfitting for service on Lake Malawi, Archdeacon Johnson had gone to his brother's home in New Zealand in an effort to recuperate from blackwater fever. Thus he did not see the new steamer until he returned to Malawi in 1903. The new vessel now at his disposal was not only much larger than the *C.J.,* it was also equipped with many desirable, even luxurious, features that the older steamer lacked. The *C.M.* carried a crew of twelve sailors with their *capitaos*, ten stokers, cooks, stewards, servants, two European officers, at least twelve or more teachers, five or six printers, a "dispensary boy," and two watchmen. In addition to the captain's and engineer's quarters, the clergy had four cabins, each with two berths. Another twelve berths for Europeans had been added by 1907, along with a new bathroom offering a douche and a hot or cold Turkish bath. Facilities also included a post office and a dormitory with thirty bunks for African students.

The *C.M.'s* upper deck contained the wheelhouse and sick bay. It also featured a combination classroom and chapel (about sixteen feet wide) with thirty desks and seats, and a printing press (installed in 1908). The chapel, fitted with a teakwood altar and Maltese cross inlaid with mother-of-pearl, aroused great pride among the missionaries and African Christians. Hung above the altar was a painting of Christ and His disciples in a fisherman's boat, being tossed on a stormy Sea of Galilee (*CA* 22 [1904]; 25 [1907]: 125; Mills 1911). The missionaries often invoked the symbolism of this scene in connection to their own labors. Initially the UMCA brought African teachers on board for a three-month course and review, with classes offered as the boat steamed up and down the lake from one village to another (Mills 1911).

The presence of the sick bay insured that the *C.M.* soon became a hospital ship. It transported the mission doctor on his medical rounds, and its accommodations permitted large numbers of seriously ill patients from the various lakeside villages to be transferred to one of the UMCA's hospitals on land. Three hospitals for Africans at Likoma, Malindi, and Kota Kota existed in 1904, and several more opened by World War I (*CA* 22 [1904]: 141).

Travel aboard the *C.M.* was considered to have health benefits. It offered abundant fresh air and cooler temperatures. And it was popularly believed that disease-carrying mosquitoes were left behind on land. To aid "run down" European staff members and those recovering from a debilitating illness, the mission doctor often prescribed a supervised, month-long rest cure aboard the noisy steamer. This was encouraged as salubrious "for all," even the "bad sailors" who experienced frequent bouts of seasickness (*CA* 28 [1910]: 247). The sick bay also served the more immediate needs of those on board, including students and others affected by the all-too-common curse of seasickness.

The *C.M.* may have been the first of a small number of "hospital ships" to operate in sub-Saharan Africa. Twenty-five years later in the Congo, the inauguration of the "Hospital Ship of Governor Lippens" was incorrectly described as a novel event. Displacing 100 tons, this vessel carried a doctor and medical assistants and regularly visited villages situated along the Congo

River and its tributaries. Its objective was to dispense medical and surgical help to "white men and black men." Plans also called for the *Governor Lippens* to have a "purely scientific section, to which will be entrusted the study of diseases of men and animals" (Smith 1926, 144).

Initially, the UMCA intended to use the *C.M.* as a training college for African teachers as a counter-strategy against politically unsettled conditions on the coast. This plan was abandoned within a few years as more peaceful conditions prevailed, and in view of the fact that the lake's frequently rough waters and sudden storms proved less than ideal for study and training.

Sailing on the huge lake was certainly not for the faint-hearted or queasy of stomach. Father Bertram Barnes, who worked closely with Johnson for many years, observed that "in some states of the Lake your only chance of keeping dry will be to climb to the top of the mast" (Barnes 1933, 95).

Later on, the *C.M.* was proudly described as a "Christian boat," as "her time-table provides for a weekly rest from Friday evening to Monday morning at one of the larger Mission stations, so that her crew may go ashore to worship on Sundays" (*CA* 54 [1936]: 208). Archdeacon Johnson's delight in the amenities and potential of the new steamer led him to call it "a fairy palace, which makes all the whites up here envious." People, he exclaimed, should "believe in the Chauncy Maples. With the Chauncy Maples we ought to be able to really deal with the problem of [establishing] a native church" (*CA* 22 [1904]: 193).

The arrival of the *C.M.* on Lake Malawi, and the *C.J.* before it, raises the issue of the ways in which the local populations responded to the arrival and capabilities of these technological marvels. How did Africans receive and understand the steamship as a form of technology, and as a representation of the projection of foreign power and change? Little is directly known about this, although the arrival and mystery of the steamers in a preindustrial society certainly fired imaginations and produced colorful additions to local folklore. The only written "evidence" of African perceptions of the encounter discovered is a condescending account based on unsubstantiated fragments of purported statements and views of Africans collected over time and ordered with the hubris in a European mindset. A reviewer of A. E. M. Anderson-Morshead's *The Building of the "Chauncy Maples"* noted that it contained "a delightful little bit re: the native mind" generally and African ideas about steam locomotion in particular:

When they had grasped the idea that the white man is not content with getting about in a canoe, but required "a house on the water," their first difficulty is as to how it moves, for its seems to obey a word of command as a soldier might obey his leader. Oxen are one of the African modes of locomotion, and it was believed that oxen were shut up in the engine, and so propelled the ship. "Was the steam their panting breath?" When shown the fire as an explanation, they expressed their surprise at the cruelty of "burning up" the oxen, even if they were worn out with work. One tribe on Lake Nyasa, wishing to express "everlasting fire," decided that it was the stokehold on the steamer, which has to burn day and night when in motion, and they named the regions of the lost "Stoko" and regarded them with favour as a warm retreat from cold winds. Their eschatology had to be slightly corrected. (*CA* 22 [1904]: 192–93)

Once in service the *C.M.* immediately facilitated the work of consolidating and expanding UMCA's evangelical, educational, and medical outreach. The steamer was operated as a "second head-station" and "the floating church of Lake Nyasa," in concert with Likoma (Mills 1911, 66). Johnson and two other European "steamer" clergy supervised the entire lakeshore ministry. For practical reasons Malindi, with its engineering facilities, became the "home" port of both the *C.M.* and the *C.J.*

Both the "steamer method of work" (Howard 1904) and the "steamer parish" are concepts that originated in UMCA concerns about missionary health. In the beginning the lakeshore was made dangerous by the raids of the Ngoni, Yao, and Arab-Swahili slave traders. The *C.J.* enabled the missionaries to maintain a safe distance from them. Early experience had also taught them that the east coast of the lake was extremely unhealthy, such that "no [European] Mission stations were to be built there" even though "the importance of isolation was not realized" (ibid., 45). Thus residence aboard the steamer shielded them from a disease they did not understand.

Dr. Howard traveled extensively on the *C.M.* and did much to develop the mission's infrastructure and system of medical care for both Africans and Europeans. He worked tirelessly to promote malaria prevention and public health throughout his ten years in the diocese. Howard emphasized the need to use great caution, based on health factors, in the selection of sites for stations and facilities. Because of its speed and mobility, he argued forcefully that the *C.M.* had a central, indeed crucial role in the provision of adequate medical and nursing care. Within a few years of his arrival in Nyasaland, Howard concluded that

it is improbable that the steamer method can ever be entirely superseded by one based on a system of European stations on the mainland, for in order to cover the same area it would mean at least three or four stations, and each would require a staff of four (i.e. two men and two ladies). It is, however, very possible that, in the future, some important mainland stations may be established to supplement the work of the steamer. (46)

By 1910, the diocese was now administratively divided into three land spheres on the eastern side of Lake Malawi. These included a large middle section under Portuguese administration, a much smaller zone in the north under German rule, and the southern end of the lake, which was under British control. A fourth, the "water" sphere of the "steamer parish," cut across these imperial boundaries and the lake's international waters.

SOCIAL USES OF MISSION STEAMERS

In addition to its unusual and instrumental role, connecting people and places and facilitating the development of a mission field, the *C.M.* also fulfilled some of the European missionaries' important social and psychological needs. It frequently served as a kind of floating health "resort" where one could repose for up to a month, armed with the mission doctor's prescription for "lake air" and recommendations on how best to recuperate from fatigue, malaria, or other illness.[22]

Once a year the steamer would make the rounds of all the main lakeside stations to collect the missionaries and transport them to Likoma for a week-long conference and retreat (*CA* 22 [1904]). Malindi staff relished the occasional invitation to tea or dinner after dark aboard the *C.M.*, either solo or with others when it was in port. Once aboard, guests might choose to enjoy a swim or play water polo, and listen to a gramophone concert after dinner before retiring to bed.[23] While not frequent, shipboard social gatherings did help to break the tedium and strain of station life.[24] In important ways the steamer was appreciated for its simple pleasures—as an island to which one could briefly escape the routine. It seemed like a piece of home, where the English flag was raised and English bachelors and spinsters could choose to be themselves in their own company.

Other steamers also helped to satisfy the missionaries' need for contact with Europeans elsewhere in Malawi. Chauncy Maples's observations vividly illustrate these concerns, and also reflect the not so subtle backdrop of race and class distinctions in mission life. Thus on Christmas Day 1894, with "the great service of the day over," he noted, "we prepared to receive our friends and countrymen from the gunboats, both the *Adventure* and the *Pioneer*" (*CA* 12 [1894]: 69). Following an outdoor Christmas service and carols with "blue jackets" and officers held under the "preaching tree," the "natives dispersed"—presumably to their own entertainment and homes. Those Europeans present—naval officers, blue jackets, and missionaries— retreated to church for their own Christmas morning service and sermon, complete with "old familiar hymns and their time-honoured associations." Numbers aside, "it was nevertheless the largest white congregation we had ever mustered at Likoma, and thankful we were to have this opportunity of joining with these representatives of her Majesty's Government" (*CA* 12 [1884]: 69–70).

Several days later, after the *Pioneer* and *Adventure* had departed, the *Hermann von Wissmann* arrived at Likoma prepared for a New Year's Eve celebration (71). Friendly relations between the British and German communities prevailed at this time. At midnight the captain "ushered in the new year with a salute from the guns, blue lights, rockets, and volleys from the rifles" (ibid.). On New Year's morning, the *Hermann von Wissmann* left with the Bishop of Nyasaland and the UMCA's doctor aboard for a two-week tour of settlements and ports around the north end of Lake Malawi. A few days' rest at the Berlin Mission's Langenburg station broke their voyage.

For the Europeans of the UMCA, the steamers represented much more than an essential means of transportation (fig. 4.10). Given the policy that the crews be Christian converts, the missionaries believed that the lifestyle and behavior exemplified on and off the ship by both Africans and whites would be fundamental to their progress in changing African culture. Curious heathen and Muslim eyes closely watched how the Christians lived. The example, the missionaries believed, "comes through the lives of a native crew, themselves so lately won from a great darkness to the Light of Christianity. May they be true and steadfast amidst the many temptations which assail them." The metaphor extends to the steamer, whereby Africans living in darkness "may be won to the shelter and safety of the true Ship" (Mills 1911, 65).

EXPANSION AND CONSOLIDATION OF THE UMCA'S
SPHERE, 1901–25

The diocese was hierarchically organized, with a growing number of headstations more or less tributary to the ecclesiastical center of Likoma. Each head-station was responsible for the development and supervision of schools, churches, and medical work in a large outlying region along the lakeshore and in a few cases for many miles inland. Malindi's tributary region, for

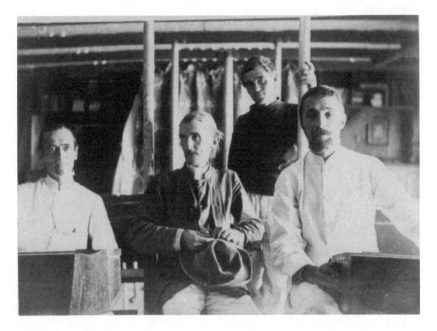

Figure 4.10. Rev. R. Marsh, Archdeacon W. P. Johnson, and European crew aboard the *Chauncy Maples*.
(Source: USPG.)

example, encompassed villages up to about twenty miles north along the coast and several miles to the south of the station. The UMCA posted resident African teachers to tertiary outstations in each region and gave them very broad responsibilities (*CA* 31 [1913]). However, UMCA and African customs relating to sexual comportment and food preparation, respectively, made it impossible to offer a post to a male teacher who was unmarried, or to a widower (Wilson 1920).

The young men whom the mission specially selected for teacher training attended St. Michael's College. The college was located first at Kanga, opposite Likoma Island on the Portuguese mainland.[25] After his posting to a village, a teacher typically conducted a local school twice daily for five days each week. He was expected to recruit children for the UMCA school, teach the "hearers" and catechumens, and hold a daily service in a small wattle and daub church. He also held services on Sunday, conducted prayers during the week, and was expected to open and maintain good communications with the villagers. It was the teacher's responsibility to live an exemplary life and to "influence the elders, as far as possible, to listen to the Christian message" (ibid., 44).

Systematic deployment of the *C.M.* from 1902 spurred the UMCA to expand its sphere of activity beyond the thirty-three lakeside villages it claimed up to that time (*CA* 20 [1902]). By 1910 the steamer parish included villages as far north as Ameila (Mbamba) Bay, some eighty miles inside German East Africa. Schools had been opened there and prayer books printed in two of the local dialects (Mills 1911).

The missionaries frankly conceded their dependence on the African teachers, and admitted that the latter performed "the greater part of the missionary work" in the Nyasa Diocese (*CA* 31 [1913]: 293). The challenge to African evangelists is highlighted by the fact that in the years up to World War I, Johnson and two other European steamer clergy had accumulated responsibility for fifty to sixty congregations, some quite large, spread out along some three hundred miles of shoreline.

The *C.M.* began its itinerary at Malindi. Five weeks were required to complete the entire circuit. In practical terms this meant that the African congregations could expect a visit from the steamer clergy, who alone could celebrate the Holy Eucharist, only once in four or five weeks (*CA* 31 [1913]; Winspear 1960).

Archdeacon Johnson had developed a system for registering all Christians in their villages according to their matrilineal kinship relations. He supervised the development of local directories for each parish and had them printed on the *C.M.*'s small printing press (Winspear 1960). Expansion of mission activities and influence continued steadily right up to World War I. This development reflected an ever-increasing dependence on lake transport and the *Chauncy Maples* station.

In 1911, the UMCA was operating ten main stations at a total annual cost of £5,688. Fully one-quarter of this budget was allocated to the expense of operating the *C.M.* in its large steamer parish in Portuguese territory (81 percent of cost) and in its smaller service area (19 percent of cost) in the German sphere of influence.[26] The UMCA had penetrated German East Africa via the *C.M.* shortly after it was placed in service. By 1908 baptism had been administered among the Mpoto peoples, the mission's first converts in the German sphere (Blood 1957).

Lake Malawi's frequent storms and rough seas often prevented the steamers from maintaining a precise schedule of arrival and departures. Generally, the steamers called at the main stations at least once every three weeks. Constrained by this time frame, the priests rotated among the four coastal districts, endeavoring to train catechumens, and to baptize and prepare people for confirmation and communion (Mills 1911, 73). Typically the *C.J.* carried one or two steamer clergy, and the *C.M.* three. When the ship arrived at a station a priest would be dropped off to make the rounds of its neighboring coastal villages. He would teach and administer the sacraments and be picked up on the steamer's return voyage. In this way the priests staggered their work in the British, Portuguese, and (temporarily) German spheres.

Both steamers carried passengers, mail, mission stores, and cargo between and among the larger European and African-operated stations. The *C.M.* also transported a collection of books from Likoma and served as a "lending library" for staff at the stations on its route.[27] During the first decade of the new century, Likoma's work had expanded to include 10 outstations and 16 schools. In contrast, the *C.M.* floating station was assigned to supervise 38 outstations and 48 schools. Overall, by 1911 the UMCA claimed active work in 133 outstations and 178 schools.[28] Between 1905 and 1910, and despite opposition from Muslims, four additional head-stations had been started up at Mtonya, thirty-five miles inland in Portuguese territory; Msumba, the largest village on the eastern side of Lake Malawi; Lungwena, fifty-five miles north of Malindi; and Likwenu on the plateau south of the lake.

Mtonya's case is of interest because it was seen by some influential members of the mission to have an altitude conducive to missionary health. It was also seen as a key link in a strategy to connect the Nyasa and Zanzibar Dioceses via a chain of stations between Lake Malawi and the Indian Ocean. Mtonya was to be the first inland station on the chain, and the mission's medical officer emphasized that "we must not stop there" (*CA* 24 [1906]: 11). Mtonya opened in 1905 following the purchase, for one hundred shillings, of about a half-square mile of land from the local chief. Access was through the coastal village of Lungwena, where the *C.J.* deposited about one hundred thirty loads of equipment and supplies. Porters headloaded these items to Mtonya some twenty-eight miles in the interior (*CA* 24 [1906]). This new station was about 2,300 feet above lake level and nearly 4,000 feet above sea level. After the rains in November it sat in an undulating sea of grass ten feet high. Weeks later the grass was customarily set on fire and burnt off. Mtonya was cool, even seasonally cold. Some missionaries saw the place as the answer to a long-desired hill station that "might be the health resort and recruiting [*sic*] ground for those who are run down and exhausted with the heat on the lake shore" (ibid., 11). Robert Howard, the UMCA's medical officer in the Nyasa Diocese from 1899 to 1909, readily embraced the theory and use of "climate therapy" that prevailed among colonizers at this time. From India's " hill stations" to Africa's highlands, Europeans celebrated the salubriousness and restorative powers of health resorts in the higher altitude tropics and sub-tropics (Sandwith 1907). In Howard's judgment, Mtonya, in Mozambique, was admirably suitable for such a sanitarium.

An additional European hospital was opened at Mponda's village in 1912. Africans had to wait until 1915 for a men's hospital and later still for a women's facility. Apart from the few hospitals, other medical work was carried on through a slowly expanding network of dispensaries at Mtonya, Mponda's, Unangu, Likwenu (fig. 4.11), and, of course, on board the *C.M.* Soon after it was put in service, the *CM.* assumed a central role in the transport and referral of patients from villages and other medical facilities to one of the UMCA's hospitals. The steamer's speed and medical resources made it possible to save or rehabilitate many of the critically ill and emergency cases that reached its sick bay. Distance, steamer schedules, poor land-to water communications, strangeness, fear, and other factors meant that only a small percentage of people living on or near the coast of Lake Malawi who became sick could or would be in a position to make use of the *C.M.*'s medical resources. Lacking access to the steamer, families sometimes sent their sick to Likoma Hospital in a dugout canoe, a journey that could require hours of paddling and involve considerable risk over open water (*CA* 29 [1911]). It was through individual and group decisions and myriad actions such as this that precolonial social and place relations in the lake region changed quite fundamentally over time. Such developments occurred incrementally and often imperceptibly (cf. Blood 1957, 25).

WORLD WAR I: COMMANDEERING OF THE STEAMERS

In August 1914, the Royal Navy commandeered the *Chauncy Maples* for war service on Lake Malawi against the Germans. The *Charles Janson* was similarly bound over to the "Lake Nyasa Flotilla" in 1916, along with several smaller mission boats. At Malindi, the government also took over the engineering shop. Neither steamer was returned to the UMCA until after the war. Lt.-Cmdr. G. Dennistoun, R.N., who was in charge of the lake flotilla throughout the war, allowed the *C.M.* and *C.J.* to be operated by the mission's own officers and crews. Both Captain Augustine Shannon, RNVR, the *C.M.*'s skipper, and his first officer, Sub-Lt. Haywood, and their "Christian crews" thus saw duty on their own steamers.[29] Shannon occasionally also served as a pilot on British gunboats such as the *H.M.S. Guendolen*, particularly in the waters of German East Africa which he knew well. Dennistoun also accommodated the UMCA by allowing the *C.M.* and *C.J.* to resupply

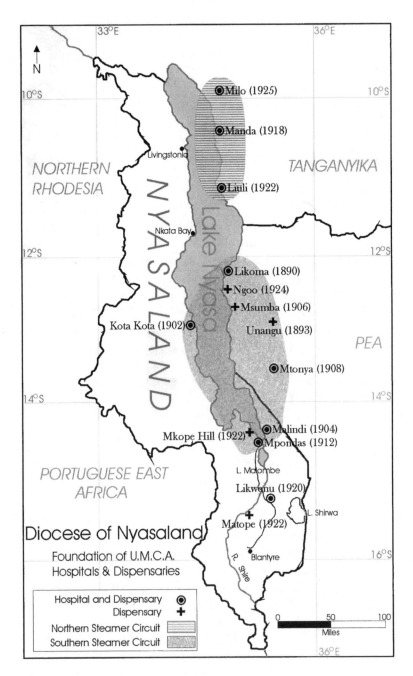

Figure 4.11. Hospitals and dispensaries

Likoma and some other lakeside settlements. Missionary work in the Tanganyika section of the *Chauncy Maples* station was temporarily abandoned (*CA* 33 [1915]). Dr. Wigan, the UMCA's medical officer, had volunteered for the King's African Rifles (K.A.R.), which greatly weakened the mission health care system. The mission staff was further depleted when seven or eight priests and laymen left to work with the British Army's African Carrier Corps, overseeing rationing and traveling with them (ibid.; Winspear 1956; Hayes 1964). By the end of 1917, only three UMCA nurses and several African "dispensary boys" were available to the entire diocese (Blood 1957, 127). During the war the Africans who had been trained by the UMCA as medical auxiliaries performed in exemplary fashion and reportedly exceeded "European expectations."

As its wartime contribution the *C.J.* towed barges and collected foodstuffs and firewood for the British forces. The larger *C.M.* was used primarily to ferry troops of the K.A.R. to various battle zones such as Karonga on the north end of the lake. Its direct engagement of German forces was limited to a skirmish or two. The most prominent confrontation began on May 24, 1915, when the 350-ton *H.M.S. Guendolen*, a patrol gunboat, left Ft. Johnston in the company of the *C.M.* and headed north for the German port of Sphinxhaven. Armed with Maxim guns, the mission steamer also carried two companies of the K.A.R. on this expedition. The larger *Guendolen* was armed with six-pounder Hotchkiss guns. Their objective was to capture and try to refloat the *Hermann von Wissmann,* the German gunboat laid up in a slip for repairs. This same boat had been been disabled by the *Guendolen* in dry-dock at Sphinxhaven on August 13, 1914, in what became known as the first naval action of World War I. It was then believed the Germans planned to get it running again. British forces had orders to neutralize the *Wissmann* as a gun platform and reduce the potential threat it posed to British steamers and coastal population centers. Around 3:00 A.M. on May 30, the British vessels landed troops south of Sphinxhaven. Most of the twenty odd defenders of Sphinxhaven, including the lone German missionary in command, withdrew into the night. The *Guendolen* commenced shelling the *Wissmann,* and captured the German boat before noon. It was then "blown up" and "completely disabled by means of dynamite charges" (Murray 1922, 269).

According to the *Chauncy Maples*'s log of May 30, 1915, after the *Wissmann* was taken the two captains guided their ships dangerously close to sunken rocks in order to enable the British forces to safely reboard the steamers from small landing craft. When enemy troops opened fire on the last unit of returning British forces, the *Guendolen* bombarded their positions, prompting two Maxims and troops to open fire from the *C.M.*'s upper deck (Hayes 1964,

21). The mission steamer returned from its engagement "bearing the marks of Maxim bullets upon her" (Blood 1957, 91).

Apart from a few minor skirmishes in 1916, practically no further naval activity occurred on Lake Malawi for the duration of the war. A one-pounder gun removed from the *Wissmann* was fitted on the *C.M.*'s deck, and a searchlight installed. She made numerous voyages as a troop ferry in actions against General von Lettow, and on one mission reportedly transported five hundred *tengatenga* (carriers of military supplies and food) to the front at the north end of the lake (Williams 1958).

Lt.-Cmdr. Dennistoun remained on duty with the Royal Navy in Nyasaland for three and one-half years. He described his wartime command on Lake Malawi as one of the "smaller sideshows . . . which were being started all over the world" (Hayes 1964, 24). Yet the war resulted in permanent changes in the UMCA's modus operandi, and in Malawi generally. When it ended, the *Wissmann* was repaired and fitted with petrol engines at Malindi. Renamed the *King George* in 1919, it was sold to the Lake Nyasa Steamship Co. in 1920, renamed the *Malonda* (trader), and refitted again with different engines and boilers. Meanwhile, at great inconvenience to UMCA activities, the *Chauncy Maples* remained out of operation until May 1921, due to boiler repairs. During part of this "down" time the *Malonda* was given over to the UMCA for help with essential transport services (ibid.). The *Charles Janson* was used for transport services during the *C.M.*'s long postwar repairs, but was an inadequate stand-in.

THE STEAMER PARISH IN TRANSITION

Loss of steamer capabilities due to the war and marine engineering problems caused the UMCA enormous dislocation and inconvenience for almost seven years. This situation forced the mission to reassess the role of its steamers and ultimately to reorganize the conduct of missionary work. Isolated at his headquarters at Likoma, Bishop Fisher complained about this "inaccessible island on a Lake constantly swept by winds, which make it difficult for steamers to be punctual" (Blood 1957, 126).

Meanwhile, the four independent sections of the vast *Chauncy Maples* station—the steamer parish—now had to be worked by just a few priests and women from four centers on land. These divisions included (1) the German coast, temporarily abandoned;[30] (2) the Kobwe Circuit, irreverently known as the "Kobwe Circus," in Portuguese territory, worked by a priest stationed on Likoma (Winspear 1960); (3) the main Portuguese section from Mala to

Msinje supervised by Archdeacon Johnson, which included villages situated one to four hours' walk away in the hills above the coastline; and (4) the British, or Monkey Bay district in the far southwest (*CA* 33 [1915]: 300–301).

During the war, a strong effort was made to carry on with the normal range of mission activities, but work was greatly hampered by the continual unfolding of new circumstances. In 1917 Johnson lamented the loss of the *C.M.*, which "becomes more and more a mere memory."[31] Hardship and suffering as direct results of military actions in Malawi were minimal compared to the heavy losses of life and property experienced in parts of German East Africa and Zanzibar. Mtonya and Unangu in Portuguese East Africa were the only UMCA head stations to suffer raids and capture by German forces. Nevertheless, business as usual was no longer possible. Loss of the steamers certainly forced the most dramatic changes, notably the reorganization of the *Chauncy Maples* station.

Transit of British and South African troops, carriers, and supplies through Mponda's and Malindi disrupted the life of those stations and interrupted normal communications between all stations. Work at the Likoma Printing Office declined sharply after the European layman in charge was conscripted by the military. By 1916, St. Michael's College, Likoma, the teacher training institute, had sixty African students in the general academic course. Included in this group were several "dispensary boys," young men who also received practical training in a hospital/dispensary on Saturdays. Another twenty-five teachers studied for advanced certificates (*CA* 34 [1916]: 225). In 1917, the college was forced to close due to the strong competition for scarce food reserves from African troops and carriers. This "terrible shortness of food," wrote Archdeacon Eyre from Mtonya station, was directly "the result of the War" (*CA* 37 [1919]: 89). It was precipitated by the government's siphon of the more able-bodied men as conscripts to carry supplies needed by the troops. This intervention withdrew critically necessary labor from the villages and, in combination with poor rains, undermined local food production systems. Many fields were left un-hoed or neglected, and hospitals struggled to remain open for lack of food. During most of 1918, Malindi was actually closed to inpatients, whereas Kota Kota Hospital managed to remain open with help from the resident magistrate (68, 89).

Immediately after the war, the Spanish Influenza pandemic reached Malawi. It spread unevenly and varied in its harshness, but whole villages and towns were infected. In some localities crops failed and the resultant food shortages greatly aggravated the suffering. The government supplied drugs to mission dispensaries, including Likwenu station, where a "whole village was down at once." Reportedly, those few villages where European medicines were still feared had the highest death rates. Requests from "Islam villages" for mission medical help raised evangelistic hopes (92). Many Africans perished, and not only in areas lacking mission or government medical help. At the height of the epidemic, Zomba, the protectorate headquarters, had become like "a city of the dead" (ibid.).

All the while the mission strained to prevent losing its tentative toehold on the Muslim frontier. At Kota Kota, the UMCA station was situated in the old slaving center on the western coast of Lake Malawi; the war years apparently brought increased medical work to the hospital and greater tolerance among Muslims and Christians. These developments triggered profound changes in the environments and societies situated beyond the immediate hinterland of the coast (Kjekshus 1977). There was even a Muslim-initiated request for joint prayers for rain with Christians during the drought of 1918–19 (Blood 1957, 128). This situation contrasted with the strongly negative perceptions of Islam held by the missionaries stationed in the Monkey Bay district, at the southern reaches of the lake. Here, it was alleged, "the [Christian] work was constantly harassed by outposts of debased Muhammedanism" (129). The war simultaneously impeded the UMCA's ability to make inroads against Islam at the same time the mission was beginning to make lasting contributions to social change. As the missionaries viewed it, their mandate to counter Muslim influence was hampered because African teachers were scarce. Also, the attraction of war-time jobs in and around Ft. Johnston, near the mouth of the Shiré River, drew many of the young men and older schoolboys away from their villages (ibid.).

Europe's inability to sustain peace on the African continent had grave consequences for its colonial subjects and missionaries. The UMCA's work shut down in a number of locations, including villages in German East Africa. Labor was drained out of entire countrysides. Government commandeering of the *C.M.* and *C.J.* forced a reorganization of the mission's work. Ultimately, this change led to a determination that the "steamer parish" concept had become obsolete. In Likoma Archdeaconry, St. Michael's teacher-training college was forced to close. Its principal was drafted to supervise the government's transport workers. Meanwhile, patients were "crammed" into those mission hospitals that remained open, and only four European nurses remained in the entire diocese.

Speaking at a UMCA meeting in London in 1918, Bishop Fisher observed that "schools had also suffered beyond belief, going down in a most pathetic" manner. In the medical work, he noted that while the Scottish Free Church Mission had a doctor at each of its stations, the UMCA had but one. While the military authorities had greatly needed support, men had been taken from their villages and given "a very rough time" in the service of a war that was not theirs. The effect of this demand was "lamentable" since "enormous numbers of carriers died . . . or came back sick or ill." Fisher also observed that while he had made good friends among European military men in Central Africa, "a certain number of them lived very much below the Christian tradition." While he did not want to throw stones, they had come from "a very wicked country . . . and the influence of many of these white men was simply deplorable" (*CA* 37 [1919]: 76). The UMCA's journal *Central Africa* published Chaplain Arthur S. Cripps's "The Dirge of a Dead Porter," a stinging indictment of the British Army's exploitation of the Carrier Corps, calling the forced labor "assuredly a sin against England's conscience" (*CA* 39 [1921]).

Mission staff strength was further reduced immediately following the war because members who had served with British forces were all due for furloughs. When they returned they found the *C.M.* still operating, but Bishop Fisher had redefined its mission. He maintained that the pioneer days were behind them. A different era had begun, and for the most part itinerant evangelism from the steamers belonged to the past. This change in the steamer's status caused Archdeacon Johnson much grief, understandably so considering his long and intimate association with the lakeside work. For the rest of his life, Johnson believed that the mission could and should have served a much larger territory by retaining the old steamer method (Barnes 1933). After World War I it was evident that the settlement pattern was undergoing a transition begun during the peace in the 1890s. More and more people from land-hungry lakeside villages shifted into the once dangerous hills back from the lake, causing the population in a number of the larger coastal settlements to shrink (ibid.).

Upon returning from furlough in 1921 Johnson, now sixty-seven years old, was "full of plans for resuming his old pre-war work on and with the steamer" (163). To his dismay, he discovered that the bishop had assigned him responsibility for the remote mountainous territory in southwest Tanganyika that the mission had inherited from the Germans. Johnson had worked parts of this large area before the war, and had cultivated excellent personal relations with the Germans. On his own, he had founded "between twenty and thirty village stations on the Lakeside worked entirely by the steamer" (177). Now, however, the steamers' "floating ministry" would be permanently curtailed. This was a painful fact of life that Johnson came to accept, although the disappointment lingered for the seven remaining years of his life. He hated to see the steamers relegated to the "donkey work" of mission transport. In 1926, shortly before his death, and physically unable to get up and down Tanganyika's steep mountain trails without help, the archdeacon still expressed frustration with the demise of the "steamer method" of missionary work. Writing to his brother on May 8, he observed that the Roman Catholic missionaries worked the northeastern coast of Lake Malawi "in canoes only, while we with two steamers leave it!!!" (153).[32]

While the sacraments could still be administered from the *C.M.*, impatience had grown over delays and uncertainty involved in coordinating these essential rituals with the steamer's sometimes unpredictable schedule. It remained true that "a certain amount of oversight" of missionary work on land from the *C.M.* was still possible. Yet Canon George Fisher's opinion that "little real pastoral work could be done" from the steamer was apparently shared by many in the mission (Wilson 1936, 193).

To Canon Frank Winspear, who arrived in Malawi in 1906 and became one of the *C.M.*'s "steamer clergy" in 1909, it had become "abundantly clear that efficient as the steamer plan had been for pioneer days the time had come when it could only be adequately worked from various centres staffed by both men and women workers" (Winspear 1960, 58–59). In a reform considered "long overdue," all of the steamer's pastoral work of training and supervising African teachers and priests, previously conducted on and from the *C.M.*, was now distributed among the various land stations. This enabled "ladies . . . to live at them and supervise women and girls' work, and the work in the ordinary way had quite outgrown the monthly visits of the steamer" (36). When the *C.M.* was again ready for service, its revised "orders" were to transport mission stores, the medical officer, and passengers, including hospital cases. Soon the steamer's sick bay got more use than its chapel.

The eclipse of the old *Chauncy Maples* steamer parish reduced staff itinerancy and permitted a more efficient deployment of UMCA priests, teachers, and health workers to the land stations. It was no longer a training school and dormitory for traveling European priests. From a missionary point of view, how much better now to be in regular contact with one's parishioners and their communities.

Loss of its parish and the establishment of permanent mission staffs on land did not marginalize the *C.M.*'s utility. Eight central stations and sixty villages continued to depend on her for supplies and for transportation to various places around the lake, not least carrying the sick to hospitals. Extraordinary expectations also frequently landed in the lap of the *C.M.*'s skipper, as in September 1930, when he was asked by the diocesan headquarters to transport six hundred bags of rice to Likoma "from a place out of the regular run of the ship" (*CA* 48 [1930]: 188). Availability of the steamers also enabled the mission to hold an annual retreat and conference at

Likoma for its staff, and parties on board while in port at Malindi. At the time, Archdeacon Glossop (who had joined the UMCA in 1893), noted that the *C.M.* remained

> so essential a part of the life of the diocese, not only because . . . "the army marches on its stomach," but because she unites the various stations in so many ways, enabling the teachers and their families to be moved easily from station to station, whether going to work, or returning for a holiday, and keeping the Mission staff in touch with one another. In the old days the S.S. *C.J.* had no timetable . . . now the S.S.*Chauncy Maples* has to supply eight central stations. The European loads delivered at these stations . . . average about three hundred a month, and the native loads about another three hundred. (187–88)

Apart from the transport of European staff and mission stores, there was continuous travel by African teachers and their families, moving to new assignments and going to and coming from their holiday leaves. The steamer also transported students from their home ports to St. Michael's College or St. Andrews College, and then returned them after term. Supply of foodstuffs essential to the running of these colleges would have been virtually unthinkable without the aid of the steamer. The bishop and the diocesan medical officer also depended greatly on the *C.M.* to make their various rounds of the head stations. In effect, the shift of all its essential pastoral and educational functions to land stations did not diminish the steamer's fundamental role of support and logistics within the UMCA's mission strategy.

For the European missionaries there was, in the Victorian sense, an aura of "romance" about the *C.M.* Many a seasoned missionary as well as visitors revealed sentimental feelings about this "noble" vessel (*CA* 42 [1924]: 161). A staff member insisted that regardless of changes in the steamers' mandate after the war, "it is difficult to exaggerate" their usefulness "or to see how we could do our work without them" (*CA* 43 [1925]: 90). In contrast to its fate in World War I, the aged *C.M.* was not commandeered in World War Two. Until the early 1950s the steamer was still seen as "the most important link in the transport system of the diocese" (*UMCA Ann. Rev.*, 1944, 34).

EXPANSION OF MISSION STATIONS AFTER WORLD WAR I

Only two other head-stations opened before the end of World War I: Matope (1917) on the Shiré River and Ngoo Bay (1917) in Portuguese territory.

Previously an outstation itself, Ngoo was the place with the longest record of work in the diocese (fig. 4.2). It had already spawned nine outstations. Ngoo's supervision was placed in the hands of the Reverend Augustine Ambali, one of only two African priests ever put in charge of a UMCA head-station in the Nyasaland Diocese.[33] By this time the locality had quite a number of second-generation Christians and, compared to other stations, a disproportionate number of senior school pupils who went off for teacher training at St. Michael's College. Entire villages around Ngoo had become main predominantly Christian (Dale 1925, 195). Its service area was primarily south of the head-station. By custom, a priest from Likoma had responsibility for working the mainland villages north of Ngoo.

In 1921 a new station was also established at Mkope Hill, at the extreme south of Lake Malawi, between Mponda's village and Monkey Bay. Before it became a head station evangelical work in the Mkope Hill district had been "overseen" from Mponda's and visited by the steamer clergy (ibid.).

The UMCA also took advantage of the war's outcome by founding three new stations in Tanganyika. Between 1921 and 1925, the mission opened coastal stations at Liuli (Sphinxhaven) and Manda (Weidhafen). Some four thousand Christians were registered in the large district formed by the hinterlands of these two stations. Administering communion to them required enormous effort by the priest because the people lived in many scattered villages. From Manda and Liuli the UMCA spread its work through Tanganyika's Songea Province, building upon and replacing the work of the German Lutherans. It also acquired control of Milo, a remote mountain station formerly operated by the Berlin Mission (fig. 4.11). Hospital work got under way at all three stations by the mid-1920s.

Named after a town in Germany, Milo was originally opened by the Lutheran Mission in 1902 (CA 81 [1963]). Abandoned by the Germans during the war, the parish and station were inherited by the UMCA in a derelict state. Johnson had worked Milo from Liuli and then Manda beginning in 1914. It was formally handed over to the Diocese of Nyasaland in 1922, via a request from the new British administration in Tanganyika and the Berlin Mission (ibid.; Wilson 1936). Milo reopened in 1925 under the supervision of four Europeans, two men and two women. Given its long distance from Likoma and need for resources, this opportunity to pick up where the Germans had left off was not enthusiastically received by Bishop Fisher at Likoma. At the same time, Archdeacon Johnson, then in his last years, was "burning to seize the opportunity of doing something for these poor Christians" (Wilson 1936, 198). Johnson's legendary enthusiasm helped sway the Home Committee to underwrite the project's cost and secure the bishop's approval. This move substantially enlarged the mission's territorial interests and responsibilities for medical services. It also added new ethnic groups, with different languages and customs, notably the Pangwa-speaking villagers in the mountains.

Under Archdeacon Johnson's lead, the UMCA undertook to proselytize and Christianize the ethnic groups within Milo's formidable hinterland. The parish sprawled "over the Livingstone mountains, ridge after ridge, rising to eight, nine and ten thousand feet, with valleys down to three or four thousand feet deep between them." In its high ridges and "blue distances," Milo offered a breathtaking highland landscape that evoked Edenic visions in European visitors (*CA* 64 [1946]: 71).[34] Situated at 7,000 feet above sea level and 5,500 feet above Lake Malawi, the station is a place of great natural beauty, set in the bracing air of the rugged mountains. Day after day during the rainy season the land is covered in clouds, while the dry season features very cold nights. Apples, plums, pears, strawberries, and other temperate-zone crops grow well there.

Re-opening the station, however, presented formidable physical and logistical challenges. It was both difficult to resupply and to have ready access to the parish's numerous, small clusters of dispersed population.

Milo was the last main station that the UMCA opened in the lake region, and geographically the northernmost. By 1925 the mission's commitments, developed over forty years, extended four hundred miles north-south and took in parts of three colonial territories. Fifteen widely spaced head-stations, including nine hospitals, plus the two steamers, accomplished the main work of the diocese (figs. 4.11 and 4.12). Land stations included seven in Nyasaland, three in Tanganyika Territory, and five in Portuguese East Africa. Seven principal hospitals, at the head-stations of Likoma, Kota Kota, Malindi, Mponda's, Likwenu, Liuli, and Milo, provided both inpatient (I-P) and out-patient (O-P) services (table 4.1). By 1938 the diocese had in addition over 350 outstations.

Statistics offer a sense of the cumulative efforts of both African and European Christians to build up and strengthen this mission field between 1885 and 1925 (table 4.2). In reality, such measures provide only pale renderings of the successes and failures, hardships and sacrifices, and changes in individual lives and society that occurred on all sides.

By the mid-1920s the basic infrastructure of the UMCA's Nyasaland Diocese was complete. Thomas Cathrew Fisher, the seventh Bishop of Nyasaland (1910–29), wrote that the missionary work now extended beyond the pioneer stage of basic "preaching to the heathen." It had by then

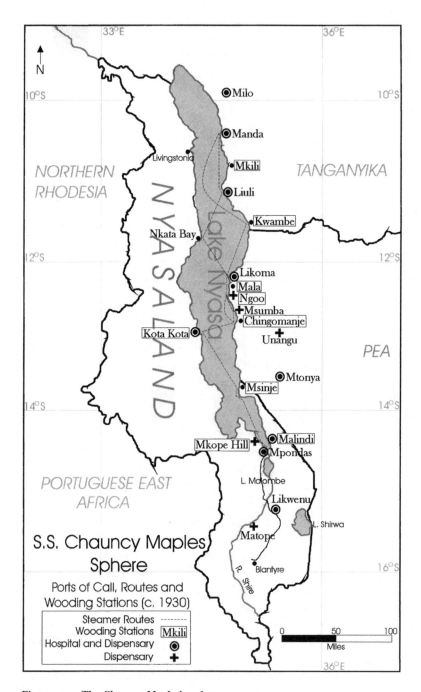

Figure 4.12. The *Chauncy Maples*'s sphere

Table 4.1   UMCA stations and main hospitals, Diocese of Nyasaland, 1925

Station	Date opened	Hospital, Date opened
Likoma (N)	1885	1890
Charles Janson	1885	
Unangu (P)	1893	
Kota Kota (N)	1894	1902
Malindi (N)	1898	1903–8
Mponda's (N)	1896	1912
Chauncy Maples	1902	Sick bay
Mtonya (P)	1905	African-managed from 1899; Jigger Hospital 1908; and World War I troop base; closed 1928; incorporated with Lungwena.
Manda (T)	1918	new hospital, 1936
Msumba (P)	1906	1920s; large outpatient center; evolved into hospital over many years.
Lungwena (P)	1906	
Likwenu (N)	1910	1919
Matope (N)	1917	
Ngoo (P)	1917	
Manda (T)	1918	previously, Amelia Bay
Liuli (T)	1921	1922; previously, Sphinxhaven
Mkope Hill (N)	1921	
Milo (T)	reopened 1925	1925; third station in Tanganyika inherited from Germans.

Sources: *Central Africa;* Malawi National Archives. Also Sims 1897; Mills 1911; Anderson-Morshead 1955; Blood 1957; Wilson 1936. For Manda, *UMCA Ann. Rep.,* 1936, 29.
   (N) Nyasaland; (P) Portuguese East Africa; (T) Tanganyika Territory.

entered the second stage, when "the care of a large number of communicants" is added to the preaching and in some places supersedes it. The third stage would occur when the mission started to function "on its own" and African clergy replaced European missionaries (*CA* 45 [1945]: 123).

Only a crude approximation of the size of the African population in the UMCA sphere of influence is possible, not least because this sphere stretched across the most remote peripheries of three colonial territories. Nyasaland's 1921 census settled on a total African population of 1.2 million, including thousands of younger men who had migrated for work to the Rhodesias and South Africa. Despite the vast distances involved in the UMCA's proclaimed service area, it probably contained no more than 10 percent of the protectorate's total population. Fewer than 80,000 people, over 80 percent

Table 4.2   UMCA census, Diocese of Nyasaland, 1925

16 principal head-stations (15 on land)
7 hospitals and several dispensaries
66 professional mission staff, incl. bishop, 24 priests (7 African), 1 deacon (African)
27 women (teachers and nursing sisters), and 13 laymen (incl. medical officer)
199 outstations, worked and supervised from the head-stations
38,350 adherents of the faith: of whom 23,712 baptized and 16,393 communicants
7,879 children in school, and 110 teachers at training college
2,058 inpatients in UMCA hospitals
216,827 outpatient attendances

Sources: *Central Africa* 42 (1924); Roome 1926, 38.

Yao and 16 percent Nyanja, lived in what was then South Nyasa District, now Mangoche District (Murray 1922). Much of the eastern sector of this district, which extended eighty miles north of Ft. Johnson (the coast beyond Malindi to Lungwena), came under the UMCA's nominal influence. About two-thirds of the population had a much stronger allegiance to Islam than the remaining third had to Christianity, a situation that caused the mission much distress. During the 1930s the Lungwena area was attracting Christianized settlers from Ngoo and other UMCA-influenced settlements much farther north along the lake side (*CA* 51 [1933]). Long before, on this same coast stretch of coast, Archdeacon Johnson had worked from the steamers to establish schools and mission posts. Now, decades later, some of the descendants of the early Christians in these same coastal villages had decided autonomously to move south on hearing of the existence of some unoccupied and moderately fertile land.

It is also possible that they preferred to live under British rather than Portuguese colonial rule. In a region dominated by Muslims, many of the new arrivals soon became ex-Christians. This provoked the great frustration and anger on the part of the UMCA missionaries. In the mission's view, the converts had succumbed to the powerful pull of the local "bastard" form of Islam (Barnes 1933, 126).

Stymied by their thin ranks and meager resources, and sometimes enraged, the UMCA missionaries had once again come up against "the bitter facts" of the still-expanding Afro-Islamic cultural frontier. An Eastertide missive singled out a former UMCA teacher who had become a Muslim convert for special condemnation, calling her "a she-devil of a woman"

(*CA* 51 [1933]: 187). In 1933 at least eight of the mission's ex-teachers were reportedly working "actively or passively . . . against us" in the area between Lungwena and Malindi, while only four Christian teachers worked to "stem the tide" (188). One missionary offered his opinion that moral turpitude led these ex-faithful to cross over to Islam: "I think in every case these ex-teachers came a cropper over the Christian marriage laws, and then turned into our most bitter enemies" (ibid.).

In the west the South Nyasa District extended far beyond the UMCA's reach, which mainly encompassed the villages of the coastal zone. Kota Kota, the former slave trade center on the west coast of the lake, was a "native town of 3,000–4,000 huts" in 1921 (Murray 1922). The town had been a Muslim stronghold since the 1850s, while the UMCA's station there had been in operation since 1894. Perhaps as many as 15,000 people in and near Kota Kota came within the mission's theoretically effective range for religious instruction and medical services.

The eastern sector of the district extended from Ft. Johnston on the Shiré north to Makanjila's and Ft. Maguire, in Portuguese territory. Some 175 miles long, this expansive strip of land and water was the original "steamer parish." Containing large villages such as Msumba and Chitesi's, this zone was home to more than half of the 38,350 "Adherents" claimed by the mission in 1925 (table 4.1). Farther north in Tanganyika Territory lay the remote head-stations and population clusters at Liuli, Manda, and Milo.

Various crude indices, including recorded outpatient use of its dispensaries and hospitals, show that the UMCA's sphere of influence was characterized by great place-to-place variations in the nature and intensity of local African contacts with the mission. Overall, in 1925 this region nominally included at least 100,000 people. Natural increase of the population had turned markedly upward, as shown in the UMCA's accounting of Africans involved in its activities. Fundamentally, the mission's physical frontiers had been reached, not least because of an unrelenting shortage of funds and European personnel.

After 1925 the primary engagement between African and missionary was more than ever ideological and religious, each side possessing and demonstrating persuasive moral authority. Divergences in spiritual matters, approaches to health, and understanding of family patterns were grounded in different psychologies, ideas, and behavior. For both Africans and Europeans, culture could be a basis for sharing, miscalculation, and confrontation as well as a refuge from each other. Intentionally or otherwise, the dialogues that emerged variously served to bridge, nullify, or reinforce the chasm of culture, race, and class. New secular influences and experiences

that penetrated into and emanated from the village complicated such communications.

ONGOING ADJUSTMENT TO UNCERTAINTY

New Steamer Mandate and Printed Schedule

After World War I, the Colonial Office, short on transport, approached the
UMCA with a view to taking over full control of the *Chauncy Maples*. When
this arrangement was viewed unfavorably by the mission, the government
offered a counter proposal with trade-offs. The mission could keep the
steamer under its control but must agree to operate a monthly itinerary
providing lake service to both government and mission ports. In return for
carrying "all Government passengers and cargo," the UMCA would receive
"a fixed monthly payment and certain allowances for service" (*CA* 40 [1922]:
214, quoting *Nyasaland Diocesan Chronicle*, n.d.).

Hard pressed as usual for operating funds, the mission accepted the proposal and quickly introduced a printed timetable, or Order of Sailing (*CA* 40
[1922]). Starting at Malindi, the 1928 itinerary shows that the *C.M.* called
at eleven different ports and settlements (table 4.3), where the anchorages
varied from two fathoms (twelve feet) to thirty fathoms (180 feet) deep
(*CA* 57 [1939]). The three-week round-trip exceeded seven hundred miles
(fig. 4.12). Manda, in Tanganyika, was the most northern port. Two stops on
the west coast, at Nkata Bay, where several villages of UMCA Africans from
Likoma and P.E.A. had settled, and the UMCA station at Kota Kota, were
on the steamer's regular rounds (*CA* 54 [1936]). Malindi, with its engineering
facilities, was the final stop on the circuit. Here, in the best of circumstances,
a whole a week might be available for refitting and repairs.[35]

Formal scheduling, routinization, and transfer of the spiritual work to missionaries on permanent land stations improved the *C.M.*'s on-time arrivals
performance. Previously the steamers' schedules had usually been ignored
and delays and late arrivals considered the rule. In 1922 one missionary observed that "during the nine months I was on the *Chauncy Maples*, I can only
remember arriving once on the date which was down on the time-table"
(*CA* 41 [1923]: 45). Over time, the mission established more congregations
and much more work than could be accommodated by a few priests alternating visits to villages. Conditions that prevailed in the pioneer days twenty
to thirty years earlier no longer guided the expectations and demands of the
Africans or the mission.

Table 4.3   Order of sailing, *Chauncy Maples*, January 1928

Day	Port call	Date in 1928
M	Nkudzi	Jan. 23
T	Msinje	24
W	Kota Kota	25
Th	Mtengula	26
F	Msumba	27
F	Ngoo Bay	27
F	Likoma	27
Sat	Likoma	28
Sun	Likoma	29
M	Nkata	30
T	Liuli	31
W	Manda	Feb. 1
Th	Liuli	2
F	Chiwindi	2
F	Likoma	2
F	Nkata	3
Sat	Likoma	4
Sun	Likoma	5
M	Ngoo Bay	6
T	Mtengula	7
W	Kota Kota	8
Th	Msinje	9
Th	Nkudzi	9
F	Bar	10
F	Malindi	10

Source: UMCA 1/2/21. MNA.

Financial Climate

Slim, insecure budgets plagued the mission during and after World War I. In
the minds of the missionaries, acts of faith and prayer must have borne fruit
on numerous occasions, considering the capricious winds that buffeted the
mission's usual sources of support. Fluctuations in the UMCA's General and
Particular Maintenance Funds, African Schools and Clergy Fund, and other
special funds in England led to real and threatened reductions in the size
of grants to the dioceses in Africa. The financial crisis that followed World
War I reduced the numbers of both African and European staff in UMCA
schools, hospitals, and dispensaries, and contributed to severe shortages of
food and drugs (Gelfand 1964). Dire warnings from London stated that the

entire mission might have to be given up unless help arrived. This theme resurfaced a decade later when the effects of the Great Depression spread directly from the metropoles to the colonies. Shrinking employment and heavy taxation imperiled the ability of the mission's British subscribers to maintain their pledges. It was believed fortunate that grants to the UMCA's four dioceses in 1931 fell only 10 percent (£6,500) overall. Certainly the retrenchment was seen in the drop in monthly cash reserves. "The Bishop cannot spare us another bean—and our Christians are turning to Islam," one missionary groused (*CA* 51 [1933]: 188).

By 1936 the UMCA was operating on an annual pledged budget of £65,275. This sum supported the work in Nyasaland, four other dioceses (Zanzibar, Northern Rhodesia, and Masasi), and Home Expenses (propaganda and administration, including eleven secretaries) at Central Africa House in London. Slightly more than a third of the total budget (£22,200) was earmarked for Nyasaland, including £1,510 for the *Chauncy Maples*. Another £4,600 went to furloughs and passages. As diocesan headquarters, Likoma received more funds for "station" operation than any other UMCA mission. However, by 1936 Likoma's increasing isolation could be seen in the fact that its total allocation for the year (£1,845) was a few pounds less than Liuli's (£1,864). Liuli's budget included 39 per cent more for African clergy and 49 per cent more for teachers and schools. Among the other stations only Msumba (£1,525), Kota Kota (£1,365), Mponda's (£1,188), Manda (£1,101), and Malindi (£1,027) received more than £1,000 for station operation, African clergy, teachers and schools, and hospitals and dispensaries. Modest additional grants to support female welfare workers could usually be counted on from the home-based Mothers' Union, but the mission received no regular assistance from any other organization. Requests for budget assistance typically took aim at public sympathies in England. It was emphasized that the grants "are not really adequate even for the maintenance of existing work [and that] there will be no possibility of extension and development until the grants can be increased" (*CA* 55 [1937]: 106).

Although the resources fluctuated, special funds such as the Mat Fund (endowed sleeping mat or bed) and the Hospital and Sick Comforts Fund proved indispensable to medical work. The latter provided all drugs and dressings for the mission's medical work, while the General Fund supported mission doctors and nurses. Additional support was raised through extraordinary fund-raising campaigns (usually special pleadings) among the members of home churches, and from the philanthropy of prominent individuals of high social standing in Britain. A persistent financial squeeze is certainly part of the reason there was little if any talk in UMCA circles of replacing the *Charles Janson* (after 1930) or the *Chauncy Maples* with modern equipment.

Over the years, the continuance of mission work often seemed to hang on a combination of pure faith and benevolence. Whatever else might be essential, strategically it was critically important to support an expanded African clergy as the foundation of the African church. The mission was hampered in that effort by continual shortages of European priests and nurses. Short-handedness was almost always aggravated by conflicts with scheduled furloughs, and produced more than enough frustration and tension to go around. English staff of the mission worked as volunteers without pay. They received an allowance of up to £20 yearly but were not expected to use it unless it was essential (*CA* 19 [1901]: 26–27). Most worked hard at their jobs, some even tirelessly, but many had a chronic sense of "running in place." When the UMCA's only medical officer went on furlough, many of his vast responsibilities devolved to the nursing sisters. His other duties simply came to a halt for a year.

At the end of 1936, the Diocese of Nyasaland counted 443 workers on its rolls. This total included nineteen European and nine African priests, twelve European laymen, ten African deacons, and thirty-five European women serving as teachers, nurses, etc. These staff members had assistance from 355 African readers and teachers (*CA* 55 [1937]). Africans thus made up nearly 85 percent of the UMCA's total complement of mission workers. Such an African-to-European ratio was not unusual among missions. It dramatically emphasizes how critically important the contribution of African readers, teachers, and later, priests, was to the fulfillment of the UMCA's aims. Twenty years earlier, in 1916, only three Africans were included among the diocese's twenty Anglo-Catholic priests.

By 1936, no European deacon remained and the African proportion had increased by two-thirds. In 1916, all eleven laymen were European. These individuals included the mission doctor, the steamer captains, engineers, carpenters, and other artisans and persons with special skills. Twenty years later, there were twelve laymen, and still no Africans. Meanwhile, the number of European women workers under contract with the mission increased by two-thirds during the period. This growth reflects the expansion of schools, nursing needs, and a trend among missions generally to give greater attention to women's literacy and domestic skills, and maternal and child health (*CA* 54 [1936]). Apparently, no African woman was as yet deemed qualified for such work.

Passing of Three Pioneers

Two of the most significant people in the mission's history departed from the scene during the 1920s. With their unique roles and personalities they perhaps came closer to being indispensable than any others in the diocese's eighty-year history. In 1926, the tireless Archdeacon William P. Johnson reached a major personal and institutional milestone when he completed fifty years of service with the UMCA. Having already received an honorary D.D. from Oxford University in 1911, in 1926 he was made an Honorary Fellow of University College, Oxford, where as a young man he had read for two degrees. Johnson chose not to retire but to continue working in and out of the Tanganyika stations until his death at Liuli Mission Hospital on October 11, 1928. Bishop Fisher, who handed Johnson deep disappointment when he terminated the steamer parish, allowed that he had "never known anyone who so obviously lived in the presence of God" (Wilson 1936, 237).

It would be an error of the first magnitude to diminish Johnson's contribution to the scope and character of the UMCA's enterprise in Nyasaland. Few men or women, living or dead, could demonstrate comparable fortitude and courage, initiate and sustain contact with as many peoples, learn as many languages, or match his mobility and resilience under such trying circumstances.

In UMCA lore Johnson ranks as "the last of the great pioneers," and it was said that his name "will always be remembered above all others" who worked as missionaries in this part of Central Africa. He never permitted his severe vision impairment to become a handicap. His reputation was that of one who never sat down or stood still, and "in early middle age he looked an old man" (*CA* 70 [1952]: 144). Because of Johnson, the mission's geographical and evangelical spheres of influence expanded much faster and farther than would have happened otherwise. At seventy years of age he was still climbing up and down steep slopes in the Livingstone Mountains of Tanganyika in order to reach villages. Long-time African associates who traveled with him in the 1920s described how they helped the weakening but fiercely determined, Johnson up and down the slopes. They would place "a long bamboo pole under each arm as a crutch, and with a man in front to pick out the best steps and another behind to bolster him up and prevent him from falling" (Barnes 1933, 193). In fact, he was responsible for opening access to considerably more area and population than the UMCA ever had the resources to effectively work. Whether or not one appreciated the type of profession Johnson represented, it cannot be denied that he was that most unusual person who comes along infrequently in the life of an institution—one peculiarly well equipped for a task that others ignore or imagine impossible.

Johnson was soon followed in death by Augustine Shannon, the former captain of the *Chauncy Maples*, who had retired from the mission after twenty years to become a game warden in Tanganyika. Shannon, like many who worked on the steamers, considered lakeside Malindi his home. He had returned for a visit and had gone off for "a shoot" with two African hunters. On their return journey he was bitten by a snake and rapidly developed severe muscle spasms and neurological symptoms. His men carried him on a stretcher about twelve miles back to Malindi, but he was dead on arrival at the mission hospital, January 13, 1929. Following a service in Nyanja with hymns in Yao, the "crowds followed him to his last resting-place: Africans, Indians and Europeans; Christians, Mohammedans and heathen" (*CA* 47 [1929]: 78).

The mission experienced another great and symbolic loss in November 1929, when the *Charles Janson* sank at her moorings at Malindi in four fathoms of water. Raised and brought to shore, she was worked on for eighteen months before being placed back into commission in August 1931. Unsafe boilers again forced the *C.J.* out of service after its first voyage following the overhaul (*CA* 48 [1930]; Blood 1957). By 1933 the vessel had not been recommissioned. Bishop Thorne was quite unprepared to place it in regular service, although it might well be used for "emergency " or special-purpose trips (*CA* 51 [1933]). Evidently the *C.J.* had seen her last voyage on the lake. In 1941 the bishop recorded that the steamer had been lying derelict "on her side" at Malindi since at least 1936 (*CA* 59 [1941]: 60).

Following discussions with the Universities' Mission Trust, who technically owned the *C.J.*, it was decided to dismantle the steamer and use the materials in the construction of small boats (*CA* 59 [1941]; Williams 1958). Thus ended the remarkable career of the UMCA's first steamer. It had served long after its task of facilitating the mission's pioneer era at Lake Malawi was accomplished, having endured innumerable repairs and several overhauls over a span of fifty-six years.

Relocation of the Mission's Engineering Port

By 1930, the slip at Malindi used for repair of the steamers had become derelict. Consequently, it was decided to shift such operations to the sheltered deep water at Monkey Bay. There was no dry dock or slip at the new site. Initially the repair work was accomplished with the aid of a makeshift pier to which the steamer was tied with the stern facing the shoreline. As the next step, Captain Haywood ordered the placement of fifty tons of sand in the steamer's bow. The sand was provided courtesy of a "daily procession" of small boys from the local village who carried drums of it aboard the vessel. Accomplished over the course of a week, this awkward procedure ultimately lifted the stern and propeller above the water. Meanwhile, the engines were stripped down and positioned forward to provide additional weight. This tough, dirty work was done by the *Chauncy Maples*'s stokers and deck hands. Captain Haywood rewarded them with a supply of fresh meat that he had personally shot in the nearby bush country. After several days of repairs and a trial run, the steamer made the four-hour trip south to Malindi. A crowd of passengers and cargo awaited the *C.M.* on its arrival. Within hours the steamer was loaded and departed on its regular schedule of calls to ports and stations up the lake (*CA* 49 [1931]).

Consequences of a Rising Lake Level

Lake Malawi's hydrology is the product of complicated patterns of geomorphology, rainfall, evaporation, and runoff in its catchment area, spread across a north-south span of 360 miles. At the Bar, where the lake flows into the Shiré, the alluvial bottom is exceptionally flat and unstable. Pronounced fluctuations in the lake's level have been the subject of much speculation about its causes. The interaction of many environmental factors has contributed to a long history of seasonal variations in water levels, with consequent periodic flooding of the lakeshore and large sections of the lower Shiré valley. Over the years these changes have impeded navigation and damaged arable land (Pike 1968).

Record keeping did not begin until 1896, although evidence pieced together from the accounts of early travelers on the lake and the Shiré suggests a distinct pattern of fluctuations in water level. For example, Lake Malawi was very low in 1830 and very high in 1857 through 1863. It was also high in 1873 but fell during 1875–78. There was a high water level in 1882. In 1890 it fell very low again, but once again rose rapidly between 1892 and 1895. A steady decline occurred over the next twenty years, the level dropping to the lowest recorded level of 1,537.8 feet in 1915. Gradually the channel of the Upper Shiré became blocked by reed-covered sandbars and remained that way until 1934, despite a steady rise in lake level. Thereafter the lake fluctuated within a range of ten feet, from 1,547.5 to 1,557.4 feet.

Exceptionally high lake levels also occurred in 1937, 1963, and April 1964, when the all time maximum of 1,557.4 feet was recorded. Thus, the historical range of fluctuation between 1915 and 1964 exceeded nineteen feet. Three to four feet is a typical seasonal variation, although six feet has been recorded. During high years, the flooding of low-lying coastal lands caused severe damage to agriculture, houses, and port facilities (Pike 1968).

These uncontrolled lake levels also had important implications for the mission. The UMCA had established important inland stations at Mtonya and Unangu in Portuguese East Africa; at Likwenu, located about half-way between Mponda's and Zomba and originally set up as a missionary health resort in the Shiré Highlands; and at Mulanje in the deep south, set amidst the plantations of European settlers. Liuli and Milo stations also lay in the interior, in the Tanganyika sphere. Yet it was the far-flung string of lake-side stations, schools, and church missions that served as the mission's long-term preoccupation. When the level of Lake Malawi began a rapid rise in the late 1920s, many stations had to be relocated.

For decades Msumba head-station had been known to be "exceptionally free from mosquitoes," but by 1930 it was hemmed in on two sides by an unhealthy "rice Swamp" (*CA* 48 [1930]: 196). By 1936 the lake at Msumba had reached its highest level in memory, and a storm drove waves against the foundation of some of its buildings (*CA* 54 [1936]: 143). Over time, water continued to penetrate and collect around the perimeter of the site, promoting malaria and other diseases.

Beginning in the 1920s, encroachment of the lake forced entire stations, or portions of them, including Msumba, Chia, Lungwena, Malindi, and Mponda's, to relocate and rebuild on higher ground (fig. 4.2) (*CA* 48 [1930] and 54 [1936]). When the priest's house at Msumba was built in 1923, it was seventy yards from the lake. During a storm in 1930 the waves washed against its foundations (*CA* 48 [1930]: 196). A visitor interested in seeing the old station at Lungwena was surprised to discover that he had no choice but to take the tour in a canoe (*CA* 55 [1937]). On Chizumulu Island, food production was affected when the lake entirely submerged some rice fields. Relocating a station disrupted routines and was costly in staff time and funds. Sites and activities at damaged or collapsed schools, houses, churches, and clinics (and Malindi's marine engineering facilities) were affected.

THE MISSION SPHERE: PHYSICAL EVOLUTION AND LEGACY

In the absence of steamers, the UMCA's mission field would have been limited to a small fraction of the scale actually attained in its Nyasaland Diocese. Even if the mission had delayed its pioneering work until the 1940s or later, without steamers its influence in the same region would have been minimal because no north-south access roads had been built along the lakeshore. Canon Winspear, looking back over five decades on his life and work aboard the *Chauncy Maples,* in the steamer parish, believed "it must be almost unique in the annals of missionary enterprise for such a vast parish to be worked from floating headquarters. There were 68 village outstations lying between what is now Mkope Hill parish in the South and Manda . . . in the North" (Winspear 1960, 51). While he is hardly a disinterested onlooker, Winspear can rightly point with a fair measure of pride to some of the extraordinary accomplishments of his lifetime with the mission. He makes a persuasive argument about the profound sense of the uniqueness of the UMCA's steamer parish vis à vis other missionary frontiers, at least those in Africa.

UMCA pioneer missionaries viewed the deployment of a steamer as their central instrument of strategy for spreading the Word. The technology was critical. No other scheme could possibly offer such efficient access to remote populations in scattered villages up and down the lake, and to interior settlements across such a vast area. For instance, in 1905 when the inland station of Mtonya (in Mozambique thirty miles from the lake) was opened, a UMCA party of four Europeans, led by Bishop Trower, relied on the *C.J.* to carry the necessary equipment from Malindi on the first leg of the journey. Dr. Howard, the diocesan medical officer who was charged with supervising the acquisition and loading of cargo for Mtonya, had "accumulated nearly everything necessary to build a new station" (*CA* 23 [1905]: 260). Once it had steamed fifty to sixty miles north of Malindi the *C.J.* could drop anchor and unload at a place on the lakeshore where there was a comparatively efficient overland route for headloading equipment to the new mission site.

From 1885 onward, the steamer's availability offered UMCA stalwarts fresh hope and renewed confidence that a mission at Lake Malawi was still possible. This was no small accomplishment in the light of memories of the Mackenzie expedition's short-lived and disastrous attempt to plant Christianity two decades earlier. In his *Nyasa the Great Water* (1922), Johnson recalls how Captain Sherriff of the *C.J.* was fond of pointing out the mission's inability, without the steamer, to contact new villages, provide emergency refuge (from Angoni marauders and slave-raiders), and transport teachers, priests, sick Europeans, and supplies. As the mission's geographical base and work-load of evangelization expanded it became increasingly difficult "to meet the hundred and one calls each village made on us, which led those on board to think of a bigger steamer" (198). Johnson claimed that the "paramount consideration" in deciding to add a larger steamer to the mission's fleet was not so much the convenience of those who would work on and from the vessel, but rather the overall needs of the diocese and existing and future stations. As it turned out, he noted "the hopes we had formed in the *Charles Janson* seemed to live on board the new and much larger steamer, the *Chauncy Maples.* The work soon doubled" (ibid.).

Quite early in its development the UMCA's self-assigned regional responsibility for medical mission encompassed thousands of square miles. That the *C.M.* might enhance this work was not unrealistic. But it also raised the bar in terms of what should (and could?) be accomplished, causing a further stretching out of available medical resources. As early as 1903, understaffing, financial shortages, and cutbacks of all kinds had become a major, vocalized concern within the UMCA. *Central Africa* asked its 11,000 subscribers, "Why should we have to appeal year after year for a doctor?" (*CA* 21 [1903]: 145). The mission also found it extremely difficult to recruit competent schoolmasters, engineers, printers, bookkeepers, and so on—men who were physically and emotionally stable, and willing to stay the course in Central Africa. Administrators in the mission's London headquarters complained that incompetent recruits had depressingly become the rule rather than the exception. This contributed to a sense that "we merely flounder along" (*CA* 21 [1903]: 145). By implication, at least, women recruits disappointed less often.

SPHERES OF INFLUENCE

The mission's steamers also had their limits and constraints, featuring political, environmental, and technical factors. Scottish Presbyterians had planted themselves firmly on the western side of Lake Malawi ten years before the UMCA's return and the launch of the *Charles Janson.* Several other mission societies had also established important programs of teaching, evangelism, and medical work in Malawi well before World War I. The four principal Protestant societies are shown in table 4.4.

Others missions in colonial Malawi included the Dutch Reformed Church Mission, Nyasa Industrial Mission (Australian Baptists), the Baptist Industrial Mission of Scotland (1890s), the Zambezi Industrial Mission (1892–), Seventh Day Adventists (1902–), and the Roman Catholic Montforts (1901–) and White Fathers (1902–).

UMCA steamers could sail anywhere on the lake. On land, informal rules of competition evolved. Disputed cases typically centered on a claim of encroachment occasioned by one society attempting to establish a school or church near the activities of another mission. Very often the charges and countercharges involved the Roman Catholics, particularly the White

Table 4.4   Profile of major Protestant missions in Nyasaland, 1921 and 1925

Mission	Date	Main stations	School population	Adherents 1921 (1925)
Free Church of Scotland Mission (Livingstonia)	1875	6	5,722	12,699
Church of Scotland Mission	1876	5	1,794	10,989 (22,839)
UMCA	1885	13	11,669	(38,350)
Dutch Reformed Church Mission	1889	10 (12)	(38,000)	(>15,000)

Sources: Murray 1922; Roome 1926.
Statistics in parentheses refer to the year 1925.

Fathers, and a Protestant society such as the Dutch Reformed Church Mission. Conflicts frequently generated a flurry of appeals to the protectorate government for mediation, irritating officials who saw them as petty and time-wasting.[36]

Gradually, a delineation of mission "spheres" evolved within which missionaries could legitimately proselytize without infringing on the territory of other missions. Among the main Protestant societies these areas were more or less strictly understood and agreed upon through their representatives to the Conference of Missionary Societies in London. On the other hand, intense conflicts involving the Roman Catholics and certain Protestant missions persisted into the late 1920s. Nor were such disputes peculiar to Nyasaland. The UMCA's Bishop Fisher complained that the Catholics "repudiate" Protestant concerns (cited in Blood 1957, 257). Governor Horace Byatt of neighboring Tanganyika, where the UMCA was beginning to take over former German mission stations at Liuli, Manda, and Milo, wrote to the Secretary of State for the Colonies, stating that the Protestant "Conference of Missionary Societies in London was still engaged in considering the division of this territory between its members. But . . . the Roman Catholic Church, claiming the world for its province, strenuously objects to the adoption of the principle."[37] Recalling the tragic history of Catholic–Protestant relations in Uganda, and the principle of missionary spheres adopted, abandoned, and ultimately reimposed by a Roman Catholic governor of Kenya, it was "obvious that, by their own logic, the Catholics must accord others a freedom no less than that which they claim for themselves."[38] According to the governor, it was regrettable that all Christian missions did not appreciate the value of territorial spheres to their own well being and pur-poses. Close interspersing of different, competing doctrines was harmful to the establishment of the Christian faith. This process, he said, led to "the complete bewilderment of the pagan native, and so played into the hands of the proselytizing Mohammedan."[39]

After World War I the Nyasaland protectorate government adopted measures to regulate "the establishment and operations of missions." On October 25, Nyasaland's attorney-general signed the Missions Ordinance, 1922, into law with the approval of the secretary of state in London. He noted that the origin of the legislation was directly traceable to a recom-mendation (No. 19c) of the Report, dated January 14, 1916, of the Nyasaland Native Rising Commission that had been appointed after the Chilembwe affair (see below). The basis for asserting such control at this point, the gov-ernor argued, was clearly set out in the recent revisions of the General Act of Berlin, 1885, and the General Act and Declaration of Brussels 1889–90 undertaken at the convention of September 10, 1919.[40]

At first some Protestant missionaries, such as Alexander Hetherwick of the Church of Scotland, raised objections to the Missions Ordinance, 1922. Hetherwick believed that existing ordinances had already secured its objects, and that it interfered with African religious liberty. The ordinance also exceeded what was needed to suppress seditious teaching, and could be used to advantage one mission over another. Finally, the ordinance would lead to grave injustices because of the delays caused by the necessity of having to report cases to the secretary of state.[41]

As time progressed and conflict with the Roman Catholics dragged on, Hetherwick conferred with the UMCA's Bishop Fisher and five other heads of Protestant missions whose opinions the governor had solicited on the matter of spheres for Christian teaching.[42] They agreed on general prin-ciple to negotiate a working agreement concerning the territorial limits of each denomination's schools. The idea was to avoid working against each other, and to preserve a sense of Christian unity among both Africans and missionaries.

Official and mission concern was not confined to Catholic–Protestant relations. "Ethiopian propagandism" that encouraged independent, break-away churches had reportedly been gaining sympathy in the territory, brought back by men who had emigrated to work in South Africa.[43] Fur-thermore, the early nationalist movement had grown dangerous, symbol-ized by the armed "Chilembwe Uprising " in 1915. This movement was di-rected against numerous European and colonial abuses and infringements on African life. They included conscript labor (*thangata* system) and harsh treatment on European estates, heavy demands on African men to serve as soldiers and carriers for the military, increased tax rates, and the undermining of institutions of traditional authority. UMCA authorities grew worried that the protectorate government, in its efforts to quell African protests because of their alleged security threat, would choose to lump all missions together and place them under strict controls (Rawlinson 1917).

John Chilembwe was a Yao and an ordained minister. As a young man he had been deeply affected by Joseph Booth, an English missionary he met in 1892 at Mitsidi Mission. He had lived and worked as a servant in Booth's house, and had served as a "nurse-companion" to Booth's children. By promoting ideas about "Africa for the Africans," Booth's then radical philosophy went strongly against the grain of colonial society. With the assistance of Booth and the National Baptist Convention, Chilembwe went to the United States and studied for two years at Virginia Theological College, a Negro seminary in Lynchburg, Virginia. There he met African-Americans and learned of their experiences and ideas (Crosby 1980, 28).

When Chilembwe returned to Malawi in 1900, he purchased ninety acres of land in Chiradzulu District, in the Shiré Highlands north of Blantyre, the protectorate's commercial center. On this land he soon established his independent, African-controlled Providence Industrial Mission (PIM). Several Black American Baptist missionaries arrived and spent five years helping to evangelize, establish cash crops, and set up mission schools for academic and practical subjects (27–30).

For the first several years Chilembwe aimed to inculcate European deportment and work habits among his African followers, believing that "if his community experienced European type success they would develop more self-respect" (28). Working with the colonial system, he sought to bring African grievances to the authorities' attention. He campaigned against low wages and increased taxes, and the long working hours and abusiveness of the *thangata* system—particularly on the three hundred square miles of land known as the Bruce Estates. But his strategy achieved little success. During World War I, with African soldiers and members of the Carrier Corps dying for the British and Germans on the front lines in northern Nyasaland, Chilembwe had seen enough. He changed tactics and in January 1915 led an armed attack on white farms in the Bruce Estates. Chilembwe and many of his two-hundred-plus followers were shot dead or hanged during the uprising and its aftermath.

British officials continued to view the doctrines Chilembwe planted as seditious and an ongoing threat to colonial rule. On the mission front, a long editorial in the UMCA's *Central Africa* decried the abuses to estate workers, and noted that the Protectorate government's Chilembwe Commission of Inquiry had found that unjust treatment of Africans "directly conduced to the rising." However, the main point was to assert that the uprising reflected the fact that no well-established churches or mission schools were allowed to operate on the estates, where the atmosphere was permeated by "unintelligent anti-clericalism" and antimission hostility. Apparently, this writer was least concerned about African exploitation and justice. His main point was that a Chilembwe would never have materialized had proper missions, such as the UMCA, been allowed to promote Christian education and enforce appropriate Christian discipline among the African workers (Rawlinson 1917).

By 1922, protectorate authorities suspected, without proof, that Chilembwe's ideas were being kept alive and reinforced through the American "Universal Negro Improvement Association" under Marcus Garvey, editor of the *Negro World* newspaper.[44] Decades later a leading authority on Chilembwe concluded that he had led "the first Central African resistance to European control which looked to the future . . . , the prospect for which Chilembwe began to fight was one of founding a nation rather than of restoring the fortunes of the tribes" (Shepperson 1958, 409).

THE OLD DIOCESE NOW

In addition to political factors, physical geography also influenced what the UMCA was able to accomplish. Lake Malawi's size and shape, and its coastline, so often hemmed in by rugged hills and mountains, imposed enormous constraints on how many interior settlements could be reached by a chronically understaffed mission. Yet the steamers also enabled the UMCA to stretch out its "topological" sphere over several hundred miles.

Today, much of the territory in the UMCA's old mission field, long vacated by the European missionaries, remains remote and largely inaccessible by land or water except for those who can travel short distances by canoe or other small craft on the Mozambique side of the lake. Since the early 1950s local populations on the eastern side of Lake Malawi have been left high and dry, without access to lake steamers except at Likoma Island. On the mainland north and south of Likoma, the fishing and farming settlements in Tanzania and Mozambique carry on in great isolation, more remote than in the colonial-missionary period. Vehicles, electricity, and running water are curiosities. Dugout canoes remain essential for local transportation and fishing. Government-owned Malawi Railways operate the Lake Service, and the diesel-driven ships *Mtendere* (1980–; 924 tons) and *Ilala II* (1951–; 620 tons) offer the only scheduled passenger and cargo services on Lake Malawi.

Steamer service today is primarily along the west coast, from Karonga to Chipoka, where there are more people and economic activities. South of Likoma, service on the eastern side is limited to Monkey Bay and the tiny southeastern ports of Makanjila and Chilinde. Among the many old ports and settlements frequented by the UMCA's *Chauncy Maples* and *Charles Janson,* only Likoma (occasionally), Kota Kota, and Monkey Bay receive boats today.

From the late 1920s road building and the introduction of motor vehicles gradually diminished the role of the protectorate government's small fleet of lake steamers. Nyasaland Railways took over the operation of these vessels in the 1930s, when the rail line was extended from the south to Chipoka and Salima (fig. 1.2). By 1935 there was an uninterrupted link from Lake Nyasa to Beira on the coast of Mozambique.

Just after Malawian independence in 1964 the pattern and standard of communication in the Lake Malawi basin was described as "a classic example of the development of communications waiting for, and consequently lagging behind, economic activity" (Pike 1968, 213). Today, unlike the colonial period, Malawi possesses a comparatively good system of hard surfaced all-weather roads built to a high standard, particularly in the south and west-central areas. However, no paved road exists along the entire eastern coast of the lake from Tanzania through Mozambique to near Mangoche (the old Ft. Johnston). There are perhaps a dozen miles of unpaved and poorly maintained secondary roads, and discontinuous stretches of rough "District" roads and tracks, all of which may be impassable from November to May during the rainy season. Considerable stretches along the east coast in both Malawi and Tanzania lack even motorable tracks. Even in the dry season it can take several hours for a car or truck to travel forty or fifty miles over rutted, rocky, or sandy tracks. Wear and tear on vehicles is unavoidable, severe, and costly in terms of spare parts, lost opportunities, and delayed communications. Much farther north, two-thirds of the lands along the coast from Liuli to Manda (forty-five miles), and from Manda to the north end of the lake (eighty miles over mountainous terrain and slopes that dip precipitously into the lake) have no roads to settlements.[45] As recently as 1991 Malindi Hospital, opened by the UMCA in 1902 and only ten miles from the district headquarters town of Mangoche, lacked such amenities as telephone service, an ambulance, and a morgue.

Today, the presence of the Malawian Anglican Church, old mission structures and customs, and new mosques in the countryside provide strong reminders of and continuity with the UMCA era. Technologically speaking, however, the region shows little evidence of progress. As the next chapter explains, maintenance and operation of the steamers was by no means a simple task. Just as their integration with so many mission activities opened the region to new possibilities through the movement of people, information, and goods, realized or not, the loss of their services when they broke down translated into great inconvenience and frustration for thousands of people. Despite such liabilities, sixty years ago the steamers provided a loose-knit linkage and identity for the lakeside villages and administrative centers that are not evident today.

NOTES

1. The lands on the northern borders of Lake Malawi are ethnically complex. Other names for peoples in the UMCA's extreme northeast reaches include Sandia, Pangwa, Mwelya. See Douglas 1950, pocket map.

2. Mills 1931; see also Barnes (1933, 11), who wrote of Johnson as a "giant "and "an example of a hero."

3. Johnson (1926, 157) believed that the religious instruction these men received on the *C.J.*, when they were a captive audience, appeared "compulsory" and was "too much like parade services."

4. McKinnon 1977, citing Nkamanga, *Likoma Diocesan Quarterly Paper*, no. 13 (Oct. 1906), 329–30.

5. S. Lyon, "The *S.S. 'Charles Janson,'*" *Likoma Diocesan Quarterly Paper* 8 (July 1905), 209. Cited in McKinnon 1977, 211.

6. Notes, *Likoma Diocesan Quarterly Paper*, no. 8 (July 1905), 192–95. Cited in McKinnon 1977, 253.

7. Evidently the Swinnys were the first and last married couple to serve in the diocese.

8. At this time the level of the water at the mouth of the Shiré was still high enough to permit the *Charles Janson* to safely pass over the bar and navigate downriver.

9. Maps of lakeside settlements, 1899 (UMCA 1903). These later maps show many of the villages Johnson began visiting in the 1880s.

10. The latter came out to Malawi first as a medical doctor and later became Bishop of Nyasaland (1896–1901).

11. Historical MS. Inventory, Vol. 1, Malindi Mission. MNA.

12. Anon., "Universities Mission," *The Aurora* 2, no. 7 (August 1, 1898): 30. *The Aurora* was a publication of the Livingstonia Mission in Malawi.

13. Ibid.

14. Dale 1925. Printing in the diocese dates from about 1893, when the *Occasional Paper for Nyasaland* (called *Nyasa News*, after its second issue) came out under the editorship of Archdeacon Chauncy Maples. After Maples's death in 1895 publication lapsed until 1902, when it was resurrected as the *Diocesan Chronicle*. In 1895 African

members of the mission created their own newspaper, *Mtenga Watu*. At first type was set on the mainland in the large village of Msumba, and thereafter transported by steamer to Likoma for printing. The *C.M.*'s printing press was not installed on the the the ship until 1908. See Barnes 1933, 105; McKinnon 1977.

15. *CA* 15 (1897): 176. These four schools ranged in size from 62 to 105 pupils.

16. Maintenance of these teachers (excluding expenses for European staff travel and messengers) cost £401 per annum (*CA* 19 [1901]: 144).

17. *Likoma Reports,* 1903. 145-DOM-10-4-6. MNA.

18. Medical and Surgical Reports, 1899 and 1900. 145-DOM-10-4-7. MNA.

19. 145-DOM-10-4-1. Likoma Diocese 1903—European Health Record. Vol. II, 1904. And Kota Kota: Health Reports and Staff, 1904–1909. Selected clinical reports on European patients. Overall annual characterizations of stations' health records by the medical officer range from "variable" to "remarkably good," "very good," and "excellent." MNA.

20. Anon. "Universities Mission," *The Aurora* 2, no. 7 (August 1, 1898): 30.

21. The official history of the *Chauncy Maples* is A. E. M. Anderson-Morshead, *The Building of the "Chauncy Maples"* (1903), reproduced in Anderson-Morshead 1991.

22. Likoma Reports, 1903, 145-DOM-10-4-6; Malindi Reports, 25-MAM-6-1-1, 1910. MNA.

23. 25-MAM-1-4, 1931. RHL.

24. Malindi Reports, 1934, 25-MAM-1-4-, 1931. MNA.

25. St. Michael's College was moved to Likoma Island in 1912, later to Malosa in the Shiré Highlands, and finally to Malindi.

26. Diocese of Nyasaland. Financial Statement and Application for Grant 1912 (Likoma: Universities' Mission Press, 1911). Diocese of Nyasaland Pamphlets, 1912–30. RHL. (The cost of operating the *Charles Janson* is not identified in this document.)

27. Letters to the Editor, *Likoma Diocesan Quarterly Paper* 5 (October, 1904): 137. Cited in McKinnon 1977, 258.

28. UMCA D8, X. RHL.

29. Reportedly the first African crew members on the *C.J.* were not Christians. Although by mission policy the men received religious teaching on board daily, few of them were converted and even Rev. Johnson thought such a requirement unnecessary. See McKinnon 1977, 268.

30. During the war a "good number" of the coastal African population in the German sector sought greater security by moving back from the lake several miles into the hills. They planted gardens there while continuing to use the lake for fishing. *CA* 36 (1918).

31. *Nyasaland Diocesan Chronicle,* [January?] 1917: 15.

32. Johnson almost certainly refers here to the Benedictines, whose self-defined sphere in southwest Tanganyika overlapped with the UMCA's work around Liuli, Manda, and Milo. The claims of each mission, particularly with respect to the location of their schools, caused recurrent friction between them (Barnes 1933, 194; Blood 1957, 58); A few scattered Portuguese garrisons and customs posts were situated in northwest P.E.A. during and after the UMCA's arrival in the area immediately east of Lake Malawi. However, there is no evidence of Portuguese missionaries venturing that far north. Despite over four hundred years of Portuguese interest in the region, their missionaries (the Franciscan's were the first to enter the territory, around 1500, followed

by Jesuits in 1560) had always confined their activities primarily to the southern coastal region and the Zambezi Valley.

33. Roome (1926, 38) observed that training of African clergy was one of the UMCA's ideals, "but it is recognized that a very full training is needed, 15 years is the minimum, and for the present it is only exceptional men who are likely to be fit for it." Such a policy seems designed to keep the priesthood in European hands indefinitely. However, the policy hardly seems discriminatory given the university backgrounds and educational standard achieved by the mission's European priests before they came out to Nyasaland. Whether a lower standard should have been adopted to speed the growth of an African clergy is another matter.

34. E.g., the visiting Bishop Thorne was enraptured, saying that he could be very happy to die there (*CA* [1946]: 71).

35. *CA* 41 (1923); UMCA 1/2/21. MNA.

36. E.g., Resident, Ft. Manning to Prov. Comm., Lilongwe, Missions, Sept. 1, 1925, NC1-18-6; Resident, Lilongwe, to Prov. Comm., Lilongwe, June 9, 1926, NC1-18-6; Resident, Ncheu, to P.C., Central Province, May 25, 1926, NC1-18-8. MNA.

37. Governor of Tanganyika to Principal Secretary of State for the Colonies, March 26, 1923. S1-2568-23. MNA.

38. Ibid.

39. See note 4.

40. Report, Attorney-General of Nyasaland, The Missions Ordinance, 1922, No. 12 of 1922. Oct. 25, 1922. S2-49-19. MNA. See also Barnes 1933, 66.

41. Alexander Hetherwick, CSM, Oct. 12, 1922. S2-49-19. MNA.

42. The Dutch Reformed Church Mission, Zimbabwe Inland Mission, South Africa General Mission, Nyasa Mission, and Seventh Day Adventist Mission.

43. Gov. George Smith, Nyasaland, to Secretary of State for the Colonies, March 25, 1922. S2-49-10. MNA.

44. Confidential dispatches from Lord Milner (1920) and the Secretary of State for the Colonies (1921) had warned that such organizations had as their goal "Africa for the African and the expulsion of Europeans. Religious teaching is made, too often, the insidious means of advancing this propaganda." Consequently, it had become "very necessary that this [Nyasaland] Government should have ample powers for controlling quasi religious movements of the character I refer to." Gov. George Smith to Secretary of State for the Colonies, March 25, 1922. S2-49-19. MNA.

45. Government of Malawi, Dept. Surveys map, *Malawi 1 : 1,000,000*, 1989.

{ CHAPTER FIVE }

Steamer Technology, Local Ecology, and Regional Economy

Coal was abundant in Europe and America, and before the mid-nineteenth century it had become the predominant fuel for steamers. Africa was a different story. Malawi proper has four fields of fair to good quality coal deposits, two in the north and two in the far south, but the seams are rent by complex faults and access is poor (Pike and Rimmington 1965). High quality coal deposits discovered in the late 1940s, around Manda in the Tanganyika part of the UMCA's territory, raised some hopes of generating new roads and an extension of the British Groundnut Scheme Railway from the port of Lindi on the Indian Ocean.[1] None of these deposits was commercially exploited. Colonial Malawi imported its coal needs from mines in Southern Rhodesia. This Rhodesian source was developed years after the UMCA established steamer operations on Lake Malawi (Nelson et al. 1975, 273).

With coal unavailable, firewood was the only fuel source for the steamers operating on Lake Malawi. Such dependence also characterized steamer operations on most other inland tropical waterways in colonial Africa, including the Congo River during the disastrous years of the Congo Free State (Troup 1890, 124, cited in Hochschild 1998, 108, 317) and the operations of the French Navy on the Senegal River (Thompson 1992). Lacking alternatives, the missionaries in Malawi procured wood into the early twentieth century through barter. Steamer captains needed assurance from African suppliers that dependable supplies would be available at specific "wooding stations" along the lakeshore. This guarantee was essential to keeping a sailing schedule to coordinate the diverse evangelical and medical activities in the diocese. For the system to function properly, African woodcutters and woodsellers tacitly agreed to work within an imposed system of periodicity, in keeping with the steamers' order of sailing and fuel needs. As the mission expanded its geographical range and activities this reliance on coordination and schedules became more formal and fixed. Yet a two-way cultural process involving attitudes toward time worked. It ensured that things would not always function like clockwork, that is, favoring the European preoccupation with subdivisions of linear time and punctuality.

Delays in wood supply, and learning how to wait, proved inevitable. UMCA personnel adapted to and probably derived benefit from the natural and social rhythms of African time reckoning—even if some did not easily accept it. Customarily, Africans tended not to rush or cut short an activity they were already engaged in just to start something new. Ironically, the delays that most severely affected diocesan operations originated not from the waiting built into more fluid, less clock-driven African concepts of time. Above all else, the most frustrating delays came in the form of "down time" brought on by boiler problems and other limitations of steamer technology. Weather and rough seas on the storm-prone lake also had significant influence on the steamers' arrivals and departures. Sailing conditions often affected fuel consumption, and plans frequently had to be revamped in deference to the continuous need to restock the bunkers with firewood (Winspear 1960, 52).

FIREWOOD PROCUREMENT

Fuel for the steamers was discontinuously plentiful on and near the coast. Negotiations for wood purchases were often complex and slow. Reliable "wooding stations" had to have supplies of dry wood ready for use when the steamers called. Up to three months was needed to properly dry firewood for use in the boilers. During the rainy season, from November to April, finding dry wood was never guaranteed (*CA* 69 [1951]).

Following his arrival at Likoma in 1885, a Mr. Young noted that "we found the inhabitants of this lovely island glad to see us and willing to help us in wooding the *Ilala*," and that "nothing could exceed the beauty of this spot." Although Likoma's land area was small, there was "room even then for pretty hills and valleys, beautifully wooded with all sorts of timber and picturesque park-like glades with numerous villages" (*CA* 3 [1885]: 171). Yet by about 1900, only fifteen years later, supplies of firewood on Likoma had become "very scarce." Giant baobabs (*Adansonia digitata*) dominated the landscape, but their soft wood made them ill-suited for fuel. Wood requirements of the island's 5,000 African inhabitants also imposed great pressure on other tree species. Constant cutting of the smaller species in the island's dry woodlands or bush forests prevented their regeneration and disrupted the local ecology (Howard 1904, 13; Murray 1922). Certainly wooding stops by the *C.J.* and commercial steamers exacted a large toll on the regenerative capacity of Likoma's tree cover.

Presumably, particular species of trees in the mixed savannas and woodlands (especially the *Brachystegia-Julbernadia* community) offered greater efficiency in generating steam and were thus favored by the steamers' engineers. Sir Harry Johnston recorded dozens of local trees and noted that both *Msumbuti* and *Napiri* (*Copaifera* sp.) make good firewood, and that *Mlombwa* makes good charcoal after partial burning (Johnston 1897). However, I have been unable to confirm the species preferred for steamer use.

Fuelwood-cutting in the uncultivated bush was generally seen as women's work, at least in the early days. Women also performed other heavy tasks connected with lake transport. For example, at the northern end of the lake it was mainly women who unloaded government and company steamers. Dressed only in a waistcloth, they waded into the water up to their knees, or higher, to receive bales of calico or boxes of stores. They then head-loaded their cargo to a warehouse on shore. At the south end of Lake Malawi one of the river transport companies preferred young women to carry passengers' hand luggage over a land route of thirty-eight miles between the Shiré cataracts. Their pay was 4½ pence, and double that if they returned with a load the next day (Mills 1911, 188). Today, wood remains the principal source of domestic fuel along the coast and inland from the lake, although general cutting in local forest reserves is illegal. Women also continue as woodcutters. Around Malindi, for instance, "professional ladies" go to the Forestry Department and pay a fee for permission to cut and sell wood obtained from the large forest reserve on the nearby escarpment.[2]

Archdeacon Johnson recalled the ritual of wooding in the mission's early years, when the *Charles Janson* was the mission's lifeline along the lake (fig. 5.1). Acquisition of wood and food often required complicated negotiations. On one occasion Yohana Hamisi, the Zanzibari *capitao* in charge of both the *C.J.*'s African crew and negotiations with Africans on land, had gone ashore to buy firewood. Immediately after landing Hamisi was drawn into a ritual of bargaining for wood. Some "twenty men and women, each

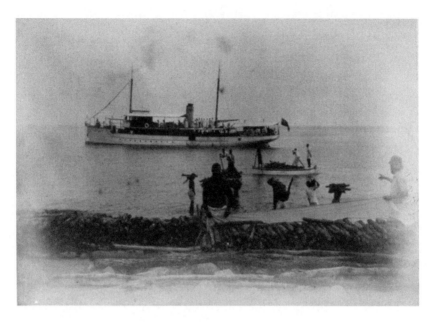

Figure 5.1. The *Chauncy Maples* taking on wood.
(Source: USPG.)

waving a good-sized stick, surrounded him. As he chose a stick he put a pinch
of salt in the owner's outstretched hand and put the stick in the boat; the
hand was still outstretched and, after buying several more sticks, he would
finally put in a supplemental pinch." This symbolic exchange of "a pinch for
a stick" signified the buyer and seller had agreed to bargain in good faith.
The *C.J.* carried a substantial supply of salt for this purpose. Payment in
calico by the yard, more fully described below, was the standard once a deal
had been struck. Johnson called Hamisi's bargaining as "a miracle of patient
work, and I only saw him lose his temper once" (Johnson 1926, 180–81).

Disputes and misunderstandings could complicate the task of procuring
firewood. For example, within a few moments of the transaction just described, Hamisi ran afoul of his suppliers and was suddenly surrounded by
twenty to thirty angry men threatening him with pieces of firewood. An
agitated crowd then captured the launch used by Hamisi and his crewmen
and carried it into a nearby village. Having lost their launch, the *C.J.*'s crew
was later "forced to hail canoes at each village to bring our firewood and to
land us" (181). How and when Hamisi was able to return to the steamer is
left untold.

A less hostile but more imaginative firewood drama had occurred fifteen years earlier in Tonga territory on the western coast at Nkhata Bay (Johnson 1922, 6). It was an event that was incredible, deceitful, and humorous, and it came at the expense of the Scottish Presbyterians of the Livingstonia Mission. On its first circumnavigation of Lake Malawi in 1875, the steamer *Ilala* called in at Mankhambira's village to purchase firewood. Contemporaries recorded that the local Tonga people, already enterprising capitalists, proved "too clever" in a scam that outwitted the Europeans. The Tonga carried bundles of firewood onto the *Ilala* at one end, got paid for them, carried them off and back onto the steamer at the other end, and sold them again for a double profit (van Velsen 1960).

After buying wood it generally took two or three hours to get it aboard ship and stowed, ready for use. The crew loaded wood into small boats, as stevedores did not exist. It was then paddled out to the steamer, which was often anchored at a considerable distance from the beach (*CA* 69 [1951]). On these occasions Africans typically surrounded the steamer in canoes, trying to sell food to the steamer's passengers and crew. Wood-loaders had to cope with the hazards imposed by this extra traffic. Firewood then was lifted onto the decks and stored in the bunkers below by the African stokers. In rough weather it was often difficult to get sufficient boatloads of wood through the surf and onto the steamer. Decades later one of the English priests remembered that wood loading was a noisy business. If loading coincided with Holy Communion being said in the *C.M.*'s chapel, "the din caused by the logs falling on the deck was quite distracting" (Winspear 1960, 52).

Stokers came from different villages up and down the lake. Their often-intimate knowledge of the coastal zone was useful during in-shore navigation of the steamers. It was also believed the stokers' social connections in their home villages benefitted missionary work. Such ties put the mission in touch with people and settlements that might otherwise have been overlooked (Mills 1911).

During a two-month period in 1889 the *C.J.* ran a distance of 1,124 miles. Operating expenses, calculated in barter terms, included the crew's wages, firewood, and stores, paid for with 360 fathoms of cloth, three pounds of beads, five soap bars, and 1.5 bags of salt (*CA* 8 [1890]: 15). In contrast, from July 1891 to July 1892 the *C.J.* covered 9,144 miles. In equivalent currency terms, the expenses for the year amounted to a few shillings over £140, including (proportionately) the crew's wages (46 percent), firewood purchased with 759 fathoms of cloth (26.5 percent), firewood purchased with 1,027 pounds of salt (5.8 percent), 60.5 gallons of English oil (14.5 percent), and 33 gallons of "native" oil (6.5 percent) extracted from groundnuts[3] that was used for lubricating the steamer's engine parts (*CA* 11 [1893]: 4). Thus the cost of firewood paid for in cloth (one fathom = one yard) and salt (257 lbs.) was 32 percent of the steamer's running costs. The cost per nautical mile was about 3s 6d. Expenses remained at this level until 1902, when the *C.J.* assumed new responsibilities following the arrival of the UMCA's second steamer, the *Chauncy Maples* (*CA* 16 [1898]: 98).

In 1884 the ALC was using calico as its main currency, and one yard of cloth brought a fixed amount of firewood for its steamer, the *Ilala*.[4] Although methods of payment evolved from bartering salt or calico to cash, as late as 1910 calico was still the medium of exchange at some wooding stations. Woodcutters divided felled trees into lengths that equaled the width of a roll of calico. Then they piled the pieces of wood into stacks as high as the width of the calico roll. To purchase the cloth, "we simply unroll the cloth along the foot of the stack to see if it is the correct height, and then cut off a length equal to the stack" (Mills 1911, 72). Often such bargaining for wood was very time-consuming and "occasionally ended in a deadlock so that the only thing to do was to leave that place and try elsewhere" (Winspear 1960, 51). On going ashore at a station the steamer hands typically tried to purchase sixteen to twenty cubic yards of wood (*CA* 57 [1939]). In the late 1920s firewood was paid for in cash at eighteen pence a cubic yard, and by the late 1930s one cubic yard varied in price from one to two shillings (*CA* 47 [1929]: 134; 57 [1939]: 66).[5]

By 1910, the mission steamers had instructions to buy firewood "in large quantities at a time" from the respective governments when operating in British and German territory. This attempt by the colonial administrations to monopolize firewood supplies evidently did not apply along the central coastal zone of UMCA operations, which was in the Portuguese sphere. On the western side of the lake, Nkhata Bay port was a major wooding station for steamers operated by the African Lakes Company and the protectorate government. The *Chauncy Maples* also called here about twice a month on its rounds, in part because Nkhata had a colony of Likoma communicants living there.[6]

"Wooding Stations" on the Chauncy Maples's Circuit

Fuelwood needs created a resource dependency that bound the steamers to people on land. Wood also required substantial storage space on the small steamers, which dictated that it was possible to take on only enough fuel for a relatively short journey (*CA* 47 [1929]: 153–56). We know from an African *capitao* (whose father had been the head *capitao* on UMCA steamers for forty years) that the *Chauncy Maples* had to "wood" at least nine times during a typical three-week voyage in the 1930s (*CA* 57 [1939]: 66–68). The route, modified from that of 1928 (table 4.3), began and ended at Malindi, with northbound stops for wood at Mkope Hill, Msinje, Chingomanje, Ngoo, and Mkili (fig. 4.10). An English layman with the mission noted that Msinje was "where we wood in great style, with some twelve or more boat-loads of wood, each boat holding some four cubic yards."[7] Loading time at Msinje was three to four hours. Southbound wooding stops included Njambe, Kwambe, Ngoo, and Kota Kota.

Prior to departure from Malindi it was customary for the steamer to take on goods for the northern UMCA stations that had been sent over by barge from Mponda's, about ten miles across the lake. Passengers also boarded at Malindi, destined for Kota Kota, Msumba, Likoma, St. Andrew's College, Liuli, Manda, or Milo. Loads and passengers might be landed or taken on at any stop. At Chingomange the Portuguese Customs Officer would board the *C.M.* and inspect the passengers and loads headed north for Mtengula and Msumba.

On Friday, after taking on wood at Ngoo or Mala, the steamer sailed on to Likoma to spend the weekend. Generally the crew had leave to stop work at noon on Saturday. Most would go ashore for a walk or to visit friends, returning at 5 o'clock for Evensong and later to sleep on the steamer. After Sunday morning church services on Likoma there might be time to visit families and friends. The next day the *C.M.* set out for Manda in Tanganyika, arriving on Wednesday. A main UMCA head station from 1918, Manda was the port for the interior station of Milo. At Manda, the captain handed over cash boxes (containing pay for teachers and other African employees) and mail boxes to waiting *capitaos* and porters, who would carry them to Milo. Southbound the *C.M.* called again at Mponda's to drop mailbags for Matope and Likwenu stations, and to disembark European passengers traveling on to England. Usually the steamer arrived at Malindi from Mponda's on Friday, more or less as scheduled, after three weeks of steaming up and down the lake with supplies and passengers. The fire in the boiler was soon put out and the steamer's crew and missionaries went ashore for a much-anticipated weekend on land, including religious observances. Early on the following Monday morning the *C.M.* began its circuit once again. A fire in the boiler was started several hours before dawn. Near dawn a whistle blast alerted passengers to prepare for boarding and a 7:00 A.M. departure. Custom prescribed that Africans board before Europeans. Two European ladies could travel together without restriction, as could any European man. Unaccompanied travel on the lake by a European woman required that the bishop personally give her his consent in writing.[8] "Month by month the steamer work is thus," said *capitao* Harry Liponde (*CA* 57 [1939]: 68).

From its beginnings the shape of the UMCA's mission field grew increasingly elongated, north and south. Lake Malawi, in the Rift Valley, and the adjacent highlands dominated the physical environment. With its territory fully traced out by the early 1920s, the mission's distinctive form reflected the fact that all the lakeside stations came to depend on the monthly visits of the *C.M.* for their food, stores, cash, and personnel movements.

Fuel Consumption

A regular round-trip by the *C.M.* covered 700 lake-miles, and required about 80 hours of steaming at an average of 8 knots per hour. Wood was consumed at 2.5 cubic yards per hour, or 200 cubic yards per trip, with the engine pressure at 100 lbs. At this rate, a mission member observed, "you can guess its does not go far, especially if one has a strong Mwera [south wind] on the bow and heavy seas running" (*CA* 46 [1928]: 13–14). Captain Haywood calculated that the *C.M.* had traveled about 280,000 miles during its first fifty years (*CA* 69 [1951]). Thus on average the steamer traveled more than 5,600 miles annually, or around 500 miles each month. These calculations include allowance for down time for repairs and its years of commandeered service in World War I. These figures yield an estimate of total wood consumption for the *C.M.* (from 1901 to 1951) of some 80,000 cubic yards, or 2.16 million cubic feet! This was enough to cover two football fields to a depth of three feet, or to cover a half square mile to a depth of one foot. Added to this was the wood consumption of the *Charles Janson,* the smaller pioneer steamer that saw service from 1885 to 1931 and was in operation for sixteen years before the *C.M.* arrived on the scene. Estimating conservatively, if the *C.J.*'s consumption of firewood was 25 percent of the *C.M.*'s, then the older vessel accounted for another 20,000 cubic yards of trees. Total lifetime consumption of firewood by the two UMCA steamers was thus in the range of 2.7 million cubic feet.

It must be remembered that when able and seaworthy the UMCA's two vessels remained almost constantly under steam. Their movements created an unceasing demand for wood from local African cutters. The mission's fuel needs probably accelerated deforestation and erosion around the eastern and southern coastlands and in the village hinterlands behind the lake. Land degradation processes almost certainly grew in intensity as the general population started to expand in the 1920s, placing additional pressure on the source areas for firewood. It bears emphasis that while the shoreline of the world's twelfth largest lake is hundreds of miles long, the bulk and weight of the firewood meant that collection areas remained relatively close to wooding stations accessible by the steamers. Also, in several areas, the topography hemmed in the populations and confined woodcutting and gathering to a narrow coastwise belt that was in some places only a few hundred feet wide. Most of the available bush forests had few trees of commercial importance except for firewood (Murray 1922). In view of these factors it is reasonable to assume that the fuel needs of the steamers placed considerable stress on indigenous woodlands.

Apart from the firewood needs of the UMCA's boats there was also the quasi-missionary *Ilala* (1875–87), the African Lakes Company's *Domira,* and the steamers *Hermann von Wissmann* and the *Vera* used by the Berlin Mission at the northern end of the lake. Between 1892 and 1899 the British administration had deployed the gunboats *Pioneer, Adventure, Queen Victoria,* and *Guendolen.* Collectively these ten wood-burning vessels must have been responsible for consuming an enormous amount of the wood extracted from the forests bordering Lake Malawi, particularly during the first forty-five years of missions and colonialism in Malawi. By the 1920s only the *C.M., Guendolen,* and *Queen Victoria* had regular runs on the lake. The *C.J., Domira,* and *Pioneer,* the old hulks, respectively, of the combined missionary, ALC, and lake fleet, had been reduced to occasional sailings (Murray 1922). Yet running the steamers would continue to exert significant ecological pressure on the woodlands until the UMCA retired the *Chauncy Maples* in the early 1950s.

Beginning with the quasi-missionary *Ilala* (1875–87) and the *C.J.* (1885–1931), "feeding" the mission steamers did more than transform communications and power relationships on the African-missionary frontier in Malawi and surrounding areas. Steamers were among the very first products and symbols of European technology aside from guns on the frontier. They demonstrated as few other things could the vastly increased power of the industrial revolution to perform work. However, this technology also had distinctive liabilities and penalties, including a potential to consume and destroy large quantities of renewable (woodlands if not replanted) and nonrenewable (soils) resources. New European ideas and technologies often led to an accumulation of incremental changes in the ways people organized their economic and social affairs. Such changes reflected or were facilitated by greatly increased ranges of movement for more people through new transportation systems. Migration had its consequences for family life. Settlement patterns were reordered. Health care was newly conceived and organized as an additive and pluralistic process. People were exposed to new influences that affected their livelihoods, sometimes greatly, and they participated in the gradual spread of a common currency. Steamers contributed substantially to restructuring in each of these areas of African life, and increased reliance on them produced a measure of technological dependency that could produce lengthy isolation, hardship, and general inconvenience to all associated with activities around the lake basin. Many of the steamer-related changes, such as greater ease and speed of travel, materialized slowly in small, imperceptible increments.

Within Britain's imperial sphere one might reasonably anticipate that technology would spread to the colonies in a somewhat lagged manner according to industrial fashions and distance from the metropole. It has been suggested that the preeminence of the British merchant shipping industry served to wed the British to steam. This preference may have led to an "unduly tardy adoption of diesel power" since the pinnacle of the diesel revolution occurred in the first generation of the twentieth century (Greenhill and Giffard 1979, n.p.). In Malawi, the first diesel-driven ship, the *Mpasa*, belonged to the railway and was not commissioned until 1933 (Williams 1958). Did the relatively late deployment of the *Mpasa* on Lake Malawi reflect an Empire-wide overcommitment to an obsolescent technology? Regardless of such debate, the UMCA's continuing dependence on a firewood-powered steamer stretched its exploitation of local woodlands over sixty-five years.

MARKETPLACES AND MIGRANTS: STEAMERS IN THE
REGIONAL ECONOMY

From an early date, the UMCA's steamers, and perhaps most importantly those operated by the African Lakes Company—the "economic arm" of the Scottish Livingstonia Mission—provided a stimulus to commercial traffic within and beyond the lake basin.[9] African traders and marketplaces also responded to the arrival the steamers in their neighborhoods. Complementary exchange was certainly not a new phenomenon on the eastern and southern margins of the lake. In precolonial days, the Yao peoples had gained a reputation for their local and long-distance trade activities, including dealings in slaves and ivory. Along the east coast there was local canoe trade in salt (made from tree ash), hoes, and fowls (Johnson 1884). Members of Livingstone's 1861 Zambezi expedition believed that Africans along the east coast of the Lake Malawi considered their European trade goods, notably poor quality calico, as inferior. Slavers had arrived first and stimulated a taste for superior American and Indian prints among the local populations. There was also a vigorous east coast salt trade via the dhows (Wallis 1956).

Harry Johnston commented on Africans' fondness for trade. He noted that both men and women made long journeys to sell their goods, and believed it "to be bad policy on the part of a chief to drive away trade by deeds of injustice or rapine" (Johnston 1897, 471). Barter remained the principal method of exchange for trade with and between Africans during the UMCA's first twenty years at the lake. Africans who worked for the mission got paid in fathoms (two-yard lengths) of gray calico known as Americano, as well as salt and soap. They in turn used these commodities for their own personal transactions. Coinage had little value to villagers who lived beyond walking distance of a store or market (Winspear 1960). While documentation is thin, it is noteworthy that the arrival of the steamers at or near customary places for markets almost always stimulated some new growth of exchange. Likewise, new marketplaces took root near sites that developed into wooding stations or other ports of call.

Given the developments above, it is also indisputable that the markets associated with the steamer traffic never attracted enough resources nor generated sufficient division of labor and local production to lift the local subsistence economies out of poverty. No investment or policy accomplished that in colonial Malawi, where the chief export was labor and the main income an unreliable stream of remittances to families left behind in the villages. Fifty years after he began his career with the UMCA in Malawi in 1906, Canon Winspear offered his observation that "in fact there has been very little increase in real wages since the early days of the century" (Winspear 1960, 48). While there is truth in the claim that the commercial steamer, in particular, was "the prime mover in the country's development" (McKinnon 1977, 234), one must still ask: what kind of development, and for whom?

Lakeside markets did take on new significance as centers for the dissemination of information, and they served to inject some money and goods into the local economy. In 1910, at the wooding station of Msinje just outside Portuguese territory, the native market was "an intensely interesting sight" and a place to observe "sailors and passengers bargaining with different groups of villagers for flour, beans, fish, tobacco, sleeping mats, fruit, etc." (Mills 1911, 62). Nearly thirty years later, Msinje was only marginally more lively than it had been in 1910. The people still produced mats and tobacco and carried these items and baskets of other goods to sell to the steamer passengers. Food staples also found a ready market at schools and for hospital patients at Likoma and other places in the steamer parish. Observing one such steamer visit, a UMCA staff member offered the romanticized and apparently unexamined conclusion that "the inhabitants never tire of this trade because they get much gain from it" (*CA* 57 [1939]: 67). Ironically, he thought that the people had to be industrious because food was so scarce in their district.

Through the steamers, Africans also gained opportunities for relatively efficient contact with totally new places, both within and beyond Malawi. By securing a passage on one of the steamers an African could now travel two hundred miles or more in just a few days. In addition to European staff moving from one station to another or going on furlough, the *C.M.*'s passenger lists regularly included African teachers, their wives and families, and their household effects. During term breaks many students from St. Michael's teacher training college returned to their homes via steamer. The *C.M.*'s sick bay had room for four cases. Bulk goods could also be moved for individuals and in substantial quantities.

Labor Migration

The steamers also offered safe and relatively efficient transport of the many migrant laborers who sought work in southern Malawi to earn cash with which to pay their annual hut taxes. Beginning in 1891, all adult males had to pay a tax of 6 shillings (British) or an equivalent in Indian rupees. Imposition of this tax was "bitterly opposed" by the missions, in part because of its inherent unfairness (there was little money or means of earning it outside the highlands of southern Malawi) and also because it would lead to large-scale emigration of labor (Pretorius 1972). This rate was soon lowered to 3 shillings because it was deemed a hardship for Africans and a deterrent to the economy (Coleman 1973). Many men gravitated to the European coffee, and later tea, estates around Blantyre and Mlanje, while others worked as porters for various commercial enterprises and the government.

The African Lakes Corporation needed 10,000 to 15,000 men daily as carriers. Smaller numbers of men worked as carriers for European traders and travelers making overland journeys (*ulendo*). Each traveler carried in a hammock (*machila*) needed about sixteen men, four at a time, for a one-day trip (Gelfand 1961, 293; 1964, 206). For whatever reason, men who defaulted on their taxes had to work for three months on European estates situated north and south of Blantyre. Their first month's wage of 3 shillings was deducted to cover their hut tax. As noted in connection with the Chilembwe uprising of 1915, widespread abuse was a hallmark of this hated *thangata* system of forced labor. Writing in November 1899, Dr. W. H. Murray, head of the Dutch Reformed Church Mission in Malawi, observed:

> Things have lately taken place that might shame any Savage, if committed by him, and that in the name and by the instruments of the Govt. Because men refuse to pay their taxes (on account of the hardships entailed in going to work 200 miles from their homes, where there is a great scarcity of food) women and little children have been ruthlessly shot down by native policemen.[10]

In the African view, whatever benefits the system produced went entirely to European landlords and a protectorate administration that offered few if any services.

For its own reasons, the UMCA did not subscribe to the government and planters' vision for the protectorate's economy. The latter's secular interests sought to create a system based on capitalist principles, including the free mobility of low-wage labor. The protectorate would be turned into a labor pool, serving the administration and local white planters' needs first, with surpluses available for "export" to the mines and factories of Rhodesia and South Africa.

In contrast, UMCA missionaries believed that male absenteeism was certain to place great stress on families and lead to unwholesome and un-Christian behavior. Much of the money men earned while away would be spent on ephemeral and worthless goods in the new economy. Material-ism would undermine the Christian base that was developing. The mission wanted to foster stable families, ensure monogamy, and promote clusters of peasant villagers who identified with local churches.

Regardless of its preferences, and its occasional efforts to communicate its views in print, the UMCA never made its ostensibly "pro-native welfare" case with sufficient authority to alter the views about African labor held by most of the white settler class and government officials. The mission had little influence on the appropriation of lands or on the use of forced labor by government and private landowners. It did not oppose obligatory taxation, and it was impotent to prevent what became an outflow of labor from Malawi to the mines and factories of southern Africa.

Large-scale emigration of male labor from Malawi started in the 1890s. Mission-educated men, including substantial numbers of Christians whose commitment to religion had been hard-won, formed an elite category of semiskilled workers. Known by the Portuguese term "capitaos," they found jobs as "clerks, 'boss-boys' and compound indunas" and were also paid a bonus of 15 shillings for each new laborer they recruited from Malawi (Tapela 1979, 72). Important destinations included Rhodesian Railways, Beira, and other ports in Mozambique; the copper mines of Katanga in the Belgian Congo; the Rand gold mines (from 1903) and other industrial centers in South Africa; and European farms and plantation zones from Tanganyika to the Cape. Some men chose to join the King's African Rifles, and received postings in faraway places that included the Gold Coast, Mauritius, and Somaliland (Read 1942, 606, cited in Kuczynski 1949, 2: 550). Other family members remained behind, with significant social and economic consequences for their well being. Eventually, Malawi annually sent tens of thousands of its male working population to subsidize mining and industrial development in Northern and Southern Rhodesia, and other territories south of the Zambezi.

Many men traveled independently and chose their own employer. Between 1903 and 1909 and after 1935 one could sign up with recruitment bureaus, notably the Witwatersrand Native Labour Association (WNLA) that recruited directly from the villages through agents laden with quotas (Boeder 1973). A conservative estimate reckoned that a "considerable percentage" of the men walked great distances, ranging from 100 up to 1,500 miles, to find new jobs (Niddrie 1954). Other recruits were transported by lorry to a railhead, while many workers also traveled to employment centers by bicycle.[11] Above all, Malawian migrants apparently walked to their work destinations. One official report of questionable reliability stated that 90 percent of those traveling south in 1935 walked from their homes because they lacked the cash for the rail fare (ibid.).

In addition to earning money for their taxes, many young men migrated to Southern Rhodesia seeking jobs that would yield sufficient savings to permit them to marry. The UMCA's Captain Haywood, aware that such young men typically had no means, was reportedly partial to them and frequently offered "free" passages on the *C.M.* In exchange the men helped load firewood at the "wooding stations" on the voyage. This practice could cut in half the time required at one stop or save the steamer an entire day on the run down the lake (*CA* 48 [1930]).

Coleman's analysis suggests that the demand for labor in the 1890s from within and outside Malawi had already "clearly outstripped the supply" (1973, 35). By 1904, the number of men exiting the protectorate for work was believed to exceed 10,000, a two- to three-fold increase in just two years. An "old Nyasa boy" who had given up work in South Africa's gold mines chose instead to work as an itinerant evangelist among the Nyasa miners. In a letter home he noted the "many Nyasas here working in the mines," among whom "I have got about 80 Christians and 20 Catechumens" (*CA* 23 [1905]: 275).

By 1921, estimates placed the number of men from Malawi working abroad at 50,000, approximately 20 percent of the protectorate's adult male population. This total increased to 120,000 men in 1935, when labor agencies from South Africa and Southern Rhodesia started recruiting again in the north. By 1953 approximately over a third of Malawi's employable adult males—about 413,000—worked outside Malawi (Nelson et al. 1975, 34). Efforts by the government to regulate rapidly expanding emigration streams included several ordinances (e.g., the first in 1894, and 1922) designed to stem excessive and abusive recruitment that could produce internal labor shortages and tax shortfalls.[12]

Unfortunately, the die had already been cast that would ensure the continued extraction of Malawi's manpower. As early as 1892 the explorer Joseph Thomson had advised the directors of the British South Africa Company in Southern Rhodesia about labor in Malawi. In a report he told them the country was "admirably endowed" and "thoroughly prepared" to meet the labor requirements of European enterprise in Southern Rhodesia. He had seen no other part of Africa with such good supplies of "eager and industrious men as yet unspoiled by gin and a too-paternal government" (quoted in Kuczynski 1949, 2: 550).

Missionary interests, the Presbyterians in particular, joined forces with European planters to try to stem the large outflow of labor from the protectorate. Some of the missionaries expressed grave reservations about the nefarious effects of migration on family life, including the spread of sexually transmitted infections (STI), gambling, and improper lifestyles (Gelfand 1961). Such concerns certainly had legitimacy, even if European minds often failed to connect the nature and inevitability of social change with the policies imposed on Africans, or otherwise encouraged, by the colonial government. Generally the missionaries vehemently opposed labor emigration, believing that it would work against building up the churches. Some missionaries reportedly also had a vested interest in preserving ready access to a pool of labor since several missions ran large estates and depended on coffee sales to finance a share of their evangelical activities (Boeder 1973, 38, citing F.O. 2/669). Planters also registered bitter opposition to the scale of outmigration, stimulated as it was by the higher wages offered south of Malawi.

A later report overflowed with criticism of the unreasonable, even prepos-terous, expectations of the material benefits available to migrant workers. It pointed to the "disastrous" consequences that work in the gold mines had on ordinary Africans from Malawi. Returning home after two years, the mi-grants should have arrived "rich men for life"; instead they appeared with a potpourri of useless articles. It was claimed that the men threw money away "senselessly" and none had saved any of their earnings. They also returned to Malawi with "absurd ideas" about pay scales, demanding the wage levels they had received in South Africa. Most unfortunately, work-ing underground had also broken their health (Decle 1906, 324, cited in Kuczynski 1949, 2: 550).

In contrast, Boeder (1973) asserted that studies done after 1935 exagger-ated the ill-effects of labor emigration on rural society in Malawi. Families appreciated whatever extra income and material goods could be realized from the worker's toil and long absences. This argument is partly based on the fact that Africans institutionalized migrancy, thereby fostering and per-petuating attitudes and values that reinforced the phenomenon. Boeder's analysis of the lyrics in a few women's songs reflects their varied and some-times ambivalent emotions about the absence of husbands and fathers for the long periods of contract labor. One song suggests that it could even be perceived as shameful if a man did not emigrate south for work. Another is a poignant cry of poverty and loneliness caused by the *machona*—the lost men who left their families for a job and then deserted them, never again to return home. Unfortunately, Boeder's assessment is flawed by an inex-plicable disregard for the health consequences of migration for the worker and his family. He ignores the fact that the circulation of labor, which varied temporally and spatially, had fundamental implications for the mission and government medical services.

Health and Social Effects

Tuberculosis was present and recorded in the protectorate in 1891, although its precolonial existence there is uncertain. Africans who acquired this dis-ease declined and died quickly (Gelfand 1964). In 1912, several years after labor agencies had been forbidden to operate in the protectorate because they had caused a harmful drain of workers away from local white em-ployers, the government reported a large increase the number of new TB cases. This was followed by another increase in the prevalence rate the following year. Doctors discerned that men who had returned home from the mines of South Africa and Southern Rhodesia carried the disease with them.[13]

Pneumonia, scurvy, and silicosis also took a high toll among the migrants. Many men fell sick when they first arrived on the Rand, resulting in a very high mortality. On the Rand gold fields in 1905–6, the death rate among Malawians was an astonishing 166 per 1,000, compared to 118 deaths per 1,000 Rhodesian Africans, 38 per 1,000 men from Basutoland, and 14 per 1,000 from Zululand. Explanations at the time strongly relied upon an environmental theory that "tropical" Africans had difficulty acclimatizing to the higher and colder environments of the south (Gelfand 1964). Acting from self-interest, Malawi's European planters and missionaries and the British House of Commons fiercely opposed the methods of labor recruitment being used to lure African labor outside the protectorate. In 1906 Winston Churchill, then Colonial Secretary, stepped in and banned labor recruitment for South Africa from tropical zones north of 22° S. latitude (Gelfand 1961, 298; 1964, 219). Such restriction remained in one form or another until 1935, but it was not intended to apply to voluntary or "independent" migration. In fact, it had little influence on absolute levels of out-migration from Malawi, and such movements actually increased. Clever recruiting agents simply set up shop just inside the Mozambique border, within easy reach of Malawian men who wanted to work outside the protectorate. In 1921, up to a quarter of Malawi's adult male population lived abroad. The Travers Lacey Report noted that in 1937 at least one-fifth of Malawi's adult males worked outside the country. Of these, about 70 percent and 15 percent, respectively, labored in Rhodesia and South Africa. Having begun in the 1890s as an internal movement of labor in response to the imposition of taxes and demands of European economic interests, migrancy in Malawi rapidly evolved into a huge southward emigration to income opportunities (Coleman 1973).

Passage of the Native Hut Tax Ordinance in 1921 drew quick criticism from Malawi's Federated Board of Missions because it extended to marriageable women as well as men. The missionaries believed that this poll tax would "press hard on unmarried girls," leading them into evil acts or to unwanted marriages.[14] Age of marriage would also be driven down to expand the tax payer base. Based on medical experience in the protectorate, the missions aimed to promote the highest possible age of marriage to protect the lives of immature girls and enhance the health of babies. They reckoned that 21 or even 25 was a favorable age for marriage, and more likely to produce women whose relationships reflected the moral codes they wished to instill. Appealing to the governor, the board asked that young unmarried girls who still slept in their parents' hut or lived under the supervision of parents not be recognized as of marriageable age for tax purposes. Widows, Christians in particular, should also be excluded from the tax to discourage them from "polygamous or otherwise unsuitable marriages."[15]

Labor export produced a high loss of life and effectively culled a substantial part of the protectorate's able-bodied manpower for the duration of the colonial era. This process continued for a decade after Malawi's independence in 1966. Tapela asserts that the protectorate government's statements of humanitarian concern were, with one notable exception, a foil meant to cover an intense, "desperate" desire to extract tax revenue from labor migration.[16]

South Africa's demand for foreign laborers, which the *Nyasaland Times* termed "The Rand Octopus," was particularly aggressive, exploiting a laborshed that stretched over a thousand miles north into Tanganyika (*CA* 40 [1922]). Both South Africa and Rhodesia systematically expelled foreign workers, typically in batches, who had been weakened by illness or injury, and the destitute. Many had been gone long enough to establish families abroad, in some cases losing touch with their relatives at home (Mufuka 977, chap. 2).

While averse to promoting the "industrial" way of life among Africans (Maples 1899, 268–75), the UMCA missionaries could not avoid being direct witnesses to many the changes within the villages that the out-migration of so many husbands, fathers, and able-bodied males generated. Also, however unintentionally, the mission quite naturally created opportunities and pressures for out-migration when it trained people in carpentry, masonry, or to operate a printing press. Individual crewmembers on the mission steamers also broadened their job prospects if they acquired navigational experience, learned about engine mechanics, or became skilled in techniques of boiler operations and stoking (McKinnon 1977; cf. Thompson 1992). Many men found employment on steamers attractive. Writing two years before the *Charles Janson* arrived, Johnson declared that "all the natives like work on board the Lake Company's steamer [*Ilala*], and will go to work on it at half the rate of wages they demand as caravan porters" (*CA* 2 [1884]: 57).

Malawi's own peasant economy lagged severely as the countryside evolved into a vast labor reserve for the "white" economies of southern Africa and British capitalism. With high male absenteeism, either temporarily or permanently, agriculture and food production declined in many areas of Central Africa (Niddrie 1954). Demographic effects of migration on the extended family were quickly felt in rural areas. For example, in the Atonga country west of the lake "hardly an able-bodied man would be found—only old men, women and children, all the men having left for South Africa" (*Report on Emigrant Labour,* 87–88, cited in Kuczynski 1949, 2:552). A report just after World War I by H. E. Munby, a priest at the UMCA's Kota Kota mission, noted that of about 680 "Christian men on my books here, some are away in Rhodesia, Congo Belge, the Transvaal, and other parts" (*CA* 39 [1921]: 200). UMCA men attracted to the explosive growth of work opportunities on Northern Rhodesia's copper belt earned somewhat better wages and generally stayed for only six months before returning to their families in Malawi (Kuczynski 1949, 2:549).

From the vantagepoint of a UMCA missionary, a primary concern was the men's tendency to backslide in the faith. Migrants faced many new temptations and had more money than ever. Few in the mining compounds remained eligible for Communion, most importantly because the "majority" of them were living with local women who by custom could never become their wives (*CA* 48 [1930]: 172).

It was impossible for the mission to avoid or shield Africans from the social and economic ramifications of the colonial system in which it grew up. The renewed threat of a labor drain to South Africa in the early 1920s prompted a UMCA spokesman to sympathetically predict a strong protest from the protectorate administration. After all, the issue was "vital to [Malawi's] existence as an [European] agricultural community" (*CA* 40 [1922]: 215). For the UMCA, this kind of identification with the colonial government was as much the rule as the exception. Compared to other missions its direct influence reached a smaller population. Thinly spread over a vast area and faced with stiff competition from the Scottish missions, the South African Dutch Reformed Mission, the White Fathers,[17] and others, the UMCA nevertheless claimed de facto status as the protectorate's Established Church.

It was not the UMCA's expressed policy to help depopulate their mission field of its young able-bodied workers, husbands, and fathers. Yet by the late 1890s the flows of southward-bound and returning migrants to southern Africa's nodes of European capitalism had become more or less institutionalized. Increasingly, the steamers supported the livelihood activities of many Africans in the general population whose purpose on the lake was business, not evangelism. Especially after World War I, public access to the *Chauncy Maples* remained important until it was decommissioned in the early 1950s. After five decades in service the steamer continued to carry "as many ordinary [non-mission] passengers as she has room for, mostly people going to and from Southern Rhodesia and South Africa, and for the last three years and more she has been the only means such people had of getting to their homes" (*CA* 69 [1951]: 206).

"UP" TIME, "DOWN" TIME: LIABILITIES OF STEAMER TECHNOLOGY

During the 1880s and 1890s cumulative efficiencies in design and materials engineering made steam technology the ultimate form of locomotion for water transport around the world. British shipbuilders had committed heavily to investment in steam, and they built almost all the small steamers found on Lake Malawi. This technological progress of the late-Victorian period clearly aided the participation of mission societies in the "new imperialism" of the late nineteenth century. Yet the benefits of steamer technology did not come entirely free and unencumbered. For its systematic dependence on the *Charles Janson* and the *Chauncy Maples,* the UMCA incurred considerable technical and human costs. Equipment breakdowns, particularly the boilers, routine repairs, such as a hole punched in the submerged part of a hull, and the need for annual overhauling had implications for all people and activities directly or indirectly connected to movement of the steamers. In addition, steamer service could be temporarily halted for varying periods of time by a lack of operating funds, the occasional unavailability of a ship's engineer, or dry-dock problems (Johnson 1926). Furthermore, in wartime the British government deemed it necessary to commandeer the *C.M.* and *C.J.*

Myriad other difficulties with the steamers caused great inconvenience and seriously impeded the mission's work. An example occurred in 1893 when the *C.J.* ventured down the Shiré River to Matope station at the end of the rainy season. Soon after its arrival, a sudden, unexpected drop in the river's level rendered it impossible for the steamer to return to the lake. It was now "imprisoned" for several months, blocked by rocks lying upstream that would rip out its bottom if an attempt were made to run over the rapids (Wilson 1936).

In March 1909, the *C.M.* was "holed" when one of Lake Malawi's notorious sudden squalls blew it onto rocks in the treacherous Bay of Papai, some forty miles north of Likoma. Only continuous pumping kept the ship afloat long enough to make the long journey back to Malindi, where numerous repairs and a general overhaul removed it from service for three months. Unfortunately, the *C.J.* was undergoing repairs at the same time. Having both steamers out of commission seriously interfered with the mission's work in general and the movement of staff in particular. For his part Archdeacon

Johnson, ever resourceful, adapted by using a rowboat from the *C.M.* and a canoe to proceed with his work on the Tanganyika mainland north of Likoma. Fr. De la Pryme managed the Kobwe district opposite Likoma on foot, while another priest based at Mponda's took it upon himself to visit "our brethren in heathenese" in the southern reaches of the diocese (Blood 1957, 25).

Other circumstances also occasionally interrupted the use of the steamers. When the *C.J.*'s engineer departed in 1904, the vessel was forced out of commission and the mission was "dreadfully handicapped . . . in innumerable ways" (*CA* 22 [1904]: 3). Tight budgets almost always obliged the mission to do the proverbial more with less. By 1909, the UMCA's geographical range and agenda had expanded far more rapidly than its supporting resources. In a cost-saving measure, members away on furlough or other business were told not to return to Malawi. In 1910, the bishop left for a new post in Australia and planning for retrenchment fell on the shoulders of Archdeacon Johnson. To cut costs a decision was made to close the carpenters' shops and the printing press, hold all stations to their allowance for the previous year, and remove the *Charles Janson* from service (*CA* 28 [1910]: 216). The *C.J.* remained out of commission for an entire year, "twisting her cables in Likoma harbour with only a watchman aboard" (Blood 1957, 59). Meanwhile, a priest in Oxford with whom the late Charles Janson served as curate managed to raise funds that enabled the steamer to be returned to service in 1911. This allowed the *C.M.* to shift to doing more parish work and less diocesan transport. Slightly more than a year later, lack of an engineer again demobilized the *C.J.* (ibid).

By the 1880s all new steamers built in Britain and the U.S.A. had riveted boilers and reciprocating engines. The bolted *C.J.* was an exception.[18] Steel, lighter and stronger than iron but still riveted, was now increasingly used for the construction of hulls and boilers (both materials are lighter and of greater capacity than a wooden hulls of the same displacement) (Headrick 1981). Rivets remained the standard method of plate assembly into the twentieth century, when welding came into use. Overall, boiler problems presented the most significant source of mechanical malfunction in the steamers.

In the cases of the *C.J.* and *C.M.*, there is conflicting evidence about the actual causal agents of boiler dysfunction and metal wear. Generally speaking, corrosion was the primary culprit in both iron and steel boilers. While the introduction of steel represented a metallurgical advance that enabled hulls and boilers to be lightened by 15 percent and strengthened, steel was actually more subject to corrosion than iron.[19] Boiler corrosion occurred when there was inadequate treatment of water with softeners and a poor system for removing the oxygen from the water. Over time corrosion acts unevenly on different types of iron or steel, weakening the parts of a boiler differently. Circulation of hard water corrodes the boiler tubes and they plug up, reducing the through-flow of water. Other tubes are then exposed to flames in the furnace and cannot properly cool. Inadequate inspection and repair of weak places in the boiler may cause it to burst. If one bit of corrosion is detected it is predictable that other spots, even hundreds, exist elsewhere in the boiler. It is thus necessary to dry the air in the boiler water to inhibit the spread of corrosion spots, as well as to allow considerable time for preventive maintenance and repairs.[20]

Rapid rusting and defective boilers proved particularly troublesome in hot, humid climates (Kubicek 1990). The Zambezi River was the first leg of the southern route to Lake Malawi in the late precolonial and colonial eras. Among the problems posed by this route was the fact that the chemistry of the lower Zambezi's brackish, muddy waters reacted with the metal hulls and boilers of steamers, exacting a heavy toll on vessels including Livingstone's *Ma Robert* and the ALC's *Lady Nyassa* (McKinnon 1977). On the Senegal River in West Africa, ships' boilers on French Navy steamers "needed constant cleaning to remove mineral deposits . . . [which] required disassembling the engine" (Thompson 1992, 289). In dramatic contrast, McKinnon twice asserts that "corrosion . . . did not affect vessels navigating the purer waters of Lake Malawi" and that "the lake water was not corrosive" (McKinnon 1977, 88 and 146). Furthermore, when the UMCA's *C.M.* was mistakenly galvanized during construction in 1900 "the missionaries were unhappy at the needless expense" (88–89). Interviewed in 1974, Malawi's Surveyor of Ships, Ernst Hansen, said that when the *C.M.* was renovated in the 1960s he had found "absolutely no rust, inside or out, when the steamer was stripped for repainting" (89). If this assertion is accurate, and if it also applies to the engines on lake steamers, there has to be an alternative but still unknown explanation for the chronic boiler problems experienced by the *C.J.* and *C.M.* over the years.

Fuels used to produce combustion and generate heat in steam boilers included mineral coal, coke, peat, charcoal, and wood. Coal was the fuel of choice for steamers in many parts of Europe and North America.[21] Since coal was unavailable to them in Malawi the UMCA relied on wood to run the *Charles Janson* and *Chauncy Maples*. The fact that they burned wood instead of coal probably had little direct effect on the nature, frequency, and severity of the steamers' mechanical problems, or their "down" time. On the other hand, wood did produce more gases and volatile matter than coal. Wood also required a larger furnace volume, and it created a creosote hazard.[22]

Structural and mechanical difficulties on the *C.J.* forced many interruptions and delays. In March 1895, Arthur Fraser Sim, the first UMCA missionary at Kota Kota, observed in a letter that the *C.J.* was often out of commission, resulting a delay of supplies, among other inconveniences. A month later he wrote, "The poor steamer, *Charles Janson,* is laid up. She wants something done to her plates and engines. Old as she is, she is still the fastest and best weather boat on the Lake" (Sim 1897, 199). The *C.J.*'s first boiler was replaced in 1900 after fourteen years' of service (Williams 1958).

Upon resuming mission work after World War I, the steamer experienced a variety of operating difficulties. Some reports indicate merely that "the *C.J.* broke down that afternoon and could not sail for three weeks."[23] In 1929 the steamer sank in four fathoms of water while moored at Malindi. It remained out of commission until 1931. After only one trip on the lake, its boilers were declared unsafe, and it was again laid up for eight months (*CA* 49 [1931]). It returned to service in 1932 at the age of forty-six years, but its days were now numbered. Since about 1936, she lay derelict on her side on the beach at Malindi, never again to steam on the lake. Finally, in 1941, the bishop was prompted to recommend that the *C.J.* be broken up and the materials used to construct a series of small boats.

In 1913, the *C.M.* was laid up so that its original boiler, then twelve years old, might be adapted and the draft of its furnace altered (*CA* 31 [1913]). News of the boiler's repair came as "welcome surprise to all workers in Nyasaland . . . but especially to the priests of the 'steamer parish' who are thankful to know they will not be compelled to trust only to the *Charles Janson* for paying their monthly visits to those Lakeside villages [50–60 congregations] which rely upon them for administration of the sacraments" (ibid., 293).

Upon the outbreak of World War I the mission was forced to make profound adjustments to its transportation system and outreach activities. First the Royal Navy commandeered the *C.M.* for use as a troop and supply carrier. In 1916 the *C.J.* was also drafted into wartime service. This blow to mission transport was cushioned slightly when the protectorate government and the navy agreed to have a vessel stop at Likoma or Malindi as conditions permitted to drop off supplies or mail (Winspear 1960). The help was appreciated and the missionaries remained loyal English subjects; but the war's demands, and subsequent down time for repairs and overhaul, effectively prevented the mission from using the *C.M.* for seven and the *C.J.* for five consecutive years. Before the war ended, and for about two years thereafter, the *C.M.* was out of commission to permit installation of a new boiler. This development forced the mission to reorganize and work the villages of the steamer parish from places on land.

Following its postwar overhaul and return to UMCA service, the *C.M.* remained a source of missionary pride. Over the years it had become a romanticized symbol of their British and especially English identity and sensibilities, and their common life of service. Nonetheless, the ship also brought continuing disappointment. Its new boiler was imported in pieces from Britain during the war. It was assembled on the lakeshore, moved around once or twice, and finally installed in the *C.M.* in 1920–21. A frustrated Bishop Fisher (1910–29) observed that this boiler

> has never been altogether satisfactory. Our engineers have . . . done everything that can be done in small ways, but I am afraid that larger measures are necessary, and the steamer will have to again be laid up and the boiler dealt with by fully-qualified boiler-makers from home. I feel rather guilty over the whole matter of this boiler. . . . It would have been much better if we had left it alone altogether. (*CA* 43 [1925]: 108)

Another development added insult to the existing concerns about the *C.M.*'s mechanical reliability. Around 1925 the government promulgated an ordinance that stipulated special qualifications for captains and engineers on all lake steamers. By custom the UMCA had always used experienced volunteers, such as Brixham trawlers, to run its steamers. It was feared that enforcement of the new regulations, which included advanced knowledge of trigonometry, astronomy, etc. would make it impossible for the mission to guarantee a succession of fully qualified men on its vessels. While recognizing that safety was the top priority, the mission appealed for a "common sense" approach to the matter, including allowances for local conditions. Surely, was not running a small steamer on Lake Malawi, where the main knowledge required is essentially "pilotage," quite different from the requirements of "the Captain of a Union Castle liner running on the open ocean," asked Bishop Fisher (ibid., 109).

During most of 1926 the *C.M.* was again unable to sail. Under Captain Haywood the *C.J.* provided back-up support and got considerable help from the *Guendolen*, a government gunboat and the largest ship on the lake from 1899 to 1951 (*CA* 44 [1926]; Cole-King [1971] 1987).

Following a string of relatively problem-free years, in 1934 "disturbing reports about the condition of the boiler on the '*C.M.*' " surfaced once again (*CA* 52 [1934]: 102). Technical advice was sought in South Africa, and in late 1934 the *C.M.* was taken out of commission for eighteen months in order to have a new boiler installed. In Archdeacon Glossop's opinion, 1935 was "the most difficult year for the diocese out of the past forty years" because the mission had neither bishop nor steamer (*CA* 54 [1936]: 132). Anonymous supporters in Britain came to the rescue with the £2,000 needed for the new boiler and repairs. Nyasaland Railways officials also lent the mission their large crane, apparently without charge, to help install the boiler in the *C.M.* Finally, on February 21, 1936, the refitted steamer arrived at Likoma. Along with many other UMCA stations, the headquarters had been cut off from most of its communications during the previous year and a half.

For Glossop, the "poor little SS *C.J.*" was doing all it could in the *C.M.*'s absence; "but she is quite unequal to doing the steamer work of the diocese today [and] no women and children are allowed on her" (*CA* 53 [1935]: 118–19). He thought it virtually impossible for the UMCA's followers in England to have a real sense of how drastically the *C.M.*'s absence disrupted the work in the lakeside stations. On top of this was the increased cost of "our heavy item of 'passages': passages for those going home on furlough, or coming back; passages for those changing stations because of the above; passages for the teachers and wives and families moving backwards and forwards for their holidays at their homes after two years' service" (118).

During the first part of World War II, the *Chauncy Maples* was occasionally used for troop transport, but it was never commandeered for government service. Unfortunately, the vessel's pattern of down time was to continue, leaving the work of the mission "sadly crippled" (Winspear 1956, 44). Thus from October 1943 to October 1946, the mission experienced "three steamerless years" (*CA* 65 [1947]: 35). The steamer was again out of action because a new boiler was needed. As was soon evident, such equipment would not be easy to find. For most of its three-year wait the *C.M.* was lying off Malindi minus a boiler, and thus "without any means of raising even one ounce of steam." On this same beach one could also see "the disintegrating skeleton of the little '*C.J.*' of happy—and unhappy—memories. . . . In the midst of the wreckage, her boiler, still in fair condition, holds high its dome and with wide-open furnace mouth gapes derision across at the upstart '*C.M.*' which consumes *her* boilers like some unnatural monster devouring its young" (*CA* 63 [1945]: 15, emphasis in original). This last, dramatic reference to the *C.M.*'s mechanical problems was published locally in the *Nyasa Diocesan Chronicle* (1944) and reprinted in *Central Africa* (1945). It unmistakably suggests that the steamer had the bad fortune of possessing boilers that were manufactured with defects or poor materials, or that steaming in the tropical setting of Lake Malawi did in fact invite boiler corrosion, or both of these factors. McKinnon (1977) never specifically mentions boilers when she refers to an absence of corrosion. In contrast, the writer above (presumably Bishop Thorne) who so graphically relates the *C.M.*'s woes leaves no room for doubt that boiler problems had remained a persistent threat to the steamer's reliability and usefulness.

Fortunately, in 1944 the government stepped in and provided the missionaries with a monthly service by the *Malonda* (vintage 1892), known in earlier incarnations as the *Hermann von Wissmann* and the *King George*. This vessel did not meet the mission's strategic needs but it did permit some renewed connections with UMCA centers and was thus gratefully received (*CA* 63 [1945]). Lake transport was even more disrupted when, on its fourth voyage, the Nyasaland Railways M.V. *Vipya* capsized and sank in a violent storm in July 1946, killing 145 of the 194 passengers and crew on board (Cole-King [1971] 1987).

To imagine that the mission could expect to secure a boiler for its lake steamer in Africa during World War II could only mean that reason had yielded to a strange ether of hope and presumption. Yet the UMCA did make the effort. By 1944, however, weariness and frustration had set in because the mission's effort to obtain a boiler in South Africa had "only succeeded in wasting six valuable months and producing a negative answer."[24] Their response was to shift their procurement efforts to England. Once again the UMCA secured the good offices of the colonial government, and "the Governor kindly wrote to the Colonial Secretary asking that the order might have priority" (*CA* 63 [1945]: 23).

In 1946, the UMCA finally located a boiler in England. It was shipped to Malawi at the beginning of August 1946, and was towed by barge from Mpimbi, on the Upper Shiré, to the mission's engineering shops at Monkey Bay. As they had a decade before, Nyasaland Railways again lent a crane with which the mission's engineering crew succeeded in the difficult task of removing the *C.M.*'s old boiler and installing the new one.[25] Following the first stage of boiler installation the steamer was towed about twenty-five miles across the lake to Malindi. Here the remaining boiler connections were made and new decking installed.

Assuming that testing of the boiler and a trial run proved successful, a target date of October 8, 1946 was set for restoring the *C.M.* to service after "three steamerless years" (*CA* 65 [1947]: 35). Finally, the steamer was back up and running. Its order of sailing was published to include Mponda's station for the first time since before 1910 and sent out to priests-in-charge (*CA* 69 [1951]: 108; Mponda's inclusion was made possible by a rising lake level). Meanwhile, the mission was turning the plates and "ribs" of the "disintegrating skeleton of the little '*C.J.*'" into "much needed hoes . . . and pruning hooks."[26]

Another technology, already decades old, was finally adopted by the UMCA near the end of World War II. A wireless service from Likoma Island was inaugurated in 1945, enabling telegrams to be received there from any telegraph office and providing the European and African mission staff with much appreciated connections to the outside world.[27] Unfortunately, disappointment soon befell this event as well. Said a correspondent for *Central Africa*, after only "three glorious weeks . . . the batteries failed [and] at the time of writing we are enjoying complete silence once more . . . it is just not functioning!" (*CA* 63 [1945]: 86). Wireless communications were again lost in 1946, because

> the engine for charging our batteries for the telegraph has died on us—it was always old and decrepit, and needed constant care and nursing—and so *we have once more been cut off from the outside world*. Messages we want to send elsewhere, news we want to hear from the outside, all seem to have increased beyond bounds since we have been perforce deaf and dumb. (*CA* 65 [1947]: 63, emphasis added)

When the *C.M.* returned to mission service, it was immediately called upon to recharge the wireless's batteries. The breakdowns of the telegraph system symbolized the liability that accompanied dependence on advanced technology, and they were undeniably a great inconvenience to the mission. Had Likoma and many of the other stations not also been so dependent on lake communications, isolation from the telegraph would not have been felt so intensely. Once again, the UMCA's perennial and systemic dependence on its ship extended well beyond its basic transportation function.

For about eighteen years after World War II the Diocese of Nyasaland operated financially in the red. Cutbacks in routine activities and services often had severe consequences and the potential to negate, or at least deeply undercut, the mission's accomplishments and perceived mandate. Acute shortages of money and supplies continued to affect Likoma's operations for several years:

> We have had a difficult time here at Likoma . . . for apart from the telegraph . . . we have been without steamers, mails, stores and money, our altar wine, incense and candles all ran out. As I write there is no money on the island, at the Post Office or in my Bank. Postal orders are mounting prodigiously, and people are demanding their money, but they cannot get it. Perhaps fortunately in a way the Mandala [ALC] store is also completely empty so there is nothing to tempt people there to use

their money, but what is most felt is the difficulty in obtaining the requisites and necessaries for marriages and the money with which to buy materials for house building. Just now is the time when people want to get on with their houses, and to get married. (*CA* 65 [1947]: 63)

In addition, education in the Portuguese sector was strongly compromised when lack of money forced the dismissal of a number of African teachers, while others resigned. Two of four schools were closed, leaving Msumba and Ngoo as the only places in a district of 4,000 square miles where young people could even learn to read and write. Both remaining schools were situated on the lakeshore, where almost all the population was Nyanja (Nyasa). The remainder of this Archdeaconry, historically the source of most of the mission's African priests and teachers, was "sinking back into illiteracy" (*UMCA Ann. Rev.*, 1948, 16). The more thinly populated hill country above the lake, inhabited by the Yao, now had no school. No new Yao priests were available, and few young Yao teachers remained to evangelize their Muslim brethren. More ominously, African congregations declined to increase their self-support. An especially drastic retrenchment of annual operating funds prompted Bishop Thorne to record that 1948 "must be reckoned as a black year the history of the diocese" (Blood 1957, 248).

In March 1947, another cost-cutting measure placed the steamer on a reduced schedule, with voyages every six weeks instead of four. In October 1947, even this plan had to be scrapped because the replacement engineer on the ship suddenly departed, leaving the mission and the *C.M.* without an essential officer. Early in 1948 the protectorate government chartered the *C.M.* to carry seed and cassava cuttings to food-short settlements in and near the coastal zone. Thus the mission was deprived of lake transport, and Likoma's connections to the rest of the diocese had been severed once again. When the wireless went dead communications suffered severely because the *C.M.* was not available for the monthly recharge of its batteries.

Finally, news arrived that the mission had secured the services of a new engineer for the *C.M.* from South Africa. Mission officials hoped that the protectorate government might charter a private vessel for famine work and return the mission's steamer by March 1948 (*UMCA Ann. Rev.*, 1948, 17). But was it foolish to continue to hold out for a reliable steamer service? What would become of the work in Malawi, now in its seventh decade? To understate the case, the missionaries had never enjoyed full confidence in the steamer's availability. Events in the next few years would provide further harsh reinforcement of this fact.

MISSION STEAMERS: SYMBOL OF THE OLD ERA

Over time, the steamers proved both a lifeline and, when laid up for repairs, a source of frustrating dependency for both the UMCA missionaries and their African followers. In the late 1940s, some seventy years after the founding of the mission, the missionaries continued to pay for, and complain about, its isolation and the high cost of their reliance on "modern conveniences." Indeed, the whole social, economic, technological, and even ecclesiastical infrastructure that had gradually been built up over the years connected the common and separate life of Europeans and Africans in myriad ways. Even in the closing decades of the UMCA's tenure in Malawi the entire system was vulnerable to collapse if one element broke down.

The most important disadvantage was the fact that the mission often had to cope without the *Chauncy Maples* and thus without its crucial international connections via the Shiré, the railway, and the tiny but growing commercial centers such as Blantyre south of the lake. Links with other lake ports such as Kota Kota, Karonga, Bandawe, and Nkata also withered. Other steamers operating on the lake called at Likoma only intermittently, or never. For Likoma and the lakeside stations, the steamer was really the only readily available source of re-supply for so many essential commodities and services.

Following its overhaul at the end of World War II, the *Chauncy Maples* saw several more years of service. In October 1951, the UMCA held a Golden Jubilee celebration at Malindi station in honor of the steamer's fifty years of existence, if not full-time service. Many of the steamer's existing crew, including Captain Haywood, had served more than thirty years (*CA* 69 [1951]: 206). Large crowds gathered on the lakeshore and saw the ship "dressed out" for the occasion. A government Public Relations Officer recorded that "the vessel, with its gay bunting whipping in the breeze, lay anchored in the blue-green waters of Lake Nyasa, overlooked by heavily wooded mountains at the foot of which lay the buildings of Malindi with animated crowds of Africans lining the white beaches" (*CA* 70 [1952]: 11). Launches carried a large number of guests, including the district commissioner and his wife, out to the ship for a reception on board. A "simple and impressive" religious service, preceded by the singing of "God Save the King" in both English and Nyanja, was held on the top deck (ibid.). A contingent of Nyasaland's Police Band "accompanied hymns and Te Deum [Laudamus]" (Winspear 1956). After attending a tea party on board, the visitors then went on shore to listen to selections by the Police Band, where they were joined by "thousands of Africans listening with intense concentration and fascination" (*CA* 70 [1952]: 12). Ceremonies continued during the next month at each port the *C.M.* visited (Blood 1957). On arrival at Liuli in Tanganyika, the steamer was met by a "flotilla of dug-out canoes," some with banners, that "accompanied her to anchorage like destroyers welcoming home an honoured and gallant battleship" (*CA* 70 [1952]: 12). Farther north the festivities included a fireworks display on the lakeshore. This was the old order, about to give way in the tensions between new demands and old constraints.

Captain Haywood advised that the ship was "beginning to show her age, and ship stores are increasing in price and difficult to obtain, and maintenance becomes increasingly difficult as she has to pass an annual survey by the Surveyor of Ships" (*CA* 69 [1951]: 206). Bishop Thorne confirmed Haywood's observations about the *C.M.*'s age and increasing running costs. It was anticipated that a new steamer Nyasaland Railways was about to commission would help to meet some of the mission's requirements for lake transport. Further, the bishop proposed to reduce the *C.M.*'s present work by half. Implementation of this dramatic stroke would occur as part of a mandate from the Archbishop of Canterbury in 1951 to divide the current diocese—over "four times the size of England"—into two dioceses. The Archdeaconry of Nyasa (Likoma's northern sphere, under German rule until 1918) became the Diocese of South West Tanganyika (ibid., 160; *UMCA Ann. Rev.,* 1952). This move spurred a change in the Likoma's headquarters function. It was now "no longer the central hub of the diocese.

As with previous bishops, Bishop Thorne had found the island too remote. He initiated the move of his headquarters to Mponda's, which had always been the administrative centre. Likoma remained the ecclesiastical centre."[28] In the context of this reorganization, the *C.M.* now appeared disposable. While Thorne preferred that "that . . . sad day . . . will be long delayed," he publicly acknowledged that "it is possible that before long [the *C.M.*] may have to be laid up, or even sold" (*CA* 69 [1951]: 206).

The diocese had reached the outer limits of its geographical expansion thirty years before the *C.M.*'s Jubilee. Its pioneer days, beginning with the *C.J.* in 1886 and continuing with the *C.M.* up to the start of World War I, had ended even earlier. As late as 1951 Bishop Thorne, facing an imminent decision about the *C.M.*'s future role, reiterated once more the fact of its integral place in the "life and affections" of the mission's field:

> All the lakeside stations depend for their food, stores, money and personnel on her monthly visits, and the two "*C.M.*" days of each month, when she

makes her northward- and southward-bound call at each station are the most important events of the month, and crowds come to the shore to greet new arrivals and learn the news of the diocese. (Ibid.)

There is nothing to dispute in this familiar refrain. Yet by then the bishop's statement was a prelude to a requiem for both the *C.M.* and the UMCA in Malawi. An acute crisis in the mission's finances just after World War II made drastic spending cutbacks inevitable.[29] Three options existed: closing an entire station and repatriating the Europeans; closing one or more hospitals and sending European staff home; or retire the *C.M.* and put it up for sale (*UMCA Ann. Rev.*, 1953–54). To eliminate primary tasks of the mission, such as evangelization, pastoral care, and caring for the sick would, reasoned mission officials, be irresponsible and a dereliction of duty. Targeting the aging steamer would greatly inconvenience the entire diocese, and bring "even greater sorrow and in some cases . . . resentment" (ibid., 13). Since the responsibilities of the Diocese of South West Tanganyika (spanning five hundred miles from northwest to southeast) included the northeast coast of the lake in Tanganyika, Bishop Thorne argued that the mission could go on without the steamer and that its disposal represented the least damaging of the three possibilities. Captain Haywood's retirement after forty-seven years with the mission, and the extraordinary difficulty of finding a new skipper and engineer to volunteer who had Board of Trade certifications, seemed to reinforce the decision to cut losses with the *C.M.* In addition, under the new scheme of two dioceses, it seemed unjustifiable to the UMCA missionaries in Malawi that they were expected to cover all costs of the steamer (Winspear 1956).

Early in 1953, when "the evil day" could no longer be delayed, the Diocesan Finance Committee reluctantly decided to save money by placing the *C.M.* on a lighter schedule, and reduced its voyages from once a month to rounds once every six weeks until September (Blood 1957, 251). It had, of course, tried this once before in 1948, exacerbating the difficulties all around in a famine year (*UMCA Ann. Rev.*, 1948). This time the odds were strongly against the *C.M.*'s return: there was a strong intent to remove it from further mission service and try to sell it.

A GROWING SENSE OF ABANDONMENT: AFRICAN RESISTANCE TO THE C.M.'S FORCED RETIREMENT

Several leading Africans in the UMCA did not take kindly to the rumors about the steamer's retirement, and they followed up with open discussion about Bishop Thorne's plans.[30] Other complaints also bubbled to the surface during 1952–53 in the contentious and racially charged atmosphere that permeated the events leading to the formation of the Central African Federation. An informal, handwritten letter from "Likoma Christians," signed by their Chairman, a UMCA Elder, was directed to the Archbishop of Canterbury in England. It presented "several complaints" relating to "destructive changes in our Mission," and requested an investigation. Major complaints included the removal of St. Michael's Training College from Likoma to Malindi; an unexplained loss of support for Likoma Cathedral's choir; the physical deterioration of the cathedral, including the embroidery and the seven big lamps of the High Altar. Most grievous was the arbitrary decision to sell the *Chauncy Maples*. The steamer, said the Likomans, "was given us as a means of conveying the Gospel on the lake."[31]

In 1952–53, Bishop Thorne had a new house built for himself at Mponda's station at the south end of the lake. He justified his move on the grounds that, the diocese having been divided, Likoma was no longer at its center. Mponda's also had the Treasurer's Office, and was considered more convenient and accessible to the political and economic centers of Zomba and Blantyre. To African church members this move, apparently undertaken with little or no discussion with them, symbolized a distinctly undesirable turn of events, even betrayal. The bishop's physical relocation and his apparent insensitivity to their concerns led the African community to interpret the move as a breach of sacred trust with them and with the legacy of Likoma. They saw the bishop's departure as ironic, since the Europeans had always trumpeted Likoma as the "see-city" and ecclesiastical headquarters of the mission.[32]

It is useful to recall that Likoma had possessed significant locational advantages during the mission's pioneer period, such as its water barrier that offered relative security from marauding Gwangwara and slave-raiders. Yet by 1910, while the diocese's administrative, medical, and ecclesiastical activities continued to concentrate on the island, the safety concerns of 1885 had melted away. Likoma's good harbor became a crucial hub of steamer activity as the *C.J.* and *C.M.* greatly facilitated the founding of mission stations, primary schools, and churches in "UMCA" villages on or near the Mozambique coast. With respect to steamer operations, however, the island was primarily a depot, and virtually all material resources had to be imported from the south end of the lake. Even the steamers' fuelwood had to be cut and loaded elsewhere. It was also of no small consequence that while the steamers serviced stations up to 140 miles north (Manda) and 75 miles southwest (Kota Kota) of Likoma, the mission's critically essential marine workshops were located at Malindi, 175 miles south of the island. Meanwhile, the nucleus of Malawi's embryonic "Western" economy and communications, technology, and administrative development was south of the lake. Over time these factors whittled away Likoma's efficiency and suitability as mission headquarters.

Likoma, the greater diocese, and indeed all Malawi and Central Africa were experiencing rapid social change at this time. To witness but not participate in this process was certainly unnerving to many African Christians. For all or most of their lives they had been intensely associated with the mission's most historic and prestigious place. Now the sinews holding these connections together had begun to unravel. A new and unfamiliar set of circumstances was emerging, shaped by four overlapping forces. First was financial retrenchment and devolution of responsibilities in the diocese. Second, political change was leading to the imposition of federalism in Central Africa, and the likelihood of African self-government in Malawi and Northern Rhodesia in the near future. Finally, the UMCA's European authorities had taken steps to restructure and redefine the mission's mandate. The legal status of Likoma Island itself, held in freehold by the UMCA since 1893, also changed in 1950 when title was transferred to the protectorate as African Trust Land (Winspear 1956). Together these developments would shake the mission's foundations, and especially African confidence. There was a palpable sense of betrayal, abandonment, and exclusion from the decision-making process.

In April–May 1955, the Archbishop of Canterbury and Mrs. R. C. Fisher toured three countries in connection with the inauguration of the Church of Central Africa Province. By protocol, Likoma was the UMCA station the archbishop visited first during a five-day tour of the Nyasaland Diocese. Upon his arrival the Executive Committee of the Likoma Association, an African body, presented the archbishop with a lengthy Memorandum (fig. 5.2). It was essentially a bill of bitter complaints directed primarily against alleged actions and inactions of Bishop Frank Oswald Thorne (1936–61).[33]

In the view of the Likoma Association, Bishop Thorne was directly responsible during his long tenure for a wanton neglect and consequent decay of facilities and Christian practice on the island in particular and in the diocese in general. The memorandum is infused with anger toward and contempt for the bishop, whose style was seen as autocratic and exclusive of consultations with them. Grievances were framed in terms of the "activities of the Lord Bishop of Nyasaland, since he came to Nyasaland Diocese."[34] The document alleged that Likoma's "village synagogues" and the cathedral

Likoma Christians,
P.O. Likoma Island,
NYASALAND.

HIS GRACE THE ARCHBISHOP OF CANTERBURY.
Your Grace The Archbishop,

We christians of Likoma Island, have several complaints to raise before you. We have seen several, destructive changes in our mission; which have disappointed every christian terribly. Here are a few of the major complaints

1 Ever since the U.M.C.A. was established on this island, the Saint Michael's College, i.e. Teachers' Training centre was situated on the island; but suddenly it was removed to another remote place for no apparent reason; yet this is the headquarters of the Diocese.

2. It is a great shame to see a mighty Cathedral, such as this of ours being deprived of its choir without a specific reason.

3. We do not really know why the S.S. Chauncy Maples has been sold out and yet she was given us as a means of conveying the Gospel on the lake.

4. The Cathedral to-day is in a very bad state. All the embroidery is taken away: e.g. the seven big lamps at the High Altar which were brought into the Cathedral by Bishop Trower.

We shall be very grateful if Your Grace, will investigate into the matter.
Your humble children in Christ,
Likoma Christians.

Figure 5.2. Letter to Archbishop of Canterbury from Likoma Christians.
(Source: UMCA Archives, Rhodes House Library.)

had been allowed to fall "into disrepair," apparently due to lack of funds for upkeep.[35] Church attendance had also dropped off considerably, and:

> All things, particularly buildings, steamers, Cathedral, and Churches, etc. which were built with the money from England have either been ruined or destroyed beyond repair. For instance: Two steamers—*C.J.* and *C.M.* The former was dismantled within a year or two he [Bishop Thorne] had spent in the Diocese, and the latter is now sold despite our protest. Apart from the destruction of churches and other buildings which in many cases are altered to his queer design, that magnificent cathedral, built with money from England *but with the sweat and labour of African Christians,* has suffered a great deal of negligence and damage, and it is just about to fall.[36]

The memorandum goes on to accuse the bishop of "having a strong desire to ruin headquarters" and of making decisions that brought "financial embarrassment" to the diocese. Evidence presented includes the transfer of St. Michael's College from Likoma to Malosa and later Malindi, and the relocation of St. Andrew's College to Makulawe and then to Northern Rhodesia, out the country. Health care for the people on Likoma and Chizumulu Islands had also been neglected: "all medicines, equipment, etc. have been transferred to Malindi [near Mponda's], his potential headquarters," and people now had to pay "exorbitant" fees for the hospital's services and few medicines. Educational opportunities beyond Standard VI had also been left undeveloped.[37]

Casting a long shadow over the local grievances, however realistic or exaggerated in the memorandum, was the great unhappiness many Africans felt about their forced integration into the Federation of Rhodesia and Nyasaland in 1953. Directly related to this was the formation, with no African input, of the new Church of Central Africa Province (CCAP) incorporating four dioceses in the Crown Colony of Southern Rhodesia and the Protectorates of Northern Rhodesia and Nyasaland. Racial tensions had intensified in each of the colonial territories involved. The complaints brought by the Likoma Association to the archbishop cannot be separated from this wider context of swirling transition.[38] Africans continued to experience racial domination and subordination in both secular politics and ecclesiastical affairs at this time. And there was a fear that further financial and spiritual losses would occur with the active support of the idea of racially segregated congregations, black and white, in the new CCAP and its four dioceses.[39] For Africans, the atmsphere was filled with a brooding, palpable sense of the coming withdrawal of much European support for the African Church.

Bishop Thorne and the missionaries knew that Africans strongly opposed many of the autocratic decisions the mission was taking. Yet there is little evidence of attempts to create a framework in which to give these concerns a genuine voice, or to try collaborative planning for change. For the Africans, the constitution of the Nyasaland Diocese was a case in point. Participation of the laity in the Diocesan Synod was disallowed, unlike the three other dioceses in the new federation. The frustrated response of Likoma Africans to their exclusion and lack of a forum was thus magnified in the 1955 memorandum. This document manifests their bitterness at being left out of the process, and is written as if there is nothing to gain from remaining quiet and deferential to the church hierarchy. It seethes with acute loss of respect for the bishop's actions, and is practically a blanket condemnation of him as a person. In the words of S. N. Kayawa, President of the Likoma Association:

> The Lord Bishop of Nyasaland, we are sorry to say, brooks no opposition nor advice. His words are first and final as evidenced on the selling of the steamer *C.M.*, and on the Formation of the proposed Central African Province.[40]

Correspondence predating the Likoma Association's accusations had been initiated with Bishop Thorne by the Likoma branch of the Nyasaland African Congress (NAC) in April 1952. It lodged a unanimous but uninflamed protest "against the sale of the above Steamer which your lordship officially announced at a meeting held with Likoma Church Elders on February 12th, 1952."[41] First, it was argued that links between Africans, Africans and the mission, and the past and present history of the diocese would be "severed." Second, since 1947 the *C.M.* had been "carrying paying passengers"; thus the need to sell it was not apparent. Finally, in 1951 the start of lake service by the railway's new steamer, *Ilala II*, which could carry 359 passengers (320 in third class), had disrupted the traditional pattern of passenger flows between Likoma and other lake ports (Cole-King [1971] 1987). Adjusting the *C.M.*'s calling schedule to include Chipoka could do much to reclaim many passengers who now used the *Ilala II*.

Thorne responded within four days to the NAC's protest over the *C.M.*'s "sale." The prelate's letter suggests that he was somewhat more concerned about losing the *C.M.*, and more constrained in terms of alternative actions, than the Likoma Association appreciated. Nevertheless, Thorne's style was to inform, not consult. He reasoned that the NAC was "misinformed," since he had not announced his intention to sell the steamer and "had formed no desire to do so if it can be avoided." There was thus no "immediate crisis."

Captain Haywood did not want to retire just then, and a chance existed that a retired Royal Navy officer might be willing to take over for him. Thorne said that as with any important matter he had attempted "to explain the position to the responsible people on the Island... well in advance so that they have time to think it over and appreciate the factors involved."[42] He outlined the extenuating circumstances, including the imminent retirement of Captain Haywood, the improbability of being able to afford to hire a new captain and engineer on the mission's noncompetitive terms of service, and declining mission income from England. Whereas, said Thorne, it cost £2,100 annually to operate the *C.M.*, passenger fares in the previous year only came to £530 and in the first quarter of 1952 only £50 had been collected. He emphasized, "I am as reluctant as you are to sell the *C.M.* and... I shall not do so unless all attempts to maintain her in service prove unavailing."[43] Furthermore, he advised that "the best contribution the Likoma Branch of the NAC can make to maintaining the *C.M.* in service" is to impress upon the African population that "they must increase their giving to Self-Support in accordance with their means."[44] While expressing a degree of empathy, the bishop made it quite plain that one of his primary responsibilities was to keep operating expenses in check with income and eliminate negative balances. This shifting of the mission's financial burden to Africans thus contributed to the panicked reaction evident in the Likoma Association's complaints to the archbishop.

In August 1953 the UMCA permanently withdrew the *Chauncy Maples*, once openly called the "The White Ship," from mission service on Lake Malawi on grounds of financial exigency (*CA* 42 [1924]: 161). In 1955, seventeen months after the steamer's retirement, transport on the lake was disorganized. For two months at the end of 1953 and beginning of 1954, the *Ilala II*, the new railways steamer, was out of commission for a long overhaul. Only two months after she resumed sailing, the *Ilala II* was again forced out of operation after hitting a submerged rock that opened a large hole in her hull. Repairs took seven months. After it returned to service the ship was soon withdrawn yet again, this time for redecking.

Thus for twelve of the seventeen months following the *C.M.*'s retirement, the mission had no means of traveling about the lake apart from the *Paul*, a forty foot, Dutch-built schooner of 1904 vintage. Purchased by the UMCA in 1938, this vessel had been rebottomed and converted with a diesel engine in 1953 (*UMCA Ann. Rev.*, 1954–55; Cole-King [1971] 1987). While invaluable in transporting mission staff and on occasion nonmission passengers, the *Paul* was far too small—it carried a maximum of two cabin and six deck passengers—to meet current needs. A goodly portion of this need originated outside of what some might construe as the mission's ordinary business. A case in point is the mission's transportation service on behalf of Malawians who derived wages from southern Africa's colonial economies. Lamenting its size, Bishop Thorne observed that the *Paul* could "do nothing to help the hundreds of Africans going to or returning from work in Southern Rhodesia and South Africa, who arrive at a port to find there is no steamer for weeks or months" (*UMCA Ann. Rev.*, 1954–55, 17).

RECKONING "DOWN" TIME AND ITS IMPLICATIONS

When the *C.M.* was finally withdrawn from service, it had sailed nearly 300,000 miles on Lake Malawi, or the equivalent of thirteen times around the earth's circumference (*CA* 69 [1951]). It had depended entirely on burning firewood for its steam generation. Since 1901, when it commenced sailing, the *C.M.* had been laid up for part of twenty-eight of its fifty-two years with the mission for reasons other than routine maintenance (table 5.1).

The longest consecutive periods during which the *C.M.* remained out of commission, or otherwise unavailable to the mission, included 84 months during 1914–21 (in Royal Navy service until 1918 and under repair 1918–21), 1934–36 (18 months), and 1944–46 (35 months). These absences alone accounted for some 137 months, or 11.5 years of down time. In the case of the *Charles Janson*, the longest absence was 18 months during 1929 to 1931. Overall, the total cumulative length of time (for all reasons including World War I) when neither steamer was available for mission use was approximately 21 years. Lengthy difficulties with the *C.M.*'s boilers in 1913, 1920–21, 1925, 1935, and 1944–46 greatly upset the mission's agenda. Ironically, considering its age, the *C.J.*'s boiler record was overall much better than the *C.M.*'s, with its most serious lay-ups limited to 1900 and 1931.

Between 1932 and 1953, when the *C.J.* was out of the picture for good, the *C.M.* was laid up for more than 60 months. It was then more than 30 years old, and its down time during these 21 years thus exceeded 35 percent. Realistically it cannot be treated as an opportunity cost; yet by almost any measure this level of unavailability was a heavy price to pay for dependence on a technology intended to facilitate mission business. The UMCA's spatial organization in Malawi had evolved with the expanding and repetitive movements of the steamers. Its missionaries could not function effectively without them. When the *C.M.* was no longer available, and its return from another episode of repair or overhaul could not be anticipated, the UMCA's work in the Nyasa Diocese began to atrophy. This decline certainly was not caused

Table 5.1   Selected chronology of steamer "down time"

1893	temporary loss of *C.J.* Caught in low water at Matope on River Shiré.
1895	*C.J.* laid up for work on engine and plates.
1904	*C.J.* laid up due to engineer's departure.
1907	*C.M.* at Malindi for repairs for 2.5 months.
1908	"Steamer [*C.M.*] running throughout the year."
1909	Both *C.J.* and *C.M.* (ran onto rocks) out of service for repairs.
1910	*C.J.* laid up for lack of operating funds. Returned to service in 1911 with funds raised in England.
1912	*C.J.* immobilized for lack of engineer.
1913	*C.M.* out of operation to permit boiler adaptation and alteration of furnace draft. *C.J.* takes up some of slack.
1914–18	*C.M.* commandeered for Royal Navy service as troop & supply carrier on Lake Malawi.
1916	*C.J.* also taken into government wartime service.
1918–21	*C.M.* laid up after World War I. New boiler installed 1920–21. Steam remains inadequate.
1923	*C.J.* breaks down, cannot sail for three weeks.
1924	Dry dock problems for the *C.J.*
1925	Continuing problems with *C.M.* boilers. New ordinance re: qualifications of captains and engineers.
1926	*C.M.* laid up most of year. *C.J.* fills in for *C.M.* with help from *Guendolen*.
1929	*C.J.* sank at moorings at Malindi in four fathoms. Out of commission for nearly one year.
1931	*C.M.* annual overhauling at Monkey Bay. Boilers declared unsafe after one voyage, and again laid up. Returned to service January.
1932	*C.J.* no longer operational.
1934–36	"Disturbing reports" about condition of *C.M.*'s boiler, followed by lay-up of 18 months (late 1934–February 1936). £2,000 expenditure on new boiler and repairs.
1939–45	*C.M.* occasionally used for troop transport but not commandeered.
1944–46	*C.M.* laid up for 35 months with boiler problems. *C.J.* still on beach at Malindi, a disintegrating hulk. In interlude the *Malonda* (former *H. von Wissmann*, vintage 1892), provided a monthly lake visit for UMCA. Lake services further crippled by sinking of Railways steamer MV *Vipya* in July 30, 1946.
1951	October 4, *C.M.*'s Golden Jubilee.
1953	*C.M.* permanently withdrawn from service as UMCA steamer. Budget and staffing problems.
1956	*C.M.* sold to fishing company headquartered in Salisbury, S. Rhodesia.
1965	*C.M.* sold to Malawi Railways and converted to diesel.
1990	*C.M.* moored at Monkey Bay unused and in poor condition.

Sources: *Central Africa; UMCA Ann. Review;* Malawi National Archives; Rhodes House Library, Oxford. For 1908: Kota Kota: Health Reports and Staff, 1904–1909. 145-DOM-10-4-1. MNA.

independently by the steamer's absence. As a European-managed institution, the mission had already begun to "wind down" with the formation of the Central African Federation, soon followed by moves toward
self-government and independence for Malawi. These changes initiated a
growing sense of physical, social, and economic isolation among the lakeside
populations.

Throughout 1955 the railway's *Ilala II* remained the only passenger
steamer on the lake. At Malindi, meanwhile, the *C.M.* was "riding rather
disconsolately at anchor," lacking an offer of purchase (*CA* 73 [1955]: 246). In
recent months two proposals had surfaced that could determine what role
she might play next, outside the UMCA. One of these was for the Federal
Ministry of Health in the Central African Federation to buy the steamer
and convert it into a hospital ship. Its task would be to make the rounds
of lakeshore regions with high-density populations but little or no access
to roads and medical services. From the mission's perspective this would
meet a profound need, and it would be "very appropriate for the *C.M.* to
return . . . to a work of corporal mercy" (*UMCA Ann. Rev.,* 1954–55, 17). If this
idea did not materialize, the Royal Naval Association of Nyasaland might
purchase the ship for use in naval training.

Neither proposal materialized. Instead, the *C.M.* was bought under-value
by a fishing firm based in Salisbury, Southern Rhodesia. She was equipped
with refrigeration and radar facilities, and designated the "mother ship,"
or "floating depot," for a fishing fleet of five boats on Lake Malawi (*CA*
74 [1956]: 205; 75 [1957]: 13). But this was not the end of the steamer's
remarkable career. In 1965 the *C.M.* was purchased by Malawi Railways
and converted to a diesel-powered passenger and cargo ship. By the time
she was overhauled, outfitted, and readied for operation in 1968 the *C.M.*
was 67 years old, and the last of the pioneer steamers still plying the
lake.

CHAUNCY MAPLES: "HULK OF MONKEY BAY"

In May 1990, having learned that the standard bearer of the old steamer
parish was still in the water, ninety years later, I visited the small port settlement of Monkey Bay to have a look at it. This government port is nestled in
a beautiful, sheltered cove. As I approached the gatehouse two hefty members of Malawi's Young Pioneers, a paramilitary organization, intercepted
me. At first they rebuffed my request for entry, despite the fact that I had
produced my research clearance document from the Office of the President

and also showed them my green Congress Party card. At the time, four years before the expulsion of the Banda dictatorship, possession of this card was necessary but not sufficient to the well being of any Malawian. I had determined that having one of my own would not be a disadvantage the next time I visited a market or other public place patrolled by the Young Pioneers. Dressed in green sweaters and berets and carrying batons, these young men seemed overcome with their own effusive self-importance. Mildly agitated at my unannounced arrival, they seemed anxious to demonstrate their protective authority. To them, I suppose, my request to enter the port complex to see the ancient and inoperable mission steamer seemed an odd and just cause for suspicion. Perhaps I had instructions to sabotage one or more government vessels, or at least gather intelligence that might be used for political-military objectives against the Banda regime. Despite the Young Pioneers' general reputation as overbearing toughs who abused people who did not carry a green Congress Party membership card, I persisted and found a way to break through the stand-off when I sensed that one of the young men was more conciliatory than the other. He had apparently decided that I had come to Monkey Bay for some reasonable, if not entirely understandable, purpose. Perhaps pulling rank, he finally reacted with that inimitable Malawian courtesy. My request for an escort to discuss my purpose with the officer-in-charge (O-C) of the Monkey Bay installation was quickly granted.

After a brief and cordial conversation with the O-C, and his private communications with a few of the officers on duty, I was given permission to board, inspect, and photograph the *C.M.* in the disinterested company of an engineer. The steamer had been converted from wood burning to diesel power in 1967. Sadly, it was laid up again and lacked generators. It still displayed Malawi's national colors of green, yellow, and black on its smokestack, but by the now the vessel was little more than a floating hulk. Decrepit and filthy, its smelly toilets polluted the atmosphere on its decks. The *C.M.* had degenerated in its envelope of water, tropical sun, wind, and rain, and was evidently long beyond redemption. Its eventual dismantling would be a costly undertaking, although surely there were no resources for this undertaking. An attractive plaque of polished brass, inscribed with President Banda's name to mark its recommissioning in 1967, remained fastened to the ship's forward main deck. It seemed one of the few elements of the *C.M.* that could endure much longer, with luck in a local museum.[45]

When the UMCA finally relinquished its use of the *Chauncy Maples* it coincided with an administrative reorganization that reduced the size of the Diocese of Nyasaland. Now there were two dioceses in three African territories. Long before this change occurred, the European missionaries together with African UMCA priests and evangelists had carried the banner of Anglo-Catholic Christianity across a span of four hundred miles on land and water. Available indigenous technology was limited to dugout canoes and crude dhows. These craft lacked the size and technical capability necessary to open and operate a mission field of such magnitude. Steam power alone made the UMCA's accomplishment possible in the late nineteenth and early twentieth centuries.

For Europeans the steamers became an integral, almost organic element of the mission field. These vessels also inspired awe among the lake region's pre-industrial peoples. African stowaways found their way aboard the Scots' *Ilala* as early as 1877 (McKinnon 1977). In the pioneer years some Africans reportedly believed that oxen powered the UMCA steamers. In the mission's early decades the *C.J.* and *C.M.*, reinforced by the presence of a number of government and commercial steamers on the lake, symbolized a prestigious, even mystical, form of work power. European missionaries could appropriate and manipulate this power to their decided advantage in their dealings with the locals. In the end their systematic reliance on the steamers led them to grasp at opportunities for evangelism, education, and health care that stretched their capabilities too thinly. From the missionaries' perspective, their inspired drive to overreach what they could reasonably manage with available resources may be explained in terms of a personal and corporate sense of duty and their belief in the "Great Commission" mandate. Against these circumstances, operating costs, maintenance problems, and down time revealed the steamers' vulnerability and helped to check the UMCA's grander ambitions.

PROSPECT: DIFFERENT FRONTIERS, OTHER TECHNOLOGIES

The mission's territorial limits also signified social, cultural and psychological frontiers. They defined where one sphere of church and mission influence ended and another began. These transition zones generally remained spaces in which there was a "tug-of-war" for new converts. In comparison to the competition between missions, the general frontier between African and European culture was also tension-filled. African cosmologies, social and cultural institutions, behavior, and spiritual life were increasingly subjected by the missionaries to unfavorable examination and intense pressure to change. Although raids by marauding Ngoni and slavers' atrocities had ceased, missionaries and colonialism brought new problems as well as amenities. Unprecedented apprehension and competition between indigenous values and those originating in Europe affected daily life.

Generally speaking, compared against their own accomplishments and values, Europeans saw little in African cultures to commend them. Exceptions might be made for such frequently observed traits as Africans' generosity, love of children, sociability, physical endurance, propensity to trade, adaptability, and capacity for loyalty. Yet many of these positive attributes remained more stereotyped than understood. Beyond the superficial level, few Europeans grasped, or apparently had the inclination to discover, the integrity, capabilities, or pragmatism of the African peoples into whose midst they had invited themselves.

In places that experienced more than ephemeral contact between the foreign and indigenous cultures, considerable cognitive distance and dissonance arose between the complex African realities and Europeans' images of Africans and themselves. Europeans and Africans each brought their own metaphysical, cultural, and psychological baggage to the frontier. Such "mentifacts" (Zelinsky 1973) could not but profoundly influence the kinds and depths of mutual understanding each could achieve of their respective civilizations. Divergence of belief, practice, and understanding was greatest in the realm of worldviews. A profound gap existed between the African and European belief structures that was never successfully bridged, with particular respect to the role of the supernatural and the integration of religious culture in healing.

Chapters 6 through 10 examine how the UMCA worked to influence health patterns, health status, and social change among Africans in its spheres of mission in Malawi, southwest Tanzania, and northern Mozambique. It has been widely demonstrated and accepted that missionaries alone shouldered overwhelming responsibility for education and medical care in early colonial Africa, and often much longer. The recent emergence of a small critical literature on medical missions notwithstanding, how and where these missionary services were provided by missionaries and received by Africans, and what changes followed, has rarely been systematically examined for a particular area.

Again, the steamers figure significantly in facilitating policies and actions that created and underpinned the new infrastructure that supported the UMCA's system of medicine and health care. Over the years, many hundreds of sick and injured people and their family members received transport on the *C.J.* and *C.M.* to UMCA hospitals and dispensaries. The steamers also carried nurses, supplies and "the doctor" to these facilities. A major aim is to determine what difference this "mission medicine" made to Africans' health, considering that it combined Western technology, science, and the art of medicine with an ethos drawn from a variety of forms of Christian witness and good works. I show how a system of Western-type medical institutions was built up, combining evangelism and reaching out to heal the sick.

More often than not Africans could be admitted to receive some medical attention regardless of their religion, beliefs, or standing with the church. Yet missionary medicine was incomplete unless it was a vehicle to proselytize and entice "the African" who received treatment into joining the Anglo-Catholic community of believers. For missionaries, the African's in-hospital experience of confinement provided unparalleled scope for sustained exposure to religious practice and propaganda. Captive African audiences offered the missionaries tantalizing opportunities to introduce unbelievers to the lost condition of their souls, guide them from Darkness into Light, and along the way instill grave doubts about the value of their own cultures. The missionary medical culture introduced new definitions of health and socially constructed ways of interpreting illness.

Next, in chapter 6, I describe what is known about the ecological and cultural patterns of health and disease in precolonial Malawi, before the missionary enterprise took root. The purpose is to create a baseline from which to evaluate the social consequences of contact between African and European ways of healing.

NOTES

1. *Nyasaland Diocesan Chronicle*, Dec. 1948.

2. Personal communication: Mr. H. M. Kangunga, Clinical Officer, Malindi, Malawi, May 24, 1990.

3. Also known as monkey nuts or peanuts. Bellingham reported buying "all the ground-nuts . . . we can" from mainland villages (Yarborough 1888, 113).

4. Fred Morrison, Diaries, 1882–87, June 19, 1882. Edinburgh University Library, Rare Books and Manuscripts, E71/36. Gen. 1803-Gen. 1809. Cited in McKinnon 1977, 179, n. 44.

5. By Orders in Council of 1894 and 1920, English gold, silver, and bronze became the official currency of the Nyasaland Protectorate. Before British rule began in May 1891, virtually all trade was done by barter, while laborers were paid in calico. In the early Protectorate years, the Indian rupee was introduced. English silver was acquired in 1894, and at an exchange rate of 18½ rupees to the pound the rupee was soon driven

out of circulation. By 1897, use of Nyasaland shillings and sixpences, pegged to the British pound, was widespread throughout most of the territory (Murray 1922, 185).

6. *CA* 34 (1916): 30–35. The colony was made up of Watonga who had returned to their homeland after a time of refuge on Likoma Island.

7. Hedley Fisher, "The *Chauncy Maples*," *CA* 46 (1928): 13.

8. UMCA 1/2/21. MNA.

9. Tapela 1979. By 1894 the missionaries through the ALC had set up Nyasaland's first labor recruitment bureau, which was then supplying some 5,500 workers to the European cotton planters in the Shiré Highlands (70–71).

10. Dr. W. H. Murray, Nov. 1899, cited in Pretorius 1972, 370–71.

11. Securing adequate cheap labor was a perennial concern in the colonial economies. The government of Southern Rhodesia, for example, offered free lorry transport for migrant workers and their families between Nyasaland and Mtoko, Southern Rhodesia, via Mozambique territory. Known as *Ulere*, the system was set up to lure workers onto the white farms east of Salisbury that produced labor-intensive tobacco (Niddrie 1954).

12. *Nyasaland Government Gazette*, Oct. 31, 1922. Ordinance No. 22, p. 1. P.R.O. File No. C.O. 626/15, vol. 2. of 1922. MNA.

13. *Annual Report on the Sanitary and Health Conditions of the Nyasaland Protectorate for the Year ended 31st March, 1912.* Cited in Gelfand 1964, 291.

14. Chairman, Federated Board of Nyasaland Missions to Chief Secretary, Zomba, May 17, 1921. 7/UMCA/1/2/16. MNA.

15. Ibid.

16. Sir William Manning, who became the Protectorate Commissioner in 1912, succeeded in getting the Union government of South Africa to ban the importation of labor originating in territories north of 22° S. latitude. This action had limited effect, especially since there were numerous calls from the Rand seeking removal of the embargo (*CA* 40 [1922]). Migrants had to earn money for taxes, at least, and the entire system of voluntary movements, including evasive routes, was already well established (Tapela 1979).

17. Protestant missions complained of "Roman Catholic aggression" and a "very determined Roman Catholic propaganda—engineered from Rome" within their established spheres of activity. The governor assured them that he would press their case in England, in person. Hetherwick of the Blantyre Mission insisted that the Catholics were set on planting a mission, school, or church next to existing Protestant Missions where they had as yet no converts, "purely with the intention of destroying already established work." A. Hetherwick to Bishop, April 15, 1926. 7/UMCA/1/2/16. MNA.

18. In his diary, William Bellingham, one of the laymen who reconstructed the *C.J.*, mentions that some of the steamer's plates were riveted, while the deck and boiler were bolted (Yarborough 1888, 56–59).

19. James B. Jones, Lingan S. Randolph Professor Emeritus of Mechanical Engineering, Virginia Tech, Blacksburg, Virginia. Personal communication, July 15, 1994.

20. Ibid.

21. Wood, a fuel readily at hand, continued to be used in rail locomotives in the Pacific Northwest until the 1930s. Bituminous coal was the fuel choice in most parts of the U.S.A.

22. Jones, personal communication, 1994.

23. Diocese of Nyasaland, Medical Officer's Report, 1923, 7; UMCA A3 143. RHL.

24. *Nyasaland Diocesan Chronicle*, Oct. 1944; *CA* 63 (1945): 23.

25. The crew was led by Bertram Haywood, the *C.M.*'s Captain, and Mr. Bell, an engineer and exceptionally able "man of the people" who was still revered at Malindi in 1990.

26. *CA* 63 (1945): 15. Reported in *Nyasaland Diocesan Chronicle*, May 1944.

27. The first telegram through the new system sent by an African clerk at Mandala store to Edwin, an African clerk in the diocesan store. It said: "Please Father, buy me a 6/6 hat." *Nyasaland Diocesan Chronicle*, March 1945, reprinted in *CA* 63 (1945): 86.

28. Historical Manuscript Inventory, vol. 1, emphasis added. MNA.

29. Continually rising costs and stationary income between 1948 and 1953 had produced deficits ranging to £1,800 annually (*UMCA Ann. Rev.*, 1953–54, 13).

30. Letter from "Likoma Christians, P.O. Likoma Island" (c. 1952), UMCA 1/2/20/5. RHL.

31. Ibid.

32. UMCA 1/2/20/5, n.d., c. April 23, 1955. RHL; Blood 1957.

33. The memo was copied to Bishop Thorne.

34. UMCA 1/2/20/5, n.d., c. April 23, 1955.

35. Contractors undertook to repair the massive roof (320 feet) and other interior and exterior elements of Likoma Cathedral in 1960. The general restoration was described as "an act of faith" in that despite a guaranteed contract price there was nothing available for maintenance. Furthermore, the diocese was not "practically out of debt" until 1963 (*CA* 78 [1960]; 81 [1963]).

36. UMCA 1/2/20/5, n.d., c. April 23, 1955, p. 2. (emphasis added).

37. Ibid.

38. I did not find a response from the archbishop to the Likoma Association.

39. Racial segregation of worship was rooted in the mission's origins. Its was viewed as an awkward ("there is no *race*" in Christianity) but necessary practice, designed as it was not to "force inconveniences and controversies on to people in connection with their communions unnecessarily." Practical difficulties for the Europeans were said to be the bad smells and an oppressive atmosphere in small churches resulting from Africans who allegedly chose not to wash their European-style clothing. One would also be likely to attract insects in joint worship and then carry them home. Moreover, the accouterments of a church intended for Europeans' worship were "utterly different" from those in a church "intended for natives." Furthermore, the "natives do not want" the type of service that is "natural to Europeans." And "the native craze for singing and sing-song at every service is irritating and to many persons who are quite sympathetic with natives, maddening." Class consciousness and ambivalence toward the "unwashed" Africans and their evolving expressions of Christianity proved decisive. The UMCA's general policy in 1917 that it was best for Europeans and Africans to worship separately "and in different buildings." To preserve the principle of "unity despite race," the bishop recommended that "occasional unions" of the races should be encouraged, in buildings suitable for the purpose. Bishop Fisher to Rev. Winspear, Nov. 24, 1917. UMCA 1/1/2. MNA.

40. UMCA 1/2/20/5, n.d., c. April 23, 1955, p. 4.

41. Chitenje, NAC, Likoma, to Lord Bishop, April 16, 1952. UMCA 1/2/20/5. RHL.

42. Bishop of Nyasaland to Mr. Chitenje, April 20, 1952, UMCA 1/2/20/5. RHL.

43. Ibid.

44. Ibid.

45. The *C.M.*, defying time and the elements, is still moored at Monkey Bay (photographs seen at the USPG, London, June 2002).

{ CHAPTER SIX }

Health in Sub-Saharan Africa
and Malawi on the Eve of Colonization

Solid evidence of African health conditions and disease patterns prior to 1900 is scarce, regardless of location. Available information is based mostly on isolated, unsystematic observations by Europeans whose primary purposes in Africa did not include reporting on indigenous health conditions. The personal journals of explorers, travelers, traders, company administrators, and military officers offer health-related observations of varying reliability. Selective use of these sources may provide useful clues about health conditions during the late precolonial period. They offer an intriguing menu of astute and wild speculations, hearsay, and meticulously recorded direct observations. Attempts to characterize African health status and ecology at the time of missionary contact require a considerable reliance on these journals and later interpretations of them.

Reconstruction of precolonial disease and health patterns is further complicated by the variability of environment, culture, and place. On the eve of colonization several important factors influenced African health conditions. They included widespread political instability, fear, and insecurity; and cultural behaviors that protected or exposed people to hazards, such as strong belief in witchcraft and sorcery. Health status was also affected by the degree of population immunity acquired through prior experience with epidemic disease, and by population density and mobility, housing quality, and other factors connected with place and relative location. Additional variables include proximity to transportation corridors and foreign populations, altitude, and isolation from or contact with introduced and resurgent diseases. Each of these factors in health ecology points to locational factors as critical determinants of a society's risk and wellness.

GARDEN OF EDEN OR WELLSPRING OF DISEASE?

Popular images of tropical Africa have long stereotyped it as inherently unhealthy. In the "absolutionist," perception, some evidence for which is drawn from non-African experiences, peoples ravaged by endemic and epidemic diseases that retarded development inhabited the region's environments.[1] However, such conclusions must be reconciled with the parallel evidence. During the past half-millennium, at least, African peoples have shown remarkable demographic resilience in the face of all manner of internal and external assaults on the social fabric. Unlike the Americas or Oceania, no large-scale die-offs of population are recorded, except in response to the contained if incalculable horrors of the slave ships.[2] However, this fact alone does not diminish the strong possibility that overall tropical Africa also had a disproportionate share of health hazards.

Blaut admits that there is "little solid evidence either way about the [precolonial] history of health conditions in Africa and among Africans" (1993, 80). At the same time he looks disfavorably on the "inherited diffusionist assumptions and prejudices" which he says have created the stereotype. His conclusion that "one cannot make a case that disease was an independent force that 'blocked' development in sub-Saharan Africa" can only mean that neither argument is viable. Blaut's historical-geographic vision is guided by a commitment to value the theoretical positions of the more "radical" Africanist and other Third World scholars whose orientations reflect a search for and emphasis on external causes of underdevelopment. His analysis and its final contradiction highlight the still unsatisfactory resolution of the question about the weight of the disease factor in African development. Evaluation of *both* internal and external forces must go on. Settling on a single theoretical vision weakens the possibilities of interpretation. New studies always seem to suggest the need to reexamine alternative macro-political or ecological interpretations.

A Pluralist View of Disease

Richards (1983) proposed a three-part schema for interpreting the ecology of disease in tropical Africa. First is the popular, "disease ridden" perception noted in the earlier discussion that flows from a universalistic approach to Africa's human ecology. Africans, the argument goes, did develop biological responses to meet the challenges to their survival (such as the sickle cell gene), but the price included very high infant mortality rates. In this perception, low population growth, underpopulation, and overall lack of population pressure underlie much of the subcontinent's technological retardation, and this was worsened by Africans' ineffectual control of tropical diseases.[3] The terrible cycle of poor health, maintained by underpopulation, low technology, and disease, has not been challenged or broken anywhere until recent decades. Even diseases with a relatively uncomplicated ecology but high human cost, such as Guinea worm, remained endemic and uncontested.[4] Recently, the examples of Ebola, HIV/AIDS, and other highly publicized threats to public health in tropical Africa and the world continue to sustain acceptance of this old stereotype.

A second view of the subcontinent's disease ecology builds on the idea that tropical Africa became a "zone of exceptional health risk" following increased contact with the outside world, notably beginning with the Atlantic slave trade. Smallpox, rinderpest, influenza, STIs, cholera, and other diseases entered the continent through ports and then spread along major and tributary trade routes. The entry and rapid spread of the jigger, or sandflea (*Tungas penetrans*), from Brazil to West Africa around 1872, and its transcontinental crossing to the east coast within a few years, is a striking and well known example of the principle. In the 1880s and 1890s (earlier in some places), colonial taxation policies and the widespread promotion of labor migration became significant vectors in the African health equation. These initiatives created a wholly new array of infrastructures such as towns, roads, market centers, and ports, giving rise to new patterns of human circulation and mobility that channeled disease transmission. Ultimately, the imbalancing and reconfiguration of natural, social, and human-environment relations expanded and amplified the potential and scope of disease spread.

Influenza was one of the most spectacular and deadliest examples of disease penetration from the outside. After the Spanish Influenza pandemic of 1918–19 entered Africa through Freetown, Sierra Leone, it spread to practically all inhabited areas south of the Sahara. Estimates of the number of Africans killed by influenza in about one year range from 1.35 million (Coquery-Vidrovitch 1988, 42) to least two million (Patterson 1981). It not only killed huge numbers, but also forced the reorganization of populations and living patterns.

The idea that it is the external world which is unhealthful, rather than Africa, has been attractive to proponents of both modernization and dependency theories. As already noted, some nationalist historians and others have adopted this perspective in reassessing the subcontinent's health record. For example, the presence of an extensive, persistent zone of low fertility in Equatorial Africa, including Gabon, northern Zaire, and the Central African Republic, may not reflect endemic health. Instead, one plausible explanation is that it is a long-term consequence of intensive colonial exploitation that included forced labor migration, destabilized family life, and rapid diffusion of sexually transmitted diseases. Numerous scenarios with similarly major health implications can be cited, including sleeping sickness, relapsing fever, and tuberculosis. Diffusion of diseases along communication networks was a prime mechanism of spread, together with contact spread in labor markets.

A third perspective of disease, the dynamic ecosystems approach, shifts attention away from epidemics that spread, for example, through larger colonial networks (Richards 1983). Instead, analysis relies upon the "triangle of human ecology" model, which focuses on the interactions of people, microbes, and environments (Meade and Earickson 2000). Scale of analysis and triangular analysis of human ecology are thus crucial elements in assessing disease emergence and risk. For example, one disease that typically emerges and spreads remains oddly quiescent, while another suddenly explodes in a place where it had never been recognized or when the population's immunity was taken for granted. An example is the unexpected flare-up of sleeping sickness in colonial northeast Nigeria in the 1930s. Western Uganda offers another case, where tick-borne relapsing fever underwent a dramatic shift from an endemic to epidemic disease during the first decade of the twentieth century (Good 1978). The recent Ebola outbreak (1995) in western Zaire, and "highland" malaria in Kenya, are among a multitude of present-day examples of emergent infectious diseases breaking out for the first time, or in new places, often explosively. These examples demonstrate the principle that ecological adjustment or adaptation is an ongoing process, with dynamic and complex interactions among many biological and cultural factors.

It is increasingly acknowledged that understanding and effective control of diseases also depends on access to indigenous environmental knowledge and cooperation with traditional medical systems (Richards 1983). Furthermore, the ecological template outlined above reflects positivist methods of the natural sciences and diffusion studies. Today, such analyses, based on observation, measurement, and generalization, may be seen as incomplete or even misleading unless the questions they address (and ignore) have also been projected through the lens of social theory. New "geographies" of health use social theory to articulate and evaluate concerns that are less readily counted and quantified (Gatrell 2002). Such work often stresses the importance of intangible, subjective, "lived" experience of illness and health-care among individuals and small groups in specific places. Dealing with the stigmatization and isolation experienced by persons with tuberculosis or leprosy is one example. There are also conceptual and practical concerns about the underlying causes of disease and inequities in health resources that are embedded in established political and economic systems. Other studies recognize the mutual effects of the interactions of social structures and social practices, or "human agency," on real people's lives. The implications of missionary-introduced maternal and child health services is a case in point. Finally, current theoretical approaches also aim at understanding how knowledge and experience of health and illness are constructed within contexts of power relations. How, for example, did medical missionaries, and the indigenous medico-religious authorities present in every Malawian village, perceive and adapt to one another's political and spatial authority?

LIFE, DEATH, AND THE ECOLOGY OF HEALTH: TROPICAL AFRICA

Demographic patterns go beyond the details of culture and religion and reflect "feedback loops" to other powerful epidemiological forces. Given its long notoriety as "one of the world's most disease-ridden regions" (Caldwell 1985, 463), tropical Africa's demographic resilience seems remarkable. While disease potential and hazards certainly varied in intensity according to location and time, pathogens and other threats to health abounded. Considering the alternate (yet not discrete) ways of evaluating Africa's health record discussed above—its in situ unhealthiness and length of human occupancy, the wrenching disequilibria caused by outside incursions, and the concept of dynamic ecosystems—the region has a strong claim to having had more cumulative experience with a greater variety of health hazards than any other part of the tropics. The reality includes four slave trades spanning centuries (trans-Saharan, Atlantic, East African, domestic), political instability and warfare, and famines, as well as the penetration (and sending) of disease carriers and microbes from epidemiological realms outside Africa. In view of the longevity and potency of some of these factors, it is not fanciful to assume that over time large areas of tropical Africa would have experienced depopulation.

Demographic evidence from premodern Europe suggests that many societies had high birth rates and slightly lower death rates. From time to time epidemics, warfare, and famine produced tremendous surges in the death rate, when mortality drew even with and surpassed births. Overall, in Europe the unstable death rate could have remained about five points below the agrarian birthrate, thus allowing for slow population growth (Caldwell 1985).

What lessons from this scenario carry over to the African experience? Caldwell, a demographer, thinks that the entire continent was subject to oscillations in population levels during the past thousand years: "almost certainly," he says, "many individual societies have experienced disastrous population decline with subsequent recovery" (1985, 462). He correctly asserts that the high birth rates found in most of today's Africa reflect deep contexts and complex causes. Ranked among the most important must be the long history of high death rates and the perpetually strong, pronatal influences of traditional culture and religious values, including the powerful emphasis on lineage preservation.

Some estimates suggest that precolonial African birthrates hovered around a more or less invariable rate of 47.5 per 1000; but it was the high and fluctuating death rate—notably very high infant mortality—that controlled population size (Coquery-Vidrovitch 1988). Reportedly, among the Ani-Ndenye peoples of southeastern Ivory Coast the natural increase of the population was practically nil. Also, group behavior "tended to minimize the value of children, regarding them as incomplete persons; only a woman's fourth dead child had the right to a funeral" (16).

It has been further asserted that growth rates of African societies in particular periods and regions could have reached 2 percent per annum, only to be restabilized at the much lower annual average of about 0.5 percent. On occasion the mortality rate might drop to around 45 per thousand, increasing life expectancy to around 22 years.

Evidence from Angola in the sixteenth century onward indicates that when demographic pressures produced higher population density on agricultural lands, shortened fallows and declining yields provoked malnutrition and lowered resistance to infectious diseases (ibid., 15). Studies in other parts of tropical Africa suggest that "the critical threshold of population beyond which the sickness ratio could become disastrous—threatening to reduce the population for decades—was remarkably low" (16).

Patterson (1993) speculated that until about 1880 the comparatively "stronger social systems" of Africa exerted a powerful role in helping communities to weather and rebound from major epidemics. Resistance to disease, a cultural focus on fertility and perpetuation of the lineage, and the arrival of New World food crops such as maize and cassava probably helped to maintain populations.

A different demographic and epidemiological scenario unfolded in the late nineteenth century as Europeans seized African territory and fashioned colonial states, and Arab and other Asian and African entrepreneurs stepped up their slaving and ivory hunting. The array of potential health influences expanded to include new patterns of population mobility, imperial "divide and rule" tactics, and disruption of the ecological balance in critical places. Colonialism brought taxation, labor migration, forced labor, and physical punishment. These conditions, coupled with changes in family structure and the organization of village labor, caused degrees of destablization that profoundly affected Africans' health and reproduction.

LIFE, DEATH, AND THE ECOLOGY OF HEALTH: LATE PRECOLONIAL MALAWI

In Malawi, at least for a time in the 1890s, some Europeans held Edenic views of the local environments. Sir Harry Johnston, Protectorate Commissioner, tried to counter this perception in a letter to the Foreign Office in 1896: "I think we may once and for all get rid of the myth that British Central Africa has the slightest pretence to be any more healthy than any other place in Africa. What deceives us here is the great beauty of the climate and the Shire Highlands" (cited in King and King 1991, 19).

Circumstances suggest that health conditions before the time of sustained European contact and the UMCA's arrival at Lake Malawi were probably fairly stable, but at levels unacceptable to any modern population or individual. Epidemics occurred at irregular intervals. Infant and child mortality probably averaged from 300 to 500 per thousand and went sometimes higher. Life expectancy was short (about thirty years or less). Longevity must have declined to a lower level with the spread and intensification of the slave trade, the Ngoni (Gwangwara) reign of terror, and increasing exposure to exotic diseases and epidemics. Dietary and nutritional patterns, differential access to foods according to gender and age, deficiencies of elements such protein and iron (the latter worsened by hookworm infection and disease) interacted with diseases such as smallpox, tropical ulcers, and measles. Such circumstances surely exerted a marked influence on the likelihood that a large proportion of the population was in poor health, either seasonally or perennially. The capability of the indigenous medico-religious health care systems to satisfy the basic needs of physical and mental health was another critical factor affecting the condition of precolonial populations. However, this aspect of health and social life will remain forever opaque and speculative.

The issues addressed above highlight important contexts—spatial and ecological, political and historical, and behavioral—that must be considered when attempting to estimate the status of African health during the 1880s and 1890s. It is essential to try to establish a health baseline for Malawi's societies just before their incorporation into the colonial state, despite the knowledge that it will be fragmentary and speculative. This effort is particularly important to the task of appraising the role of medical missions, which for at least the first twenty-five years of European contact offered virtually the only Western-type medical services available to Africans.

Regional health patterns in precolonial Malawi reflect processes described in each of the three perspectives of Richards's typology of disease ecology. Ecological adjustment or adaptation of societies and disease is a balancing act that is always a work in progress. Regardless of their ultimate cause, debilitating endemic diseases and violence contributed to very high death rates. As contact with the east coast and Europe intensified, new structures of communication and destabilized ecologies facilitated the arrival of new health hazards from the outside and also more virulent forms of known pathogens. These confrontations often caused deadly epidemics among populations with little or no immunity. In the case of smallpox, which reportedly "marked many" in 1859, the consequences ranged from scarring, disablement, and blindness to death (Kirk 1965, cited in King and King 1991, 55).

CULTURAL ECOLOGY OF DISEASE

Endemic and Epidemic Malaria

Malawi's peoples lived in a variety of ecological settings. They ranged from the hot, low-lying floodplains of the extreme south, to the extensive plateaus and plains 3,000 to 4,000 feet above sea level, to the Lake Malawi coastal zone above 1,500 feet, and to the high plateaus and mountains, ranging from the Nyika in the north to Mlanje in the south. A markedly wet-dry climate prevailed across the entire area (chap. 2). Health hazards, including debilitating helminths, varied environmentally and often spanned several altitudinal zones. The risks and intensity of disease also differed according to human practices, age and gender, productive tasks, age and density of settlement, and severity of the dry season. For example, *Falciparum* malaria was intense in the hot and humid zones of the lake basin and the Rift Valley, and practically everywhere else below 4,500 feet during the single rainy season. In the coastal zone of Lake Malawi, the UMCA's

Dr. Howard reported that native children under ten years old were universally infected with malaria, which was a major factor in the high infant mortality rate (Howard 1910, 66). Malaria was typically not endemic above an altitude of about 4,500 feet. Epidemic malaria affected all ages, not just children. It must also have occasionally occurred in the higher zones when infected people unknowingly transported the parasite upslope from lower elevations. There locally uninfected *Anopheles* could bite the human transgressors and begin a seasonal cycle of malaria in the resident, low-immune population.

Helminthiases: Water and Schistosomiasis

Schistosomiasis, or bilharzia, is a water-dependent disease complex that was and is endemic in the coastal zone of Lake Malawi, slower-moving stretches of the Shiré River and other tributary streams, and adjacent lakes such as Malombe and Chilwa. Human sanitary practices play a critically necessary role in maintaining the cycle of this complex disease. The real distribution, rates, and stability of schistosomiasis in the nineteenth century are, of course, beyond knowing.

Malawi's current high rate of bladder cancer is but one of schistosomiasis' many complications (King and King 1991, 101). Both the urinary and rectal forms of the complex are present. If the Great Lakes region is the original source of this insidious malady—an intricate complex involving flukes, their eggs, larvae, snail hosts, and humans (especially youth)—it is not unreasonable to think that the disease has been present in Malawi for many centuries. Eggs discovered in a 5,000 year old mummy indicate that schistosomiasis was an affliction of the ancient Egyptians (ibid.). Dr. Robert Howard reported in 1910 that schistosomiasis was "very common" in some of Malawi's lakeside villages, with about half of the males and a lesser proportion of the female population (who also had less marked symptoms) infected. Howard observed that people of all ages, male and female, were "extremely fond of bathing" and thus prone to infection. Paradoxically, he also noticed that although a large percentage of the population passed urine that was alkaline and contained "blood and abundant ova," at any given moment most of them did not manifest ill effects (1910, 68). For many, the dual opportunity to enjoy water recreation and maintain external hygiene must have been offset by the distressing, sometimes painful burden of internal parasitism acquired through ignorance of the schistosome-infested inshore waters.

Schistosomiasis had long been a chronic "disease of living" in precolonial Malawi. Parasitism by helminths was a "normal" and even expected part of people's lives. Howard (1910) reported on the high prevalence of Lekop, or cystitus, caused by the urinary form of schistosomiasis. He believed that it took "preeminence" among parasitic diseases in the UMCA's mission sphere.

Fecalized Environments: Helminthiases and the Parasitic Norm

If the local ecology did not favor schistosomiasis, the presence of other helminths in the human body was a certainty. Roundworms (*Ascaris*) grew nine to twelve inches long at maturity. Hookworms (*Ancylostoma*) and tapeworms were abundant and could be highly debilitating, especially in combination with undernutrition and other types of parasitism or infection. Dr. D. Kerr Cross, the government's Medical Officer in British Central Africa in the mid-1890s, identified threadworms as "the most common of all worms," particularly among people of younger age who were "poorly clothed and fed" (Cross 1897, 39). Curiously, Howard's (1910, 66–71) findings concerning the lakeshore peoples differ from Cross's. Roundworm was seen in only "a small number of cases," tapeworm ova had "not been seen at all," and "mild infections" of hookworm were "fairly common." The UMCA's Medical Officer observed that "the comparative immunity of the natives from intestinal parasites is probably attributable to the fact that they generally drink pure water from the lake" (68). Possibly the two views reflect different places and cultural ecologies. While the quality of drinking water could be expected to affect the transmission of roundworms, it would not explain lower levels of hookworm or the absence of tapeworm.

Parasitism by several organisms concurrently was the norm. As a rule, host and parasite adapted to one other. Schistosomiasis did not kill quickly or very often, although its debilitating course and infestation of organs ranging from the lungs to the rectum and bladder ultimately brought suffering to many that lived long enough. Hookworms, parasites of the duodenum, caused blood loss and anemia, and energy loss through depleting bodily reserves of iron. This in turn could amplify the potential harm of malaria and other diseases. Additional complications included bronchial inflammation and occasionally growth stunting, mental retardation, and death. In Malawi, as in the southeastern United States, hookworm remained endemic long after the means of controlling it was readily available. Referring to conditions prevailing around 1925, UMCA nurse Alice Simpkin wrote that "ankylostomiasis is perhaps the greatest scourge" and that it was claiming hundreds of Africans every year (Simpkin 1926, 28).

Contamination via feces was a significant environmental health problem everywhere, particularly in the case of hookworm. Risk heightened as population density increased and where topography made safe disposal of feces difficult. There is no evidence that any society in Malawi customarily used latrines or some other system of separating people from their waste. Consequently, "fecalized" environments (and rapid reinfestation by hookworms) were the norm around settlements.[5] Hookworm and various agents of diarrhea and dysentery spread most rapidly during the wet season, when surface drainage readily carried undetected fecal-borne parasites into closer human contact. While everyone was at risk, young children often bore the brunt of fecal-oral disease because of their contact with the soil. Overall, contact with human and animal excrement played a large role in keeping indigenous health at a much poorer level than was necessary.

Dysentery

Dysentery, a term embracing numerous diarrheal disorders marked especially by inflammation of the colon and loss of fluids, was probably always a concern of African populations.[6] It was a common hazard where domestic supplies of water were polluted. Epidemics often followed ethnic lines, one group suffering extensively while another would be spared (Headrick 1994). British colonials often called it the "bloody flux" (Cross 1897, 35). Howard claimed that it was uncommon on Likoma Island and "anywhere where people drink the [purer] lake water" (1910, 69). However, communities whose locations obliged them to rely on dirty water holes were at great risk, particularly towards the end of the dry season. Both the amoebic and bacillary forms of dysentery were present. UMCA hospitals used "emetin" to treat this condition (CA 40 [1922]: 71).

In the 1890s the social construction of dysentery among Europeans in Africa linked it to epidemic malaria. Causative factors typically included "great fatigue, under a blistering sun, together with badly cooked food, worse water, and tinned meats" (Cross 1897, 35). Colonial authorities reported the spread of acute forms of dysentery in the protectorate by the mid-1890s. A health report for the Ft. Johnston area in 1898 indicated that among Africans dysentery was more common than any other illness (Gelfand 1964, 298).

Tropical (phagedenic) Ulcers: Pervasive Disability

Tropical ulcers of various kinds were a common affliction that caused enormous disability, suffering, and even death in precolonial populations of Malawi, Kenya, and elsewhere. Only rarely do these problems receive even passing mention in historical accounts of disease, except in the medical or missions literature. In French Equatorial Africa tropical ulcers took an inordinate amount of doctors' and nurses' attention. In Gabon, for example, villagers and loggers were disabled for many weeks or months. Tropical ulcers required more hospitalization (an average stay of 48 days in Libreville) than any other disease. including yaws, dysentery, and respiratory ailments. During construction of the Congo-Ocean Railway (from 1922) tropical ulcers made up at least 40 percent of the sick cases, and nurses were heavily fined if a man arrived for work with an ulcer larger than a one-franc piece (Headrick 1994, 215, 307–8).

D. Kerr Cross (1987) devoted three pages to the subject in his manual. He observed that the sores, or degenerate tissue, occurred most often on the "legs and dependent parts." However, they could occur on any external or internal part of the body including mouth, stomach, bowels, eyes, nose, and skin. Ulcer etiology varied because an injury, poor circulation, or "a constitutional cause, such as syphilis, or trauma," could trigger it. A smelly discharge known as "ichor" was one of the telltale markers of the grayish, sloughing ulcers (125).

Chronic or callous ulcers were oval in shape, about 3.5 inches long, and outlined on the margins by a pale ring, hardened like gristle (ibid.). They tended to develop on the legs and signified those most commonly called "tropical" ulcers. Africans frequently endured them for years.

After European contact, ulcerated lesions became a key marker of the "unhealthy native." Their frequency and slow rate of healing, if left untreated, were linked to a poor diet and weakened constitution. The UMCA's Dr. Robert Howard, in "Some Types of Tropical Ulcers as Seen in Nyasaland," noted that a type known as Tropical Phagedaena was common on the Lake Malawi coast, "especially in those whose vitality is depressed by lack of food, or illness" (Howard 1908, 248). Acute septic ulcers, possibly starting with a boil, could affect any part of the body but commonly emerged on the leg. While less severe than Phagedaena, the infection and ulceration of the edges was reportedly worsened if the sufferer followed the local custom of tying leaves on the affected area to keep flies off. Since the leaves were usually not changed more than once weekly, the effect was a build-up and confinement of pus under a nonabsorbent covering. In four to six weeks of this procedure the ulcer's diameter would grow from 1.5 to 3 inches. By then the wound had become "intensely foul, and the surface covered with semi-liquid pus and small [grayish or yellowish] sloughs" (249).

There is no doubt that ulcers rank among the most important health problems in precolonial Malawi, and later, and that they have not received the attention they deserve in the history of tropical health. Arthur Fraser

Sim, a lone missionary isolated in the former slaving town of Kota Kota, expressed shock at the high percentage of the African population with ulcers. His diaries are peppered with references to them. In October 1894, he recorded that the prevalence of ulcers among women was particularly high. In another entry he observed that they are "many and dreadful, and my dawa [medicine] is giving out. . . . The people who come to me are those who have ulcers and wounds of every description. I am using permanganate of potash and Vaseline" (Sim 1897, 145, 154). On February 12, 1895, he described the ulcers he saw as "mostly of such long-standing, that even a doctor could not do anything more than dress them and make them keep the place clean" (183).

After nine years in the steamer parish, Dr. Howard (1908) wrote that ulcers remained one of the major reasons for performing surgery, under chloroform. Novarseno-benzol was the topical treatment of choice against various infections that spread through ulcerating lesions (*CA* 40 [1922]: 70). In her memoirs years later, Simpkin recalls the scene of a nursing visit to the large Nyanja settlement of Ngoo on the east coast of the lake. She was greeted by a group of eager school children, teachers, and the African Canon. Another group stood to the side: " . . . a pitiful sight: it comprises men old and young, women and children. The majority of them are disabled by large, sloughing ulcers, a deplorable condition, some uncovered, some with leaves tied over them with a string made of bark. One or two people are paralyzed, another nearly blind with a growing cataract, some are in the later stages of ankylostomiasis and can hardly walk" (Simpkin 1926, 14–15).

Since they affected such large numbers of people, there is little doubt that ulcers had anything but a profoundly debilitating effect on the quality of African life in precolonial Malawi. Their prevalence may have increased during the early years of colonial administration in connection with upheavals associated with taxation, migratory labor, and hiring of men by the protectorate administration. Stress and poor diets promoted malnutrition and susceptibility to ulcers in workers. The infections slowly tapered off under the influence of improved therapy and nutrition.[7] The point here is that ulcers were an endemic, pervasive, and systemic health problem, and a terrible cause of disability and suffering.

The Treponemas: Yaws, Syphilis, and Endemic Syphilis

Biologically, yaws is caused by the spirochete *Treponema pertenue*. Virtually indistinguishable from syphilis (*T. pallidum*), the agent is transmitted primarily nonsexually by direct person-to-person contact in unsanitary conditions. Scarring of the face and other parts of the body is typical. Years of chronic infection establish a cycle involving destruction of tissue, bone changes, and a shortening of toes or fingers that could be mistaken for leprosy (Miller and Keane 1987, 1352).

The weight of evidence indicates that yaws was very widely distributed throughout precolonial Malawi and the rest of tropical Africa. However, Western diagnostic techniques often failed to identify yaws cases as such, and colonial government and missionary doctors in more than one territory mistook the high incidence of yaws for widespread venereal syphilis. In her account of the situation in equatorial Uganda, Vaughan (1991, chap. 6) writes that, with the advent of British overrule, medical and church authorities became consumed by what they believed was a massive wave of epidemic syphilis. Diagnostic practices suggested that almost every African carried the infection. The social construction of syphilis took shape as a lengthy medico-moral debate ensued, beginning in the *Lancet* and the *British Medical Journal* in 1908. "Epidemic" syphilis was attributed to a breakdown of Ganda society and morals that was propelled, depending on one's opinion, either by the recent arrival of Western Christianity, or by a pitiable absence of European-style Christian values among the Africans. Women were singled out because it was believed that "syphilis" was clearly related to their growing sense of freedom from traditional social controls under the new colonial order. The dominant view that emerged was that with male authority over women now somewhat diminished, the latter acted on their new sexual autonomy. Construction of this problem was based on the belief that a flood of untamed passions was enticing women into promiscuity, with its prospect of venereal disease. Ganda chiefs and the male elite, sensing a loss of power, actively supported the colonial regime's public health campaign against syphilis. Many Ganda chiefs apparently believed that their people faced extinction if the syphilis epidemic persisted.

Uganda was subjected to a lengthy Venereal Diseases Campaign, but the "syphilis epidemic" persisted in one form or another until the late 1930s. By then new evidence indicated that for decades syphilis and yaws had been persistently misdiagnosed and misrepresented throughout Ugandan society. In 1938 the Medical Department admitted "many conditions previously considered to be syphilis are now being diagnosed as yaws."[8] Later on, Davies (1956) persuasively argued that the epidemiology of syphilis and yaws was a much more complex story than previously recognized. In his view, syphilis in Uganda had been misinterpreted from the start. In addition to its confusion with yaws, health personnel had too often confused "syphilis" with endemic syphilis—a chronic treponemal infection "indistinguishable from *T. pallidum*" (Miller and Keane 1987, 1200)—which mainly infected children and was not sexually transmitted. Davies suggests that what the early doctors in Uganda actually saw was both yaws and endemic syphilis, and a hybrid form of a more recent arrival—venereal syphilis.

In 1910, the UMCA's Dr. Howard observed that yaws was "very common in the villages along the eastern shore of the lake and in some parts the mothers seem to encourage infection in their children." In contrast, syphilis was "not common in the country districts and when it does occur it is mild, especially the secondaries, which seem to subside readily with native medicines. Congenital syphilis is rarely seen" (Howard 1910, 67).

Syphilis apparently existed at a low level in precolonial Malawi, but began a steady increase with the formation of towns and the loosening of customary social controls within kin groups. Since it was probably a relative late-comer to tropical Africa and was often introduced by Europeans,[9] syphilis entered a region where yaws (the two agents offer cross-immunity) was already deeply entrenched and nonimmune hosts were scarce. Yet within a few years of Howard's survey his successor, Dr. William Wigan (1911–47), indicated that "a very large proportion of the work was treating ulcers, chiefly of the legs (tropical), yaws and syphilis, and we had no Salvarsan or bismuth injections" (Gelfand 1964, 26, citing a letter received from Wigan in 1956). By then cases of STI, including syphilis, were steadily growing among the local Europeans and Africans alike.[10]

Unlike Uganda, yaws was apparently not confused with "syphilis" in Malawi. By 1920, nearly thirty years into British colonial administration, yaws seemed to be increasing in Malawi, particularly in the eastern and western lakeside villages (King and King 1991). Armed with syringes containing arsenic-based Neosalvarsan, missionary doctors, nurses, and African dressers could claim significant success in reducing the incidence of yaws during the 1920s and 1930s. Yaws persisted as a major public health problem and a cause of great misery for thousands in Malawi until the 1950s.

Leprosy

Leprosy, wrote Commissioner Harry Johnston in 1897, "is very common all over Africa," although rarely before puberty (Johnston 1897, 475). Both the lepromatous and tuberculoid forms of this ancient and often disfiguring and severely disabling disease, caused by *Mycobacterium leprae*, were endemic to central Africa. Between the two polar types there is a broad spectrum of clinical disease. Aerosol spread through inhalation of infected droplets and the discharge from lesions of persons with an active case serve as the prime methods of transmission. Sustained close contact with household members through blankets and other bedclothing, food, household objects, dust, arthropods, and mother's milk are among the factors strongly implicated as sources of infection (Hunter and Thomas 1987; Miller and Keane 1987, 701). One of the least contagious of diseases, leprosy gained the early attention of the UMCA, White Fathers, and other missions in Malawi (chap. 8).

Dr. Howard reckoned that the prevalence rate in the UMCA's sphere was about 1 leper per 1,000 of population (1910, 67). Later information would show that this rate grossly underestimated reality. Serological studies indicate that the majority of living Malawians over six years of age have been exposed to *M. leprae.* The actual prevalence level today has dropped below 20 per 1,000, and it is unlikely the leprosy rate in precolonial Malawi was lower (King and King 1991).[11] Hunter and Thomas (1987) hypothesized a degree of antagonism, or cross-immunological reactions, between tuberculosis and tuberculoid leprosy. Under African conditions of rapid urbanization, leprosy contracts while tuberculosis expands.

Smallpox: Uninvited Migrant, Feared Guest

Smallpox had traversed the Sahara and entered in the western Sudan by A.D. 1000. Reports of epidemics the late seventeenth and eighteenth centuries indicate it had spread to the West African coast and locations farther south. Circumstantial evidence for the mode of transmission southward points to sea transportation, although there is no reason to assume that smallpox had not been present earlier (Headrick 1994, 33). Infected crew members and passengers traveling aboard ships that called at Cape Town initiated smallpox epidemics there in 1713 (introduced from India), 1755, and 1767. These outbreaks seriously compromised the viability of the Cape's European colonial population. For the local Khoi pastoralists, already under great stress, smallpox spread with "terrible swiftness." It became a health and demographic disaster, "the survivors fleeing inland and carrying the disease with them" (Herbert 1975, 553).

In eastern Africa, the dhows that carried crews, passengers, and goods into and out of Lamu, Mombasa, Zanzibar, Kilwa, and other ports also helped to circulate pathogens among the varied epidemiological environments in which trade occurred. Trade with India was probably a key conduit for the spread of smallpox, although hard evidence of its presence before substantial European involvement in the region is scarce. Portuguese sources report a serious epidemic in 1589. One hypothesis is that smallpox spread from the coast into the interior of East Africa later than in West Africa because of the east's less-developed trade networks, and that the virus may not have arrived before 1800 (Patterson 1993).

Smallpox disfigured and killed. Some societies practiced forms of variolation or inoculation against it, and under certain conditions the benefits of doing so may have outweighed the risks (Herbert 1975; Headrick 1994). Smallpox was probably the most feared of all diseases in east-central Africa after the mid-nineteenth century. It spread deeper and deeper into the interior of Tanganyika and into the Congo Basin and Malawi along the caravan routes used by African elephant-hunters and coast traders. When smallpox struck a caravan, dying people were generally abandoned along the route. Kjekshus (1977) draws on Burton's observations, which captured the plight of a trading caravan in Tanganyika's Usagara Mountains that had been visited by epidemic smallpox. Burton witnessed its ravages in "the clean-picked skeletons, and here and there the swollen corpses, of porters who had perished" (Burton 1860, 1:165). Later on, Stanley noted that "the bleached skulls of the victims to this fell disease which lie along every caravan road, indicate but too clearly the havoc it makes annually" (Stanley 1872, 533). And he added, significantly, that smallpox's depredations were not confined "among the ranks of the several trading expeditions, but also among the villages of the respective tribes" in contact with them. Between 1875 and 1893 endemic smallpox epidemics erupted around the Arab-African town of Ujiji on Lake Tanganyika. Mortality rates reportedly reached 50 to 70 percent. Ujiji's base population was around three thousand in 1876, when Stanley estimated that smallpox was killing fifty to seventy of the population each day (Coquery-Vidrovitch 1988). At this rate, without vaccination and high herd immunity, everyone in Ujiji would have been dead within about two months.

Precolonial slave-raiding, ivory collection, and general commercial intercourse with the Indian Ocean coast, the Tanganyika interior, and the Zambezi basin offered efficient modes of transmission for the spread of the mild and major forms of epidemic smallpox that occurred around Lake Malawi. According to early European doctors, Africans in the Shiré Valley traditionally inoculated their children (on the web between the thumb and index finger) at the start of an epidemic, which conveyed lifelong immunity when it worked. People continued the identical practice into this century (Howard 1910). No one has identified its provenance, which suggests that smallpox has had considerable longevity in the region.

Reportedly, the cultures of Malawian tribes such as the Chewa, Ngoni, Tumbuka, and Tonga, commonly believed that it was a group's moral state that determined who survived a smallpox epidemic.[12] People in some societies showed awareness of the contagion principle and avoided going to funeral feasts during epidemics. Sim was more impressed by the lack of avoidance behavior at Kota Kota: "The careless way in which these people go in and out of the house and to other people's houses is enough to spread the disease to the whole town" (Sim 1897, 171). This alleged casual attitude might indicate a response to available information, and the fact that the town had had only one or two cases up to that time. Sim was alarmed because he had just been informed, correctly, that smallpox was already north and south of them on the west coast, at Bandawe, Ft. Johnston, and Blantyre.

Tick-borne Relapsing Fever

Tick-borne relapsing fever was endemic and occasionally epidemic close to the lake, but the vector was "rare or absent" in the hill country above it (Howard 1910, 67). Livingstone, who had been bitten by a "tampan" tick in Angola in 1857, was possibly the first to describe a potential relationship between the tick's bite and the fever.[13] The tick *Ornithodorous moubata* (nkufu) was the vector of this very serious and potentially disabling disease caused by the spirochete *Borrelia duttoni*. It infested the cracks and crevices in the walls of African dwellings and other unplastered structures. This tick added to the misery caused by mosquitoes, bedbugs, fleas, and other pests that invaded African dwellings. Together these pests often brought nightlong torture for the people on the inside. Alternatively, the health and security risks of trying to sleep outdoors were probably unacceptable to most people.

Early medical reports commented on the high prevalence of relapsing fever, noting that in certain localities blood slides often revealed that spirochetes were more commonly present than malaria parasites (Gelfand 1964). The tick passes the pathogen on to its progeny, and if necessary a single tick can live up to twenty years without its next blood meal. As people migrated, carried on trade relations, or relocated for security reasons the tick went along in their bedding and clothing. Adults typically acquired total or partial immunity through frequent exposure, or their relapses were not severe. In contrast, local children up to about sixteen and nonimmune visitors from beyond the lakeshore villages formed special risk groups for whom relapsing fever could be fatal.[14]

During the latter half of the colonial era relapsing fever received considerable attention from Medical Departments because the disease spread so efficiently along migratory labor routes and with urbanization.[15] One report for Malawi claims that a majority of cases occurred in the Northern and Central Regions, with a case-fatality rate of about 5 percent. Apart from

Howard's report in 1910, the UMCA's medical records show little evidence of this disease on the eastern side of the lake in the early 1900s. Significant progress in controlling and treating relapsing fever did not begin until after World War II, when the residual insecticide BHC ("Gammexane") and powerful antibiotics became available (Good 1978).

Respiratory Infections

Peoples of precolonial Malawi were also burdened with respiratory infections, including the common cold, bronchitis, and pneumonia. These illnesses surely affected most Africans, although there were undoubtedly important variations in risk and distribution based on the seasons, the density of human settlements, altitude, ethnicity, age, gender, and occupation. Infants could quickly progress from a simple to a dangerous respiratory ailment if they were not kept dry and warm. High numbers of premature babies probably also added to the mortality (Headrick 1994, 149). Smoke from fires burning inside poorly ventilated huts and kitchens would have contributed to respiratory problems. In addition, chronic eye irritation, possible endemic trachoma, and higher rates of blindness might then be predicted sequelae.

Recruitment of men for work in the mines of South African and Southern Rhodesia exacerbated, as never before, the risk of pneumonia and other diseases. For example, during an eight-month period in 1908, 113 of 774 (146 per 1,000) Malawian recruits died in Southern Rhodesia, principally from pneumonia.[16]

Epilepsy

Many other health-related factors conditioned the quality of individual and village life, including accidents (burns, drownings, injuries by wild animals), tetanus (Gelfand 1964, 41), epilepsy, and polio. Cross (1897) reported that epilepsy was "very common," and Johnston observed that "falling sickness is very common, strange to say. Very often it is seen in children and young people" (Johnston 1897, 477). Epilepsy was a common disease of the nervous system with frequent hysterical symptoms. In Howard's (1910, 69) view, the African population generally linked epilepsy to ideas about bewitchment or poisoning. Stigma could push an epileptic into the status of a *masikini,* a person without home or possessions.[17] Seizures near fires have probably always been a virtually unpreventable risk for epileptics. As survivors attest today, many who fall into a fire bear the scars and added disability of that terrible trauma (cf. Simpkin 1926, 27).

For more than three decades Archdeacon Johnson's life was one with the mission steamers. During the early days (1885–1900) he observed that villages in the UMCA's sphere "often [had] bad cases of epilepsy" for whom help was tenuous at best. Sometimes the sufferer "had lost his kindred or may have originally been a slave, and often the wretched man becomes through suffering quite unable to control himself" (Johnson 1926, 144). Epilepsy, it seems, was not an affliction others could accept with equanimity. Johnson pitied one impoverished epileptic man who was being pestered by some young males. "In a weak moment, perhaps, I took him into my house for safety, but his enemies were not beaten off lightly. They got a long bamboo and were poking at him with it between the poles which formed the outside of the house, which had not been plastered with mud" (ibid.). Finding it difficult to "defend" the epileptic and also manage the school, Johnson put him on the steamer and accompanied him to Likoma. He proved "unmanageable" aboard the steamer and even more at Likoma. In the end, there seemed no alternative than to "put him on a small island in the harbour and send him his food daily" (145). The epileptic, perhaps sarcastically, named this place *Sikuwa-po* ("I am not all here"), a designation still known to some in the 1920s.

Cancers

By all accounts malignant neoplasms were uncommon or even rare in pre-colonial Malawi. Dr. D. Kerr Cross reported that he had observed one case of breast cancer, this in a woman who had allegedly traveled over 450 miles to see him (Johnston 1897, 474). Bladder carcinoma occurred in association with chronic schistosomiasis infection. It was frequently seen in the Lower Shiré Valley during the colonial era, and in principle it would have been common among adults in Lake Malawi's coastal settlements before colonialism (King and King 1991). However, aside from the unusual case, colonial medical accounts typically dismissed cancers as an African health problem. It was "undoubtedly rare" to find malignant tumors in the UMCA's sphere. During his tenure, Dr. Howard operated on one patient for "sarcoma of the eyeball," and another had a sarcoma of the skull. In a third case, "sarcoma of the upper jaw," Burkitt's lymphoma was implicated (Howard 1910, 70).

King and King (1991) draw radically different conclusions from evidence of cancer available today. They maintain that the attention of pioneer doctors, whether in government or mission service, focused almost entirely on infectious diseases, trauma, and environmental sanitation.[18] They had little time to assess the incidence and prevalence of cancers. Moreover, microscopical examination of tissue was not available until 1928. When medical schools such as Makerere in Uganda opened after World War II, cancer research capabilities expanded significantly.

Several types of cancer undermined the health of many Malawians before 1890. Sites included the liver (strongly associated with the Hepatitis B virus and cirrhosis),[19] cervix (linked to early births, multiple pregnancies, genital herpes [HSV], and human papilloma viruses [HPV], uncircumcised male partners), and probably Kaposi's sarcoma. HPV is sexually transmitted and reportedly leads to 20 to 35 percent of all cervical cancer in women sub-Saharan Africa. Carcinoma of the penis is also common, primarily in uncircumcised men with poor hygiene and HPV infection.[20]

Liver, bladder, esophageal, and cervical carcinomas have been recognized as "African tumors" for several decades, with high rates in all populations studied and higher rates for the same sites than in North America and Europe. Carcinomas of the cervix and liver are in general the most important causes of cancer deaths in Africa.[21] Liver cancer is the most common malignancy south of the Sahara and is almost always associated with cirrhosis. Several studies, beginning in the 1930s and particularly from the 1960s, have uncovered a wider distribution and a more complicated spectrum of cancers than previously recognized (Hutt 1991).

There was almost certainly a burden of *in situ* and earlier-onset cancers in Malawi long before the territory's exposure to colonialism and new environmental factors. Today, for instance, the incidence and mortality rates for esophageal cancer in Malawi (male-predominant) rank among Africa's highest, and it appears to have increased over the past half-century. To assume that esophageal cancer (as well as the other carcinomas already identified) was insignificant or even nonexistent in precolonial Malawi is unwarranted. Beer brewed with maize—a widespread practice in east and central Africa today—has come under strong suspicion as an etiological factor in cancer of the esophagus (Cook 1971).[22] However, alcohol or contaminants in it evidently are not obligatory for this cancer (Vogel et al. 1974, 385). Thus other factors may have been present also, especially since maize is thought to have gained the status of a staple in Malawian diets quite late—"after Livingstone's visits in the mid-1800 and before 1910" (Miracle 1966, 155).

Burkitt's lymphoma is distributed across tropical Africa in a broad belt that extends south from Uganda and Zaire into Zimbabwe, Malawi and Mozambique. Its spatial association with altitude, temperature, and rainfall produced the hypothesis that the tumor is connected to endemic malaria (Burkitt 1970). This argument is buttressed by the theory that Burkitt's lymphoma is "triggered" by infection with the herpes-like Epstein-Barr virus in young children who have experienced "early and heavy [malaria] infection" and whose immune responses have been compromised (Hutt 1991, 230). An opportunistic infection produced by interaction of the virus and malaria apparently creates the tumor.

Evidence gathered since the 1960s makes it reasonable to postulate that Burkitt's lymphoma, as rapid-growth tumor(s) mainly located in the jaw of children under fifteen years of age, was also common in precolonial Malawi. Today it accounts for around 30 percent of all tumors in Malawian children. All African children with the tumor also present Epstein-Barr antibodies, and the virus remains widely present in their communities. Vincristine, a cytotoxic drug derived from the flowers of *Vinca* spp., grows around houses in many of Malawi's villages. It reportedly offers an effective treatment that kills cells and shrinks the tumors (King and King 1991).

Skin cancer also illustrates how disease is usually multifactoral, where health is even more compromised by secondary and tertiary factors. As previously noted, tropical ulcers, especially on the lower leg, had caused widespread, incalculable suffering among a large proportion of the pre-colonial population of Malawi. Factors favoring the development of ulcers include persistent irritation around a break in the skin, coupled with lack of hygiene and malnutrition. Timely treatment produces healing without secondary complications. On the other hand, chronic tropical ulcers can become cancerous (squamous cell carcinoma) when there is cyclical break-down and rehealing of the tissues in and especially at the edges of the wound. Erosion of shin bone by the malignant ulcer may even make it necessary to amputate the foot or lower leg (Hutt 1991, 230; King and King 1991, 145). Otherwise gangrene was usually a "rapidly fatal disease" (Howard 1910, 67).

Circumstantial evidence suggests that effective indigenous therapies for tropical ulcer did not exist in precolonial Malawi. Pioneer mission and government doctors can perhaps be forgiven if they did not recognize that skin cancer was a public health problem in the melanin-rich populations of tropical Africa. On the other hand, they did not fail to see the ubiquitous and disabling tropical ulcer.

Eye Diseases and Sight Loss

Blindness, brought on by trachoma, conjunctivitis, cataracts, smallpox, measles, leprosy, or other causes, exacted a terrible toll of suffering and lost human potential. Writing at the end of his tenure in Nyasaland, Howard saw very many "old perforated corneal ulcers," and estimated that about half were due to smallpox (1910, 70). In 1904 he set up a school for the blind at the UMCA's Kota Kota station, and around this time the government began a

systematic vaccination campaign (compulsory from 1908) using African vaccinators (King and King 1991, 56). Trachoma infections, which drove many
people to pull out their eyelashes, must have been widely implicated in the
causes of blindness. Ophthalmic neonatorum, spread via gonorrhea, may
have been another substantial contributor to the level of blindness (Kiple
1993). Old people with cataracts ran the risk of neglect. Iliffe asserts that
unless they had stature in village affairs, many elderly probably died from
concurrent maladies before their cataract was ready for removal (Iliffe 1984,
250). Rates of blindness in the southern third of colonial Malawi ranked
among the world's highest. The colonial administration choose not to make
blindness one of its concerns, preferring by default to treat it as a missionary
activity until a few years before decolonization (272).

   Three blind males were learning Braille at the Church of Scotland Mission at Bandawe in 1899. In 1905 the UMCA responded, teaching Braille
and handicrafts at its Blind School in Kota Kota. By 1908 the Kota Kota
had around twenty blind males of different ages in residence as "Children
of the Mission" (*CA* 23 [1905]; 24 [1906]; 27 [1909]). Private (secular) voluntary assistance did not arrive until the 1950s, when a branch of the British
Empire Society for the Blind was set up. Later projects included handicraft
and skills for farming; but as Iliffe (1984, 272) emphasizes, they touched only
a small fraction of the blind population.

Wildlife and Human Safety

One of the more important threats to public health came from human encounters with wildlife. Sometimes missionary accounts allegedly sensation-
alized the dangers of wild animals in order to play to the "Darkest Africa"
fantasies and sympathies of their home constituencies. There is undoubtedly
some truth in this perception. However, there is also abundant documentation that maiming and serious accidents, including fatal encounters with
dangerous animals such as crocodiles, hippopotomi, lions, hyenas, leopards,
and snakes, and occasionally buffaloes and elephants, exacted a toll far beyond anyone's imagination or threshold of tolerance today (Simpkin 1926,
29; in their index, King and King [1991] reference "animal injuries" twelve
times). Fatal and crippling injuries caused by teeth, claws, and shock were
commonplace. Sepsis worsened many casualties.

   Injuries caused by human contact with wild animals continued long into
the colonial period. Europeans in Malawi did not have to invent such stories
from romantic impulse. In 1903, a nurse at Kota Kota emphasized that the
"crocodiles here are dreadful. There is about one death every week." In

1911, Aldwyn Cox, a UMCA priest at Kota Kota, said "There is no question at all that our natives live in constant danger from wild beasts and suffer terribly." He added, in contrast, that "attacks on Europeans are of the rarest occurrence. . . . You are as likely to be killed in a railway accident in Europe than by a lion in Africa" (*CA* 38 [1912]: 23). Near the end of his tenure in the steamer parish, Dr. Howard published a surgical report of twenty nonfatal cases admitted to his hospital, including leopard (7), lion (5), hyena (4), crocodile (3), and hippopotamus (1). He noted that "fatal injuries from wild beasts are common, but death generally occurs rapidly, or the patient does not live to reach hospital, or his friends make up their minds that he will die and refuse to bring him there" (Howard 1909, 334). Lions killed at least forty people during a three-month period at Kota Kota (*CA* 36 [1918]: 44).

Alice Simpkin wryly described the risk from wild animals as "a group not found in England." She emphasized that men, women, and children were normally in considerable danger of being mauled by animals. In a single day at the UMCA's Kota Kota Hospital, Simpkin witnessed one man who had been mauled by a lion, two by crocodiles, and another two by leopards (Simpkin 1926, 29). Amputation was a common procedure. Certainly among precolonial Malawians the threat posed to life and limb by wild animals was real.

EXOTIC MICROBES: CORRIDORS OF INFECTION AND CONTAGION

Afro-Arab traders and European explorers and military personnel and their more numerous African, Indian, and other subordinates, such as porters and conscripts, brought accelerated contact between African populations and exotic disease. This process had begun decades before Europe's great nationalistic "scramble" to control all African territories in the 1880s and 1890s (Kjekshus 1977). Eurasian diseases, including typhoid, cholera, whooping cough, and tuberculosis, though possibly still "rare" in 1900 (Howard 1910, 67), had almost certainly reached Malawi's lake region by 1890, and in some cases long before. Cross (1897) observed that whooping cough was an increasingly common disease among African children, and that no special treatment was available. Cholera is curiously absent from his lengthy medical handbook.

As the following examples illustrate, substantial evidence favors the validity of the second element in Richards's typology of African epidemiology (see above). From the mid-nineteenth century onwards growing numbers of traders, adventurers, troops, slaves, and others rubbed shoulders with peoples in the interior and coastal areas of East and South-Central Africa. These contacts virtually guaranteed the introduction of new health hazards. In this prelude to colonialism many kinds of nascent infrastructures were changing the human geography. Both intentionally and unwittingly, a process had begun that would dramatically increase the variety and severity of health risks in many parts of the wider region.

Christie's (1876) well-known investigation of cholera diffusion from Zanzibar into the vast East African interior is perhaps the best-documented study of its time. A medical officer at Zanzibar, Christie interviewed caravan leaders and European missionaries, and used European reports, including Burton's eyewitness accounts of the 1858–59 epidemic in Tanganyika. He mapped some of the trade routes that spread the cholera inland in four major epidemics: 1821, 1836–37, 1858–59, and its "devastating" return in 1869–70 (Hartwig 1978).

Burton (1860) reported that "we lost nearly all our crew to cholera." It had decimated the eastern coast of Arabia and Africa, including Pemba and Zanzibar Islands—which by then had key roles in the Indian Ocean commercial empire controlled by the Omani Arabs. Cholera killed some twenty thousand people on Zanzibar within a four-month period in 1858–59 (Hartwig 1978, 28). From there it moved to the mainland coastal settlements, including those in southern Tanganyika, and many towns were almost depopulated. The epidemic then spread radially into the East African interior, where it was propagated in small settlements along hundreds of miles of trade routes. It moved north into Kenya, causing heavy mortality. It also spread northwest into the Buganda Kingdom, where it was a known killer before Speke arrived at Kabaka Mutesa's court in 1862 during his second quest to locate the Nile's source. Other trade routes fanned out to the west from Indian Ocean towns, stretching more than seven hundred miles across Tanganyika's central plateau and the Nyamwezi country to Ujiji on Lake Tanganyika. Farther south on the Tanganyika coast other trade corridors ran southwesterly and reached the northern and western coasts of Lake Malawi. Several routes from Kilwa Kiswani and Kilwa Kivinje connected with slave ports and markets on the eastern side of Lake Malawi, raising the real possibility that cholera was known though unrecorded as such.

Plague's extension into Central Africa was apparently part of a pandemic that originated in China in 1894. In his *The Lake Regions of Central Africa* (1860), Burton noted Arab reports of plague (*Yersina pestis*) in Karagwe in northwest Tanganyika. Plague may have existed in Malawi before colonial rule, although a recent study claims that the first recorded introduction was in 1917 (King and King 1991, 67). The earliest record of plague cases near Malawi reportedly occurred in 1905 at Chinde, a trade center and entry port for British Central Africa on the Mozambique coast. It was first identified within Malawi in 1916 at Karonga, where a campaign in 1917 trapped and killed over three million rats in an attempt to wipe out the plague host (ibid.). At the time a doctor noted that "trapping is carried out by small boys, and to some extent by women, who day after day troop in with their catches, and at the end of the month . . . it was a common sight to see a small boy of about 10 year of age receiving as much as 16–25 shillings" for his rat tails.[23]

Trade and pilgrimage routes have always provided efficient channels that microbes have used to disperse into nonimmune host populations. The situation in East and Central Africa was no exception. In this context Kjekshus's (1977) caveat about "the persistent error of talking about the trade route" has great epidemiological importance. There was not a single and permanent route leading, for instance, from Bagamoyo to Ujiji, or from Tabora to Mengo. Such termini were connected through a network of roads and pathways centered on all the viable communities found in the general trading direction:[24]

"This opened the possibility for temporary adjustments of itineraries to local events affecting the supply problems. . . . Several parallel routes existed inland from Kilwa where supply problems were in evidence. . . . Caravan transport operated on very different principles [from mechanized transportation]. It was human porterage working along an infrastructure of local opportunities for provisioning of barter commodities, food and water resources, and the hiring of substitute carriers. Practically all the major caravan routes of the late nineteenth century fell within the likely trading radius of centres of industrial production [iron, salt, cotton weaving]. (Kjekhus 1977, 122)"

These trade routes and networks connected and stimulated intercourse among near and distant towns and villages. They also readily circulated disease agents, including such sources as bacteria in food; fecally contaminated drinking water; bedding and clothing infested with ticks and lice; and close human contacts producing exchanges of aerosols, body fluids, and mites. Caravans frequently numbered hundreds of people, sometimes more. Local and regional trade networks informally tied into the long-distance trade routes, some of which extended more than 1,000 miles from the coast into Zaire and Zambia. During the many months of a caravan's journey it would come in contact with numerous settlements and therefore, at least indirectly, thousands of people who were potentially at risk for infections imported from the Eurasian, New World, and African pools.

Greatly expanded long-distance commerce in slaves, ivory, and trade goods provided a potent mechanism for the contagious and hierarchical spread of new microbes throughout the vast interior of east-central Africa. Trade served as an epidemiological "bridge" for vectors and disease agents. It facilitated the emergence and linkage of interconnected populations of microbes and people in Zanzibar and other coastal locations with interior zones of Tanganyika, Malawi, Zambia, Uganda, and eastern Zaire (with Rwanda and Burundi).

Events in Malawi further illustrate how, in the two centuries before the colonial conquest, both internal and external stimuli helped to reshape the disease environment through unwitting human design. A case in point is the Maravi Confederation of the seventeenth and eighteenth centuries, which developed from a focus on the southwest coast of Lake Malawi. With access to important sources of ivory, the confederation gradually extended its influence beyond modern Malawi into Zambia and to the Mozambique coast via the Zambezi Valley.

Sleeping Sickness: Upsetting the Environmental Balance

Kjekshus (1977) illuminates how "ecological control" was consciously manipulated and maintained by precolonial societies in Tanganyika. He theorizes that in East Africa ecology-control was "the crucial variable in the history of the nineteenth century" (67). Indigenous herders and cultivators forged an environmental contract "out of centuries of civilizing work of clearing the ground, introducing managed vegetations, and controlling the fauna" (181). Adjustments to these time-tested relationships had produced what Ford termed an "agro-horticultural prophylaxis" (Ford 1971, 474). The prevention effect came about through a combination of synergistic management techniques that over time helped to neutralize the risks of exposure of people and livestock to *Glossina,* the tsetse vector, and to the trypanosomiases. This enabled them to carry on well-developed and articulated economic activities with the threat of epidemic sleeping sickness greatly reduced. Tragically, these complex ecological arrangements were widely disrupted with the advent of an often harsh German occupation in the 1890s and, from 1919, British colonial rule. Early colonialist interventions against sleeping sickness proved dangerous, based as they were on a profound ignorance of delicately balanced tsetse-environment-health relationships. Later colonial attempts to manipulate the landscape epidemiology, including land abandonment and population relocation, often had the primary goal of exploiting African labor for the benefit of the colonial economy (Kjekshus 1977). Tanganyika's hypothesized "ecological collapse" in the 1890s was the product of evolving, convergent, and interactive health and environmental traumas, complicated by the loss of indigenous control.

In addition to the demographic and social effects of smallpox, jiggers, and plague, a catastrophic rinderpest epizootic broke out in Somaliland in 1889. The Italian military had imported infected cattle from India, Aden, and South Russia to feed their troops at Massawa. Local herds of cattle, sheep, and goats had no prior exposure and quickly died as the disease spread southward and across most of East Africa and into southern Africa, its virulence increasing. Buffalo, giraffe, and eland in its path, as well antelopes, warthogs, bushpigs and forest hogs, were also killed off. Contemporary observers estimated that mortality among the region's tens of thousands of cattle exceeded 95 percent (Reader 1998, 589–90, citing Davies 1979, 16). Among the pastoral Maasai the resulting famine killed two-thirds of the human population. Kjekshus (1977) asserts that rinderpest was the leading edge of what became nearly a generation-long period of unusual vulnerability to natural and human-caused disasters in East Africa.

Loss of ecological control and negative feedback—exemplified by depopulation of cattle and people, the breakdown of barriers separating people and tsetse, and the incursion and rapid diffusion of rinderpest (which tremendously amplified the collapse)—demonstrate a basic principle. It is imperative to recognize the existence of multiple pathways when interpreting disease processes and patterns. Rinderpest is clearly an epidemic disease of exotic origin that capitalized on ease of entry via the emerging corridors and networks of a nascent colonialism. In contrast, the dynamic ecosystems in Richards's (1983) typology help to conceptualize and explain the interplay of microlevel processes of disease ecology. Critical interrelationships that exist in the bushlands, Brachystegia, and other light-forest zones occupied by both humans and tsetse provide a good illustration of this approach.

Tsetse and sleeping sickness undoubtedly also figured in Malawi's precolonial ecology and disease potential. Yet a sense of how the flies, trypanosomes, and human and animal populations involved were distributed and interacted must rely heavily on speculation. Information available in the 1890s indicated that extensive areas of this region, outside the highlands, were infested with tsetse. Later on the flies were identified as primarily *Glossina morsitans*, vectors of both human and animal trypanosomiasis, as in Tanganyika.[25]

The first confirmed case of sleeping sickness was identified in the far north of Malawi at Karonga in 1908 in a man who had traveled to, and had presumably been infected in, Tanganyika. Subsequently more systematic collection of blood smears revealed the presence of *Trypanosoma rhodesiense* in individual and clustered cases in central and southern parts of the protectorate. Given the catastrophic epidemic of human sleeping sickness around Lake Victoria in Uganda, and Tanganyika's problems, in 1910–11, the Royal Society sent one of its several Sleeping Sickness Commissions to investigate the disease in Malawi (McKelvey 1973). Sick people had been showing up in West Nyasa, Kota Kota, Mvera (Dutch Reformed Mission Hospital), and other locations mainly west and south of the lake, and by 1913 a total of 163 cases had been confirmed. Ultimately a discontinuous, primary tsetse-belt was delimited in parts of the modern districts of Kota Kota, Dowa, Mangochi, Dedza, and Machinga/Liwonde.[26] Sporadic cases of sleeping sickness continued during and after the colonial era (King and King 1991, 114–16).

Europeans' experience with the tsetse and its protozoan companion led to the construction of a disease whose associations with Africa's perceived dangerousness was rivaled only by malaria. Unfortunately, much of the African experiences with tsetse in Malawi's precolonial past will remain in the shadows. Nonetheless, one can argue reasonably that the Malawi region did not experience anything that remotely resembled the kinds of epidemic assaults and ecological disturbances (e.g., bush-intensification and tsetse invasion induced by depopulation of humans and livestock on the heels of rinderpest) visited upon its northern neighbor at the start of the colonial era. It avoided the vast disruption of livelihood patterns, and it escaped large outbreaks of sleeping sickness and the compulsory herding of tens of thousands of people into sleeping sickness settlements.

Fortunately, Malawians also did not have to contend with *G. palpalis*, the "waterside" tsetse, and its deadly collaborator *T. gambiense*, which joined forces to kill hundreds of thousands of Ugandans at the beginning of the twentieth century. We also know that sleeping sickness was not a preoccupation, and rarely a concern, of the UMCA and other medical missions. It is indicative that in his survey of human diseases on the coast of Lake Malawi Howard (1910) mentions albinism, geophagy, and varicose veins ("rare"), but makes no reference to tsetse or sleeping sickness.

Jiggers

The coming of sand fleas, or jiggers (*Tungas penetrans* or *Sarcopsylla penetrans*), presented another widespread health threat to both Africans and Europeans. In a classic form of diffusion through human mobility, these insects entered

Africa at the port of Ambriz in Angola. They had been transported there in the sand ballast of a British ship bound from Rio de Janeiro. Spreading along caravan routes, it took only twenty-five years for the sand flea to migrate completely across the continent and then leapfrog to Zanzibar, and thereafter to Malawi.

Impregnated sand fleas deposit their larvae under the toenails or between the toes, or beneath the fingernails. The eggs cluster in sacs that grow to pea size. After incubation the sand flea is ejected, scattering thousands of eggs on the ground. The insects emerge a week later, ready to invade human tissue. Profound suffering may result, brought on by sores that easily form in the cavities created by the sand fleas (Cross 1897, 17). If neglected or improperly treated, the open sores become infected and can progress from painful ulceration, blood poisoning, and gangrene to loss of toes and feet, and even to death. The organism can also migrate to other parts of the body, erupting as boils on a leg or arm.

Removal of sand flea eggs was best done with a needle, followed by treatment of the wound with carbolic acid, iodoform, and glycerin. Egg extraction became an art form. For many Europeans in early Malawi, "it was part of one's morning toilet to have jiggers removed from one's feet by native experts" (Cardew 1955, 63). In neighboring Tanganyika, Baumann, the noted German explorer and ethnologist, observed in 1894 that Africans who had learned and practiced daily jigger extraction, and kept their feet clean, could avoid this "plague." Otherwise, the consequences could be tragic, including lameness. Particularly in areas where the sand flea occurred for the first time, and where its treatment was unknown, its impact was devastating. Said Baumann, "We saw people in Uzinza whose limbs had disintegrated. Whole villages had died out on account of this vexation" (Baumann 1894, 72, cited in Kjekshus 1977, 135).

In Malawi, European reports state that jiggers were unknown in the coastal villages bordering the lake until 1892, when the flea arrived from the Arab-run slave center of Karonga in the far north. From there it spread south to Ft. Johnston (near Mponda's and Malindi), spanning the lake's entire length, in less than a year. By 1906, jiggers had infested virtually the entire sphere in which the UMCA was pursuing its evangelical, educational, and medical activities. It had become "the scourge of the Yao Hills" on the eastern side of the lake, and sufferers had a characteristic "jiggers walk" (King and King 1991, 69). The UMCA's medical landscape now acquired "Jigger hospitals," erected at Mtonya (1908) and Malindi, to cope with this seemingly intractable pest.

Tuberculosis

The presence of tuberculosis (TB) in precolonial tropical Africa has not been established (Koch first identified the bacillus in 1882). Reportedly, it was not native to Malawi, and not introduced into sub-Saharan Africa until the nineteenth century (Rodriguez 1991, citing Budd 1867). King and King (1991, 78) note that the "first named death from TB in the country" was an African missionary from South Africa who had been working with Robert Laws and the Scottish Presbyterians at Cape Maclear. The UMCA's Howard asserted that TB was "a rare disease" in 1900, essentially confined to "villages along the slave and trade routes, whither infection was carried from the coast" (1910, 67).[27] But by 1910 colonialism had opened the territory and exposed the population to TB and other debilitating conditions as never before, especially through the thousands of men already migrating to Southern Rhodesia and South Africa for work. Malawians in general had no immunological experience with TB, or "phthisis." It did not take long to enter Malawi once migrants became exposed. Although the true incidence of TB remained unknown, the number of cases increased threefold between 1928 and 1948, and "relentlessly" thereafter. Just prior to independence the disease had begun to overshadow other health problems, with TB patients occupying 800 hospital beds in 1962 (King and King 1991, 79).

Following World War I, some Europeans, including medical missionaries, spoke frankly about exotic diseases like tuberculosis that whites and others in the colonialist advance had introduced into Africa. Health conditions had deteriorated, they confessed, "under the influx of civilization," and labor demands had created conditions enabling men to spread diseases from place to place as never before. African diseases quickly sought advantage wherever European activities and dictates had upset ecological balances, often affecting the food supply. Speaking at the International Conference on "The Christian Mission in Africa" in Le Zoute (Belgium) in 1926, Dr. Broden from the Belgian Congo admitted that "our ignorance of the exact nature of many of the tropical diseases and their mode of transmission favoured their extension by the progress of civilization" (Smith 1926, 75). In the end, these disruptions and costs were a "lamentable" price to pay, yet they had to be judged against "the new discoveries and the strenuous efforts now being made to rectify past errors and grapple with disease" (76).

LOCAL DEMOGRAPHY AND WELL-BEING

Population in nineteenth-century Malawi was probably in decline for several decades prior to the establishment of the British protectorate (Kuczynski 1949, 2:638). High birth and death rates, high infant and maternal mortality, and low life expectancy dominated African demography. Malaria, always a threat below an elevation of 5,000 feet, and frequent pregnancies contributed to low hemoglobin levels among women. Large elements of the population could not avoid the depredations of the Arab-African slave trade, nor the highly mobile Ngoni (Gwangwara) marauders who caused so much violence and social havoc during the 1870s through 1890s.

From around 1860 onwards the mounting incursions of missionaries and traders into the lake region made political conditions even more insecure, and often bewildering. During the first thirty years of colonial rule deaths probably exceeded births, and population continued to decline. In 1921 the first census counted 1.2 million people. At 76 : 100 males to females, the sex ratio for persons of marriage age offered dramatic evidence of profound changes that colonial policies had already fostered in the organization of family life and labor patterns (van Velsen 1961). Thereafter a small but slow natural increase was observed up to 1945 (Gregory and Mandala 1987).

In the nineteenth century, few Africans living in what is now Malawi would have met the minimal standard of what today are called "basic human needs." Iliffe asserts that debilitating "material poverty was the lot of virtually all nineteenth century Malawians," while smaller, particular populations such as refugees from Ngoni raiders qualified as the "notoriously impoverished" (Iliffe 1984, 250). They had fallen into the state of *umphawi*, a Chewa word meaning dire poverty. A dictionary from 1892 translated the same term to mean "misery, slavery, friendlessness," while a later Nyanja vocabulary defined *umphawi* as "the state of being without relations." Structural poverty also produced many orphans, including half-caste children.[28] Most were castaways from the slave trade and other violence that persisted unchecked through the nineteenth century. Some orphans appear to have been enslaved. Not a few found eager acceptance into the embrace of the pioneer missions. Sim observed that most of the children attending the UMCA's new school at Kota Kota were the poorer ones, "and strangely too most of them are without parents—these have died or been killed. We could form an orphanage here for little castaways, whose people [presumably not the parents] do not care two-pence about them" (Sim 1897, 202).

Dr. John Kirk, who in 1861 accompanied Livingstone along the malarial west coast south of Kota Kota, near today's Salima, reported that the population was sickly and poorly nourished: "Disease is frequent; we see many cases of leprosy and other skin diseases, diseases of the eye, club foot, and other deformities of the limbs" (Kirk 1965, cited in King and King 1991, 10). The infant death rate was high, and many people had been scarred by smallpox. Livingstone, who trained at Glasgow Medical School, also reported seeing numerous skin diseases, including leprosy and elephantiasis (filariasis) on this same coast. In addition to the sources of illness already noted, many Malawian peoples were at risk for mumps, chickenpox, *chikuku* (a milder measles-like disease), and possibly whooping cough. Babies and younger children surely suffered from frequent episodes of gastroenteritis with its life-threatening risk of dehydration.

Endemic goiter, produced by iodine deficiency, was reportedly "common" in 1912 in villages in Dedza District. The zones affected ranged from the lakeshore to the top of the dramatic Rift escarpment, some 3,500 feet higher (King and King 1991). One authority asserts that it is now generally accepted that goiter, while endemic in much of Africa today, "did not occur anywhere on the African continent until the nineteenth or twentieth century" (Hanegraaf 1974, 395). Such a view is questionable in light of the continent's geology. However, goiter was possibly a disease that noticeably worsened in some places due to the economic and social effects of colonialism, such as forced resettlement and dietary changes.

Seasonal hunger, probably often accompanied by significant loss of body weight, was the norm between November and February when crops were growing. Sim (1897, 107) identified April and May as the "unhealthy months" along the west coast of the lake, around Kota Kota. Food deficits were then greatest, nutrition poorest, and resistance to disease was at its lowest. Food shortages occurred almost every year in the Rift Valley at the southern end of the lake (Linden 1974, 31).

The nineteenth century's most devastating hunger struck Malawi during 1861–63. In 1863 a member of the UMCA's first pioneer missionary team recorded that "the famine brought starvation to virtually all sections of the [Shiré] valley's population" (Iliffe 1984, 251–52). In time, the imposition of colonialism brought greater political stability and, sometimes, limited assistance during hungry seasons. Unfortunately, the Pax Britannica also instigated a new and pervasive structural poverty that alienated many resources Africans had controlled, particularly labor and the soil (250). This process also affected nutrition, and could only have had a deleterious effect on family and community health.

Precolonial Malawians generally displayed remarkable resilience in the face of adversity and a wide assortment of health insults. However, the contents of table 6.1 counter any mistaken assumptions that precolonial African societies, including Malawi's, "enjoyed an idyllic life free from endemic disease" (for further critique of this idea, see Arnold 1988, 5). Against depressing odds, most of the time enough people survived myriad assaults on their immunological systems to maintain fertility at levels sufficient to reestablish their lineages and descent groups. Despite the endemic high mortality rates, successful reproductive strategies ultimately enabled most societies to transcend the hunger episodes, endemic and epidemic diseases, violence, and anomie that promoted and exploited social weakness and demographic weaknesses. Yet such success came at an enormous cost in human life and potential.

"EMPTY VESSEL"?

When medical missionaries arrived on the scene in Malawi they did not find an "empty vessel," or medical care vacuum, waiting for them to fill. Systems of indigenous medicine had long been in place in every ethnic group, created over time in each society to serve peoples' many physical, mental, and spiritual needs (Kappa 1980; Peltzer 1987; Morris 1989). Traditional medical practitioners (*asing'anga*) included various kinds of herbalists as well as diviners and other ritual specialists. They fulfilled integral roles that were inseparable from the functioning of each society. Every man, woman, and child came under their collective influence for life. *Asing'anga* provided divination (*maula*), treated physical disease, dispensed herbal and other medicines, and performed essential rituals. They gave advice to help people cope with the mind-body illnesses and conflicts that could disrupt interpersonal and social relations. Midwives delivered babies. Other specialists provided supernatural means of protecting personal and family resources, including young children; protected against or relieved the consequences of witchcraft and sorcery; and interceded between the living, their ancestral spirits, and God. Traditional medicine was first and foremost a reflection of the society's religious beliefs and worldview. It included a sizable pharmacopia (*mankhwala*), consisting of plants selected for their pharmacological properties, ritual power (accessible only through a specialist through whom it was believed God could act), or both. Knowledge and use of medicinal plants was also widespread among the general population, including children.

Today, a strong curiosity perists concerning the effectiveness of "precontact" medical care. Questions about the efficacy of indigenous materia

Table 6.1   Categories of health hazards in precolonial Malawi

Type or source	Representative diseases and health conditions
Nutritional	Marasmus, P-C malnutrition, gastroenteritis, seasonal hunger
Vectored pathogens	*P. falciparum* malaria, relapsing fever, filariases, (Rhodesian) sleeping sickness, bubonic plague, jiggers (late introduction)
Non-vectored infectious (viral, bacterial)	Smallpox, measles, mumps, cholera, typhoid, chickenpox, tropical ulcer, treponemas/STIs, leprosy, respiratory: common cold, bronchitis, whooping cough (?), pneumonia.
Intestinal parasitism	Helminthiases: hookworm, anemia, roundworm, threadworm, tapeworm
Environmental	Goiter, tropical ulcers, Burkitt's lymphoma, trachoma, wild animal encounters, scabies, ringworm, burns, snakebite, wounds, trauma
Water-associated	Schistosomiasis, helminthiases, cholera, typhoid, diarrheas
Poor-sanitation, fecalized environments	Hookworm, dysentery, cholera
Sexually transmitted infections	Syphilis, Hepatitis B, gonorrhea (?)
Other *Treponemas*	Yaws, endemic syphilis
Eye diseases	Trachoma, conjunctivitis, opthalmia neonatorum, cataracts, blindness (associated with smallpox, measles, and leprosy)
Neurological	Epilepsy, cerebral palsy
Psychiatric and psychogenic/somatic	Psychoses; "madness"—temporary and chronic
Risks to newborns	Gastroenteritis, opthalmia neonatorum, neonatal tetanus (?)
Neoplasms	Cancer of liver, cervix, penis, esophagus, bladder, Kaposi's sarcoma, skin cancer—sequel to tropical ulcer
Conflict: political and ethnic, interpersonal	Trauma, disability, death
Imports from outside Africa, mid- to late-nineteenth century	Cholera, jiggers, tuberculosis (?)

Sources: *Central Africa;* Malawi National Archives; works referenced in the text, including Howard 1908, 1910; Cross 1897; Kjekshus 1977; King and King 1991; and others.

medica and methods continue to be asked of both the pre- and post-contact eras. Certainly the core of traditional medicine was its all-encompassing religious, supernatural quality. This truth should never be discounted, lest whole cultures be trivialized beyond recognition. At the same time, it is naive to assume a pervasive, unbroken continuity between precolonial healing systems and today's praxis. As is true of virtually all health systems today, market values, the cash nexus, and cultural borrowing have deeply and unavoidably penetrated African healing.[29] However, to assert that traditional medicine and its practitioners have changed in time and place is not to imply that its core religious and psycho-social concepts and practices have been eroded away and superseded by a biomedical model.

Quantitative measures of the extent to which precolonial *asing'anga* succeeded in reducing human suffering and mortality are beyond access. Even today it is exceptional to find documented evidence of the efficacy of traditional healing, at least in the Western, rationalistic sense of establishing case-controlled, verifiable events. The current level of understanding about African herbal remedies is certainly not because it is already known that they do not or cannot "work."[30] Instead, elite and powerful shapers of biomedical ideology and opinion typically look upon tradition-based systems as archaic and inappropriate. There is little interest in producing scientifically acceptable evaluations of traditional therapeutic practices, not least because illness and therapy are conditions and processes that are not detached from but are instead embedded in complex social and cultural environments. In the scientific sense, controls are difficult and certainly expensive to establish and manage. Also, many indigenous therapies depend on unique characteristics of particular practitioners, and the power of discrete places.

Some of the therapeutic measures that precolonial people relied on undoubtedly produced genuine symptomatic and palliative relief from disease, trauma, and social discord, at least. Malawian traditional healers offered treatments for ailments such as fevers and digestive tract disorders, including diarrhea, dysentery, and constipation. Based on his personal observations and an account provided by Edward Nemeleyani and Raphael Mkoma (the first trained dispensers in Nyasaland Diocese), Dr. Howard observed that healers treated sprains with heat, simple fractures with splints, and bronchitis, among many other maladies. The methods used included bleeding (*kutema likole*), cupping (*kulumika*), and counter-irritation (*kutema mpini/chirumi*). Howard also noted that massage (*kunyasa*) with hot water and herbs was frequently used for sprains: the procedure was "often very intelligently done and the results are often quite satisfactory." There was "a whole host of remedies of the 'dandelion tea' class decoctions of leaves, roots, and beans." They included various laxatives and astringents "which are probably more or less reliable." These measures were complemented by the ubiquitous use of charms, particularly in young children, and the poison ordeal (*CA* 26 [1908]: 328–29).

In Howard's opinion, Africans had little understanding of the biology and natural history of diseases. Treatment of disease was "purely symptomatic." They did not realize that a disease might have multiple symptoms and causes. Yet he added that Africans shared this fallacy "with most exponents of popular medicine at home, and with the whole tribe of homeopathists" (ibid., 327).

When Dr. Howard came to Malawi as the UMCA's first Medical Officer, he encountered severely stressed and socially disrupted populations. Many individuals suffered from multiple illnesses such as ulcers and yaws, hookworm infection, and chronic malnutrition as well as apparently new diseases such as smallpox. Poverty was widespread, as in most of Africa (Iliffe 1987), and seasonal hunger was a common occurrence. The infant mortality rates ranged from 30 to 50 percent, and life expectancy was between thirty to forty years. Traditional medical institutions and treatment modalities appeared to be no match relative to the scope of the health challenges they confronted. In this situation, Howard and the other medical staff probably could see no real indigenous alternative to Western medicine. Whether there ever was a therapeutically effective system of curative medicine in Malawian societies in the era before contact with Western missionaries and colonialists, and prior to that, the African and Arab slavers, is an open question.

Presently there is renewed interest in examining the case that many African societies had naturalistic systems of contagious disease recognition that actually paralleled Western theories (Green 1999). Certainly, one can speculate that, given traditional medicine's pervasive holism, at least some of the time it coincidentally interacted with other related systems and processes (e.g., food types and food security, political alliances, and other cultural means of adapting to adversity) to produce health and social benefits. In this sense traditional healing may have contributed to the relative demographic success and resilience of Malawi's precolonial peoples. Having said this, it is inevitable that the scope of this truth will forever reside with those ancestors of modern Malawians. One point is clear regarding both practice and theoretical issues: it is necessary to approach African healing, in the precolonial era, and today, as a real, functioning system of social control.[31] It also represents a varied body of beliefs and behaviors that influence public health for better or for worse. Whereas certain general traits such as the ritual use of herbs and belief in witchcraft have an essentially pan-African distribution, uniform "African" or national, "paradigmatic" medical cultures are absent (Last 1986). At a minimum it is necessary to distinguish areas and peoples with and without:

(1) "organized medical "guilds" with highly systematized theories of anatomy, illness, and therapy, or other specialist groups that offer services over a broader region;

(2) complex herbal traditions based on observation and experimentation, or on highly evolved symbolism;

(3) complex psychiatric conditions, which often use "spirit possession" as the medium of therapy;

(4) cultures "where sickness is a matter of such paramount concern that it is the idiom for articulating disaster and conflict, quite irrespective of the local epidemiology of disease"; and

(5) cultures where sickness is typically deemphasized (also without reference to the epidemiological context), and other outlets are used to express illness and conflict. (Ibid., 4)"

The Malawian and African reality is one of many ethnic and regional medical subcultures with their own organization and characteristics, but often with considerable overlap and borrowing. Thus traditional medicine is not static, as numerous recent case studies have demonstrated. It also continues to evolve and integrate new ideas and practices, including biomedical procedures and symbols. Today in Malawi and the rest of Africa it is widely complementary with Western medical services, and because it is generally community-based, it has a demonstrable capacity to enable and strengthen biomedical efforts in public health, including STI/HIV/AIDS amelioration. Building a modern hospital or health center in a place does not cause the decline there of local traditional healing. For various reasons, many people will use one or the other, or both systems serially or simultaneously, in their quest to find an effective therapy during the same episode of illness. As such, biomedicine and traditional medicine remain complementary institutions, a process that began with the arrival of the first medical missionaries.

The penetration of African cultures by European imperialism and colonialism opened a profound struggle with indigenous institutions over health and social behavior that the invaders frequently cast as a tug of war between light and darkness. This contest was another "frontier" phenomenon that produced distinctive spatial relations, social behavior, and consequences for human health. It is rooted in distinct and powerful worldviews. Conflict and struggle became inevitable once the protagonists had met. The resulting competition among these systems of belief and praxis that originated in nineteenth-century Malawi will persist long into the twenty-first century. This theme is revisited in the next chapter.

By 1900, building up and staffing an infrastructure of hospitals, clinics, and medical outreach had become essential to the UMCA's perception and performance of its overall mandate. Mission medicine had started to gain influence in the politics of local cultures, weighing in with propaganda and some success against powerful African belief systems. For small numbers of Africans, personal experiences with certain procedures of mission medicine, including laboratory analysis and clinical training, expanded their intellectual horizons and vocational choices. These developments have great interest in and of themselves. However, one of the most problematic aspects of the UMCA's medical work was how their system of values, technology, hospitals, and dispensaries could be used to improve the health of the general African population. Many missionaries and Europeans generally seemed to take the outcome for granted: Western medicine was the superior system and would readily displace if not totally eclipse an inferior indigenous system.

Yet a majority of Malawians had little or no access to the resources of the medical mission. Others chose not to use them, especially conservative Muslims, although after a few decades there was a noticeable lessening of the fears and feelings of alienation among those of Islamic belief. In reality, the UMCA had little choice but to offer medical services to Muslims, not least because they offered the best hope for gaining converts. This is not to diminish the fact that the majority of missionaries seemed to believe that it was un-Christian, and against their calling, to deny medical services to anyone in need.

Always short-handed, the mission's European doctor and nurses came to rely heavily on a small cadre of African assistants they had trained. Patients in UMCA hospitals had many opportunities for exposure to Christian prayer and teaching. Ideally, and as a widely practiced rule, Africans grew to anticipate that as part of the healing process they would receive liberal doses of Christian compassion and empathy from mission caregivers who were still strangers in the indigenous social scheme. To this day, for most Malawians the humanitarian values that typify church-based health care remain a primary reason why it remains superior to government medical services. But was the UMCA able to make a qualitative difference in African health and thus in their quality of life? Chapters 7 through 10 address these controversial issues.

NOTES

1. See Blaut 1993, 76 and 79. Blaut's "absolutionist school" of historians include Philip Curtin, *Economic Change in Pre-colonial Africa: Senegambia in the Era of the Slave Trade* (1975); Joseph Miller, *Way of Death* (1988), whose work is singled out because he writes about "savagery" and "cannibalism"; William McNeill, *Plagues and Peoples* (1976). The absolutionist school of Eurocentric Africanists "absolves Europeans of most of the responsibility for slavery and the problems of modern Africa by finding explanations for such matters within Africa itself, often in the African environment." These arguments have been adopted by the "European miracle" historians (Blaut 1993, 76).

2. The hypothesis that the depredations of the slave trade produced significant depopulation in some locales and also increased the transmission and prevalence of disease in large areas is essentially indisputable. See Blaut 1993.

3. High-yield agriculture was apparently more the exception than the rule in tropical Africa. This kept population densities well below their potentials until higher-yielding food crops from outside, such as maize and cassava, began to be adapted by African cultivators around three hundred years ago. This hypothesis was contributed by James W. Newman, Department of Geography, Syracuse University (personal communication, November 6, 2000).

4. A viable program to eradicate Guinea worm disease was initiated during the 1990s by the Carter Center at Emory University, Atlanta.

5. In some rural areas even today only 30 percent of households have a pit latrine (King and King 1991, 100).

6. Today various causative agents are recognized, including bacteria, protozoa, chemical irritants, viruses, and parasitic worms (Miller and Keane 1987, 384).

7. The problem persisted long after World War I. The Dutch Reformed Church Mission reported treating 75,000 patients in their hospitals, one-third of them with ulcers (King and King 1991, 130).

8. Uganda Protectorate, *Annual Report of the Medical Department for 1938* (1939), 28. Cited in Vaughn 1991, 138.

9. According to Headrick (1994, 36–37), in Equatorial Africa "the only exception to European transmission is middle Chad, where communities tied into the cross-Saharan trade already had high infection rates."

10. The increase of Europeans with STIs was remarked on in 1900–01 and again in the *Annual Report on the Sanitary and Health Conditions for 1912*. The STD case-rate among Europeans in Blantyre, the largest town, was 6 percent (Gelfand 1964, 297).

11. By comparison, leprosy prevalence rates in French Equatorial Africa in 1935 ranged from a low of 3.5 cases per thousand to a high of 27.2 per thousand in the most affected departments (Headrick 1994, 164).

12. King and King (1991, 56) quote Cross's distinctly European interpretation of the practice: "Whereas on the other hand, if the village does not possess a good moral tone but is given to adultery and other sins, the smitten one will die both young and old." I could not find this quotation in my copy of Cross 1897.

13. Livingstone 1857, 382–83 and 628–29. Relationships of the tick vector with the agent, host, and disease were confirmed by J. E. Dutton and J. Todd (1905) and by the

simultaneous researches in Uganda of Albert Cook (1904) and P. Ross and A. Milne (1904); see Good 1978.

14. Symptoms and effects of relapsing fever include high fever and up to eleven relapses, with cerebral complications and possible optic atrophy; liver and spleen enlargement together with frequent jaundice, bronchitis, and pneumonia; and circumstantial evidence of a high rate of stillbirths.

15. In neighboring Tanganyika reported and confirmed cases of tick-borne relapsing fever swelled from a few hundred cases in 1927 to nearly 6,000 cases in 1946. See Good 1978, fig. 7.

16. Gelfand 1964, 227. Gelfand incorrectly states that the death rate was 218 per 1,000.

17. UMCA. UX 92A, Diocese of Nyasaland, Likoma Hosp., 1953. (Typed cards). RHL.

18. While not recognized at the time, some cancers such as Burkitt's lymphoma were almost certainly due to infectious agents.

19. King and King (1991, 143) report that HBV "is over 10 times more common" in Malawi's than in the United Kingdom's population.

20. Of the common cancers in Africa at least six are directly or indirectly linked to viruses: Hep. B with hepatocellular carcinoma (HCC); Burkitt's lymphoma and nasopharyngeal lymphoma with Epstein-Barr; carcinoma of cervix and penis with HPV; and forms of Kaposi's sarcoma with HIV (Hutt 1991, 231).

21. AIDS-related Kaposi's sarcoma has recently superimposed itself on the preexisting endemic form (Hutt 1991). Varieties of KS now must rank among the most common African cancers.

22. The tumor is rare in localities where malaria is controlled, such as Zanzibar (Hutt 1991, 230).

23. Poison was also used, and rat-catching was eventually stopped. The standard pay for a common laborer at this time was 4 to 6 shillings a month (King and King 1991, 67–68).

24. This important feature is partly recaptured in Rochus Schmidt's map of "East African trade routes ca. 1890" (in Kjekshus 1977, 123).

25. Several species of wild animals indigenous to the savannas and woodlands provided a healthy reservoir for *T. rhodesiense*, which *G. morsitans* could then transmit to both cattle and people.

26. In the early 1960s, tsetse fly belts covered an estimated 12 percent of Malawi's land surface (Pike and Rimmington 1965, 196).

27. TB, or pthisis, is a notable and curious omission from Cross's (1897) large medical handbook on the diseases of British Central Africa. As already noted, TB had been documented in Malawi twenty years earlier.

28. Linden (1974, 83, n. 33) maintains that "the care of half-caste children in the Protectorate became entirely the work of the [White] Sisters. For this reason many girls, today women, brought up in their orphanages speak French."

29. Ityavyar (1992, 43) claims: "The social forces which determined the dominance and autonomy of indigenous African healers and medicine men [and women] are no longer present in contemporary Africa, where the social relations and modes of production are those of capitalism. The belief structures which existed in precapitalist Africa have now been replaced by scientific rationality characteristic of the capitalistic

mode of production." While the full argument is starkly ideological, romanticized, and in need of historical perspective, the ideas are broadly expressed in the great diversity of African life today.

30. For example, there is strong evidence today from Tanga region in Tanzania that three herbal remedies developed and supplied by traditional healers are efficacious against opportunistic infections associated with AIDS. These herbs promote "increased appetite and weight gain, stop diarrhea, reduce fever, eliminate oral thrush, resolve skin rashes and fungus, cure Herpes zoster and clear ulcers." These herbs are distributed by the Tanga AIDS working group (TAWG), a NGO that fosters collaboration between traditional healers, doctors, and local communities. According to the government's regional AIDS control coordinator, TAWG now treats over 10 percent of all confirmed AIDS cases in Tanga region. See "Combating HIV/AIDS. Experience of the Tanga AIDS Working Group" (http://www.worldbank.org/afr/ik/tawg/tawg3).

31. See Feierman 1986, 206; Good 1988; Olumwallah 2002.

CHAPTER SEVEN

Medical Services for Missionaries and Africans

MALARIA: AN ENDEMIC THREAT TO PUBLIC HEALTH

From the mid-1890s the missionaries' lifestyle grew less ascetic, at least for those based on Likoma. Permanent housing materials gradually replaced their crude reed huts. The use of stones and brick helped to reduce termite destruction and contact with other insects and rodents, as well as the threat of disastrous fires, such as those that destroyed the missionaries' houses in October–November 1892. This conflagration forced "the withdrawal of the ladies" from Likoma and brought "a time of great hardship for the men" (Howard 1904, 18).

Better diet and greater variety in the commissariat also slowly helped to reduce high rates of morbidity and mortality. A setback in missionary health occurred during 1893–95, "an extremely bad period . . . [in which] a great deal of alarm was caused in England, and Likoma came to be regarded (quite erroneously) as an essentially unhealthy station" (ibid.). In his retrospective report of 1904, Dr. Howard cited cases of beri beri, neuroses, malaria, black-water fever, exhaustion and hyperpyrexia, and accidental deaths (including Bishop Maples's) as major causes of missionary illness and suffering, death, and invaliding to England during these three years. He further emphasized the missionaries' poor housing and "disregard for hygienic precautions," and their gradualness in adopting sound health measures. Implementation of new, "reasonable ideas" was often slow, even after 1896, due to "a great deal of carelessness and foolhardiness" (18–19). Following the founding of Likoma station in 1885, more than a decade passed before the UMCA missionaries accepted key health principles and showed sufficient motivation to guard their own health.

Dr. Howard's arrival as Medical Officer in 1899 enabled the mission to benefit from his knowledge of the latest public health practices. Howard was quickly and widely respected. He sparked rapid change in the way the missionaries viewed and coped with their own health risks, and he established the mission's first plan for African medical services.

A report on Malawi in the mid-1890s (Cardew 1955) identified some factors that contributed to the high death rate prevalent among Europeans in general. Strangely, they did not practice boiling their drinking water, and apparently suffered unnecessary gastrointestinal distress. Most significant for missionary health was the fact that the crucial discovery of the mosquito-plasmodium-host malaria link was still a few years away. It would also take additional time, and vigorous promotion by Dr. Howard, to integrate the new epidemiological knowledge into the mission's own public health praxis. Quinine was generally available, but some mission staff did not take it as a prophylactic but only after an attack of fever. Properly maintained, mosquito nets offered protection from the dusk-to-dawn feeding habits of the female Anophelines. Unfortunately, the nets also efficiently block air movement and could be stifling if not unbearable, especially during the hot season.

Between 1885 and 1896, thirty-eight UMCA staff members each spent more than six consecutive months at Likoma. Their health record was extremely poor. Eight missionaries (21 percent) died, and fifteen (40 percent) were invalided home, including the first Bishop of Nyasaland after only eight months in his diocese. Malaria, other fevers, and diarrheas combined with physical and mental exhaustion to exact a heavy price on health. Eight staff suffered a combined twelve attacks of blackwater fever ("haemoglobinuria"), and four died. During this same time span Likoma's annual invaliding rate (mainly to England) was 197 per 1,000, while the death rate was 105 per 1,000 (Howard 1908, 6). Six of the thirty-eight workers had previously spent an extended period in Zanzibar or on the east coast. All six reportedly enjoyed "very fair health" during their stay (1885–92) in Malawi. The explanation, it was believed, lay in their "acclimatisation" experience, which gave them an adaptive advantage over newcomers to the tropics (ibid.). In other words, it is possible they acquired resistance through repeated re-infections with the same strain of plasmodium, causing attacks to become less severe. On the other hand, such protection, or premunition, would be expected to diminish rapidly once the person left the area, was exposed to foreign strains (as presumably would have been the case in Malawi), or received effective treatment (Vogel et al. 1974, 310).

From the beginning, the UMCA was anxious to find a way to reduce the missionaries' exposure to malaria and blackwater fever. The strategy adopted emphasized the management of both social and natural environments. It closely followed lessons of the new malaria epidemiology, including such practices as residential segregation of human hosts and destruction of Anopheline breeding grounds. Malaria was endemic among the African lakeside populations and an ubiquitous threat to the health and survival of all the missionaries who worked among them. Weeks or even months might be necessary to recover one's strength after a bout with the plasmodia. Death from blackwater fever, or malignant malaria, was an all-too-common sequel to standard falciparum malaria.

Missionary deaths were more than individual tragedies. To the mission enterprise, it meant the loss of an experienced and often invaluable missionary or layman. Years of effort had been invested in a sacrificial calling to medical care, teaching, or evangelism, without benefit of material compensation. Knowledge of one or more African languages might suddenly be lost. By the 1890s, for example, many UMCA staff had acquired proficiency in the local Nyanja and Yao languages. Such skills were admired and highly respected within the mission station as well as among Africans. Proficiency in local languages became a desideratum of the mission's subculture and continued for many decades (see, e.g., *CA* 45 [1927]: 90).

Creation of an antimalaria strategy for the UMCA in Malawi fell to Dr. Robert Howard, the talented public health-oriented doctor who served with distinction as the UMCA's first full-time medical officer from 1899 to 1910. Oxford-educated, Howard joined the UMCA precisely at the time when the links in the transmission of malaria had finally been worked out by Ronald Ross, Patrick Manson, and others. The principles of malaria prevention and control that Howard introduced in Malawi in large part reflected Manson's influence. They became the foundation of public health policy in all UMCA dioceses. A key feature of this policy was the spatial separation of European residences and the mission station proper from local African villages, with their presumed high prevalence of parasitism. Some modern scholars have interpreted this practice as an example of thinly veiled racism. However, this politically correct view is oversimplified, since the first UMCA missionaries actually believed it was important to live simply and closely intermingled with Africans. Residential segregation was evidently not the prevailing prejudice in the pioneering days of the mission. In his *Report to the Medical Board of the Universities' Mission on the Health of the European Missionaries in the Likoma Diocese*, Dr. Howard (1904, 45) noted that in Bishop Smythies' time (1883–92) "it was assumed, as a matter of course, that the Mission station would be right in the middle of the native village."

Changes in the residential location of the missionaries began in the 1890s, initially in response to the new understandings and perceptions regarding disease ecology and professional medical concerns about sanitation, hygiene, and poor missionary health. In Howard's opinion the public health value of practicing and maintaining the principle of residential segregation was an "unqualified benefit" since it provided a barrier to the transmission of plasmodia by Anophelines from many African hosts to the tiny European community. Howard observed that malaria was "universal" among African children and that, then as now, it was a major contributor to infant and child mortality. Children's' spleens remained almost constantly enlarged until the age of five (Howard 1910, 66; *CA* 29 [1911]: 260).

Fortunately for the missionary mandate, the Anopheline ecology did not add risk to social intercourse between Africans and Europeans during daylight hours. Other important control measures included the draining and avoidance of swamps and sluggish watercourses where mosquito larvae breed, appropriate and systematic use of a prophylaxis such as quinine, and use of window screens and mosquito netting over beds at night. Howard's *Report to the Medical Board* remains a brilliant description and analysis of the regional medical ecology and the principles of malaria epidemiology and control.[1]

Dr. Howard's introduction of essentially regular, mandatory quinine use among European mission staff, and the environmental alterations he instigated to combat Anopheles mosquitoes, did much to preserve health and spare missionary lives. However, even if adequate supplies of quinine could have been locally obtainable, distributing it to the entire African population would have been a logistical nightmare. Moreover, Africans who survived their early childhood years built up degrees of immunity through repeated exposure to malaria. Encouraging younger and older adults to adopt a systematic regimen of prophylactic quinine would almost certainly have increased their susceptibility to virulent strains of malaria.

Howard's proposals for malaria control received widespread adoption as UMCA policy. To avoid contact with infected people and mosquitoes, he prescribed that a mission station should be built at least one-half mile from any place where Anopheles breed and a similar distance from an African village. However, at the same time Howard also conceded that social attitudes toward segregation along ethnic lines had also changed "a good deal" during the mission's first twenty years. He observed that "some degree of isolation from the village with its beer and dancing, and heathen life, is an advantage, even from the Mission point of view, and would probably now be advocated by most Missionaries" (Howard 1904, 75).

Malaria concerns reinforced 1890s medical opinion about the health advantages of using the steamers to conduct the mission's work. In 1895–96 and again in 1899–1900 the *Charles Janson* needed repairs and had to be taken out of service for lengthy periods. During these periods the missionaries, lacking a mobile, floating headquarters, tried itineration among the villages from the land. Howard concluded that this method was ill advised and unsuccessful in terms of the missionaries' mental and physical health, and productivity. It always required

> sleeping in the lakeside villages, and hence increases the risk to health, while there is the added strain of constant land traveling, with its frequent wettings in the rainy season, uncertainty about the supply of stores, absence of any home, and, in short, a return to the condition of the pioneer days. Naturally this causes a bad health record, and is not to be recommended except where unavoidable. (1904, 45)

Medical missionaries did, however, have more than one model of prevention to choose from in coping with malaria. Whereas "physical separation" of white from native settlements was the generally accepted "British" procedure, Professor Ronald Ross of the Liverpool School of Tropical Medicine took a very different and more socially progressive position on malaria control. He much preferred the system adopted by the governor of Lagos in Nigeria. Basically, this strategy aimed for improvements that would benefit both Africans and Europeans. In practical terms, it recognized that the two races could not really live or work apart, and that they should not try to do so. Separation would mean that little, or at least less, would be done for the native, and therefore the acknowledged source of infection would remain perennial.

Within just a few years of Dr. Howard's arrival the UMCA missionaries' health took a permanent turn from awful to better. While malaria was always a risk, environmental and behavioral measures, and regular use of quinine, made it less life threatening. Howard's moral and professional authority was a crucial factor in his persuading the local missionaries to adopt better practices for personal and public health. He also persuaded the mission to institute regular home furloughs. Among its other priorities, the mission could now devote more attention to African health needs. While they appreciated the improved living standard that came with better housing and a better commissariat, necessary lifestyle changes that brought measurable improvements in the UMCA missionaries' own morbidity and mortality evolved slowly.

For many, not least the European nurses, heavy workloads and stress became an all too common aspect of their lives. By 1897, the mission's understaffing and financial exigency had already strained mission workers. In London, the UMCA's Medical Board declared that "everywhere there is stress, and stress brings illness in its train almost inevitably." The "real root of the mischief" [high missionary death rates], wrote the Medical Board's Dr. Oswald Browne, "lies in the fact that the Mission is seriously *understaffed* for the work that it has in hand." In this fortieth year since Livingstone's appeal to the universities, the mission was "crippled for workers, and forced by financial stress to cut down in every direction instead of progressing" (*CA* 16 [1898]: 2–3).

The first dispensary for Europeans opened at Likoma in 1889. It was a crude structure, "well stocked with drugs" and with space for a few patients. By now a qualified doctor, the Reverend J. Hine (later bishop), had arrived on the scene, raising the missionaries' hopes that his surgical skills would attract some of their "native friends" (*CA* 8 [1890]: 5–6). Thanks to the *C.J.*'s presence, until 1894 UMCA missionaries who became seriously ill sometimes sought medical help across the lake from the highly respected Presbyterian physician, Dr. Robert Laws. Such a decision would not be undertaken lightly, as fifty miles of deep open water lay between Likoma and the Scottish Mission at Bandawe.[2] At about the time of Dr. Howard's departure from Malawi in 1909, the mission again relied on "Scottish Mission kindness," sending five surgical cases, including amputations, to Bandawe (*CA* 28 [1910]: 238).

Given enough rainfall to allow navigation, the UMCA missionaries could also sail south on the Shiré River to collect stores at Matope. Such movement reflected the UMCA missionaries' growing sense of mobility and the "security of communications" offered by the steamer.

While the missionaries appreciated the improved living standard that came with better housing and a better commissariat, necessary lifestyle changes that produced measurable improvements in their own morbidity and mortality evolved slowly. Deaths of staff members occurred at horrific rate during the 1890s. Later on, the death rate lessened but the amount and pace of work increased. Stress, perhaps reinforced by unspoken standards of "duty," became a common malady of missionary life, particularly among the European nurses.

IMPLANTING MISSIONARY MEDICINE: NATURE, PROCESS, AND CONSEQUENCES

Original drawings show the layout and features of the UMCA's main station (from 1885) at Likoma (fig. 3.4) and those opened at Kota Kota in 1894 and Malindi in 1898 (figs. 7.1 and 7.2). These detailed maps reflect the missionaries' primary purposes, notably to introduce and nurture Christian education and Christian religious practice among the local African populations. All three places had distinct disadvantages of site and relative location. Each site also reveals evidence of the mission's efforts to build up an infrastructure of small hospitals and dispensaries for Africans. There was no permanent doctor on the scene until 1899, fourteen years after the first Anglo-Catholic priests had arrived at the lake. All three of the stations proved "successful" in that they operated more or less continuously throughout the colonial era.

Likoma Island

Whereas Likoma offered missionaries and followers a comparatively safe haven from Ngoni marauders or slavers in the 1880s, most of these security concerns had abated by 1900. However, without the *Charles Janson* and later the *Chauncy Maples,* Likoma was far too isolated to have been allowed to become more than an outpost of a main station. In good weather it was accessible from Portuguese East Africa by dugout canoe. With the steamers, Likoma was only somewhat less isolated from most other stations in the diocese (fig. 4.12).

Evidently, about the time the Likoma missionaries had begun to feel safer they had grown to accept the false notion that the island was sufficiently central to serve as diocesan headquarters. This was a romanticized view that impeded efficient conduct of mission medical and other functions. As noted earlier, other liabilities included the substantial interruptions for steamer repairs (done 160 miles away at Malindi), and the island's lack of fuelwood and food-producing potential (fig. 3.2).

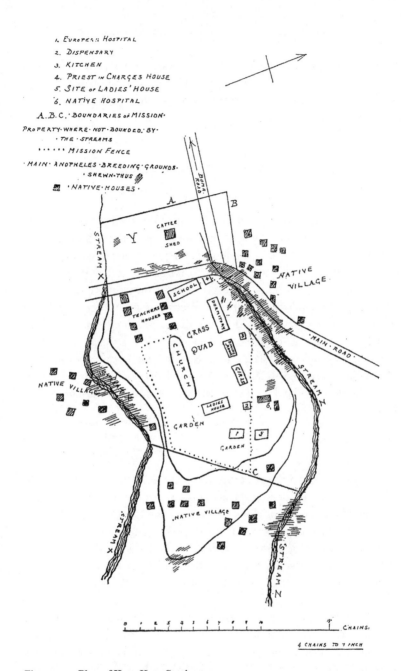

Figure 7.1. Plan of Kota Kota Station.
(Source: Howard (1904). From the archives of the USPG. Reproduced with the kind
permission of the American Society of Tropical Medicine and Hygiene.)

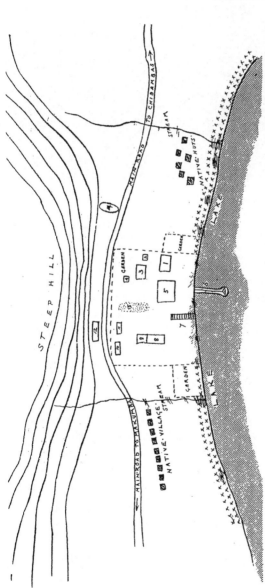

PLAN OF MALINDI STATION.

(1) Ladies' house; (2) dispensary; (3) dining room and store room; (4) kitchen; (5) engineering shop; (6) pier;
(7) slipway of C.J.; (8) European sickroom; (9) priest-in-charge's room; (10) boys' dormitory; (11) native hospital;
(12) school; (13) probable site of new church; (14) present church; × × reeds on lake shore; --- Mission fence;
/// anopheles breeding ground.

Figure 7.2. Plan of Malindi Station.

(Source: Howard (1904). From the archives of the USPG. Reproduced with the kind permission of the American Society of Tropical Medicine and Hygiene.)

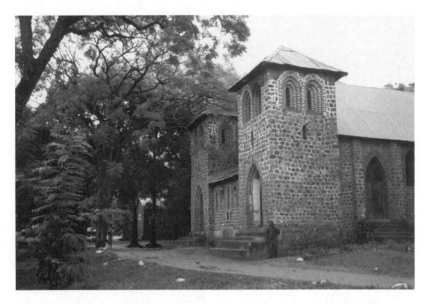

Figure 7.3. St. Martin's Church, Malindi.
(Source: Author's photograph.)

Shortly after he arrived at Likoma in 1899, Dr. Howard determined that whatever medical records the station once kept had been lost. He immediately instituted regular dispensary records and oversaw the construction of two small in-patient hospitals designed to accommodate six African males and three African female patients, respectively (below, fig. 7.4) Howard's records of his clinical experiences alone during his first seven months at Likoma suggest a hectic pace of work (770 cases per month), and they offer glimpses of the mundane and unusual conditions seen in the pioneer period (tables 7.1 and 7.2).

Howard performed several operations at Likoma in 1900, including one on a woman with obstructed labor who died from infection. He also started the practice of short-term "vaccinating tours" on the mainland. A deadly smallpox epidemic had spread into Malawi from German East Africa, and there were also severe outbreaks of whooping cough and mumps. Using human lymph and, later, glycerated calf lymph obtained from England, the UMCA vaccinated 4,350 people against smallpox in 1899–1900. Cooperating with the Blantyre Mission (Church of Scotland), they reportedly created a successful a "vaccination barrier" against the southward spread of the epidemic.[3]

Table 7.1   Likoma Dispensary: Cases, May–December 1899

Month	Total cases)	Examples of conditions reported
May	829	Spleen below umbilicus (babies); severe diarrhea; traumatic cataract; ulcer due to maggot
June	570	Ulcers; sodoform rash; cataract; also *ulendo* (medical safari) cases (8)
July	988	—
August	—	—
September	942	*Ulendo* cases (5)
October	953	Warts treated w/carbolic acid; hornet stings
November	681	Acute conjunctivitis w/small corneal ulcers
December	422	Yaws; sebaceous cyst
Total	5,385	

Source: 145-DOM-10-4-7. MNA.

Kota Kota

Kota Kota, the notorious slave-port on the lake southwest of Likoma, was closed to Europeans until 1892. By then its population had swelled to about 10,000, but with the gradual cessation of the slave trade the town's population declined to about 5,000 people in the late 1890s. A skeleton UMCA station was opened there in 1894, amidst a dense, predominantly Muslim population spread along the lakeshore and up to about a half-mile inland. Eventually, Kota Kota became the diocese's largest station (fig. 7.1).

Much of the station's environs adjacent to the lake consisted of low-lying, seasonally swampy, and poorly drained land. Heavy gales frequently destroyed African houses. Distinctly seasonal rainfall meant "for four months of the year any pit remains filled with water" (Howard 1904, 47). Kota Kota was a notorious breeding ground for mosquitoes, particularly Culex ("an intolerable nuisance") and the nocturnal Anopheles. This sprawling village had no sanitation facilities. Africans used the lakeshore and streambeds as latrines. The residents had also failed to control jiggers, and sand-fly infestation remained heavy. Dr. Howard noted that the native population "seldom bathes, and they wash very little." Poor hygiene, he believed, was a primary factor in the great prevalence of "bugs, fleas, and ticks" on their bodies. On the other hand, bathing in the lake was, in fact, a risky venture. Crocodiles abounded in the large shallow lagoon that served as Kota Kota's harbor, prompting Howard to observe that they discouraged many would-be bathers (48).

Table 7.2 Likoma Dispensary: Selected short reports of special cases and medico-legal cases, June–December 1899

Date	Patient	Diagnosis
1 June	18 mo. baby	Extensive superficial suppuration of legs.
2 June	Schoolgirl	General superficial dermatitis. Yaws?
3 July	Man	Assault victim; general bruising.
13 July	Carpenter	Acute traumatic synovitis of knee from a fall.
20 July	Teacher	Abscess; sodoform rash.
8 August	Man	Ulcer, grafting.
9 August	Man	Very large ulcer on left leg nearly encircling ankle.
17 August	Child	Ascites; large spleen.
August	Man of 40	Nodular leprosy. Ca. 10 yrs. Much oedema and thickening of skin of feet. Nodular ears, eyebrows, and nose. Leprous ulcers on lips and tongue. Fingers wasted. Lost voice due to ulcer on larynx. Lives alone. Wife left him. Relations give him food.
September	Man (seen at Msumba during doctor's *ulendo*)	Leprosy–Griffon Claw in one hand; other hand bent back and dislocated. No nodular growths. Principally nerve leprosy. Many scars of old ulcerations on body. No treatment attempted.
12 October	Man	Two large blisters on palm from spit and prick of insect (*Namkojela*). Contain seropurilent fluid.
November	Man	Variocele. Self-treatment with native medicine for some time. Right testis lower than left.
December	Arrived from Kota Kota four months ago	Anaesthetic leprosy. Perforating ulcers. Feet bitten by rats while he slept. Much nodular thickening about nose, eyebrow, and ears. Stunted fingers, feet, toes; scars of old ulcers.
December	Woman of 25	Chronic eczema of nipples and areolae. Covered with scabs, weeping and very septic.

Medico-legal cases, 1899

13 March	Man	Professed to have taken *pande* (ordeal medicine) to prove his innocence. Obviously fraudulent. Fined one goat.
24 May	Relations of deceased	Wanted to bring accusation of poisoning. In all such cases the doctor must be called at once. No *mlandu* (case) heard.
11 September	Man	Claimed to have eaten *pande* to establish innocence. Chewed only small amount and attempt was not genuine. Fined one goat.

Source: 145-DOM-10-4-7. MNA.

The mission's plot (1894) at Kota Kota was about twenty acres. It occupied a space that was situated on the brow of a hill overlooking the lake and surrounded by African huts. Dr. Howard was based on Likoma, but in 1903 he moved to Kota Kota temporarily to supervise the building of a European hospital (20 × 20 feet) and a native reed hospital (17 × 12 feet) (*CA* 19 [1903]: 9). Howard's future wife, nurse Kay Minter, served at Kota Kota. Upon their marriage, the mission's inflexible stance on celibacy obliged both of them to leave their work in Malawi. This left a great chasm and affected medical care for both Africans and Europeans, setting the work back for a year and a half.

The first permanent UMCA building at Kota Kota was Ladies' House, built in 1899. A brick dormitory for African males and a large stone church followed in 1900 and 1901, respectively. A dispensary for Africans along with a European sickroom opened in 1902. The missionaries' houses were mosquito-proofed with screens. Unlike Likoma, enough areas of good soil existed around Kota Kota to produce plentiful food supplies. Staple crops included wet-rice on low-lying, peaty soils, and maize. Local water supplies (water holes, streams, lagoon) were polluted, and by 1897 the mission obtained all its drinking water from a hot spring (70°C, and naturally sterilized) located about two miles outside the town. From 1900 water for kitchen use and European bathing was also obtained from this source.

Malindi: Site, Ecology, and Landscape

Malindi Mission (1898), situated in Muslim Yao country, is on the far southeastern shore of the lake (fig. 7.3). It was first conceived as a marine engineering station where the *C.J.* would be repaired and the *C.M.* outfitted for lake duty. Two or three engineers worked there alone for about eighteen months, and in 1899 a priest and two women, including a nurse, joined them. Within a few years an African dispensary (1902) and European sickroom (1903) opened to serve as the nucleus of local medical services. In 1908 new stone native hospitals (grass thatch roofs) and a brick dispensary, or *dawa*, were put up.[4]

Malindi has no harbor, but its section of the lake is relatively shallow and sandy. Until 1904, the site possessed a steep, clear, and sandy slope into the water, which of course was an asset in servicing steamers. Dr. Howard observed that this end of the lake "swarms with fish [and] crocodiles and hippopotami are plentiful" (Howard 1904, 60). Nearby streams normally remain dry for more than half the year.

Malindi started with considerable locational disadvantages. Its nucleus of buildings was wedged into a shelf-like strip a mere 100 to 150 yards wide (figs. 7.2 and 7.3). There was barely room for a narrow earthen road to pass between the mountain and the mission fence (Dale 1925). For about twenty miles north along the lakeside a "teeming population" inhabited "a continuous string of large villages." In the hill country to the east there were large villages inhabited by thousands of people (*CA* 30 [1912]: 142). Directly behind this strip the Rift escarpment steeply ascends in a series of wooded hills to a plateau about 1,500' above the lake. African villages hemmed in the station on its north and south perimeters; the escarpment and lake squeezed it on the east and west, respectively. Within five years of Malindi's opening the lake level had already begun a marked drop. As a result the shoreline was flattened, which encouraged the spread of reeds and undergrowth and formation of many anopheles pools. Mosquitoes thrived in abundance during the dry months, particularly July and August.

Alarmed by the increase in malaria risk, and "with a view to maintaining the [epidemiological] isolation of the station," the mission bought two acres on its immediate south and rented twenty-eight acres from the government on the north. Some old houses in the mission's African village were demolished and new ones put up on the newly added land away from the station's center.[5] Yet Malindi's physical qualities and the immediate proximity of African-controlled land gave the mission little maneuverability for future expansion. Population density had increased and, by the 1930s, the rising lake level was to bring severe flooding problems.

By 1929, Dr. William Wigan, the Medical Officer, complained that the amount of arable land the mission could claim at Malindi "will support just one person for a year!" (*CA* 48 [1930]: 213). North and south of the UMCA plot, Africans held most of the land. There was virtually no new unused or unclaimed space for the mission to occupy.

EUROPEAN INTERVENTION IN AFRICAN HEALTH AND HEALING

Wherever possible, the political architecture of European state imperialism was designed to minimize, if not avoid altogether, direct investment in the basic needs of subject peoples, including health care, education, and food production. With the General Act of the Brussels Conference, signed by all colonial European powers on July 2, 1890, the governments intentionally left the provision of social services to private agencies. By default, they delegated such concerns to missionaries, who thereby received a virtual carte blanche (but without grants-in-aid for at least the first three decades) to employ medicine and schools in the service of African evangelism (Warren 1967, 92). In taking up the slack, the UMCA and other missions interpreted medical missionary work as "a pioneer force, as a lever to open doors closed to direct evangelistic effort, e.g., Mohammedan and Zenana. . . . So the work of every medical missionary must be in a sense sacramental; they, through their art, become a channel by means of which Christ may reach their patients" (*CA* 30 [1912]: 227–30).

COMPLETING THE TRIAD: OPENING HOSPITALS AND DISPENSARIES FOR AFRICANS

Between 1890 and 1925, the UMCA built nine small hospitals, ranging from twenty to fifty beds, in its Nyasaland Diocese. Outpatient dispensaries also operated at each of these locations. Additional, freestanding dispensaries were built for outpatients in several population centers situated beyond the hospitals' hinterlands (table 7.3). During the 1920s, some dispensaries

Table 7.3   African hospitals and dispensaries: UMCA's Nyasaland sphere

	Date opened	Distance from Likoma Island (in miles)
African hospital		
Likoma	1890	—
Kota Kota (west coast)	1902 (district of 2,500 sq. m.)	~65
Malindi (also marine engineering)	1904 (Muslim Yao core)	~155
Mtonya (P)	1908–1928	~120
Mponda's (Muslim Yao stronghold)	1912	~170
Manda (T)	1918 (new hospital 1936)	~100
Likwenu (incl. leper colony)	~1920	~220
Liuli (old Sphinxhaven, T)	1922	~80
Milo (Livingstone Mts., T)	1925	~170
Outpatient dispensaries without hospitals		
Unangu (P)	1893 (Germans capt. 1915)	~75
Msumba (P)	1906 (maternity hosp. 1938)	~38
Ngoo Bay (P)	1924	~25
Matope (N)	~1922 (on Shiré River)	~245
Mkope Hill (N)	~1922	~150
Lundu I. (Leper colony: south of Liuli, T)	1924	~60

Source: *Central Africa;* Malawi National Archives.
(N) Nyasaland, (P) Portuguese East Africa, (T) Tanganyika Territory.

occasionally temporarily closed down until a trained African medical assistant (then a dispensary or *dawa* "boy," regardless of age) could be found to staff them.

After World War I, the UMCA gradually took control of the hospitals at Liuli, Manda, and Milo stations, in what became the Archdeaconry of Southwest Tanganyika. These facilities had been established by the Berlin Mission before World War I and vacated before its end. Ultimately, a north-south line of hospitals and dispensaries was created that extended for more than four hundred miles, mainly along the eastern side of the lake (fig. 4.11).

Likoma Hospital, the first and largest facility, eventually with fifty beds, or "mats," was a reed structure that opened in 1890 (figs. 7.4, 7.5, and 7.6). Years later, the opening of a new cathedral created space in the old one, and the hospital was relocated there. The last new UMCA hospital was built in 1920 at Likwenu, situated south and inland between the lake and Blantyre. Its postwar take-over of the three former German missions in Tanganyika, in what became its northernmost territorial sphere, also signified the end

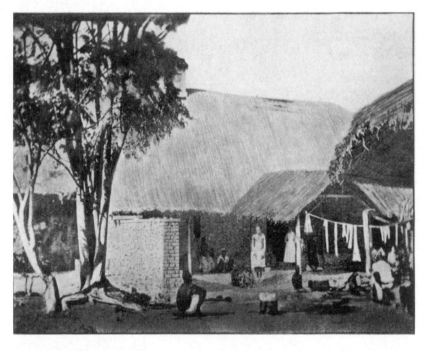

Figure 7.4. Likoma Hospital.
(Source: Mills (1911), facing p. 114. From the archives of the USPG.)

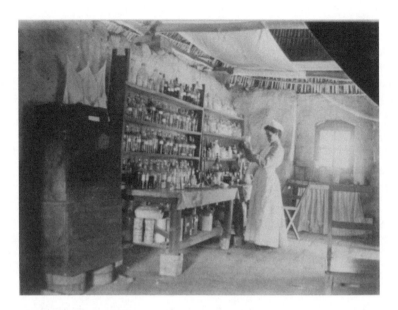

Figure 7.5. Likoma Dispensary.
(Source: USPG.)

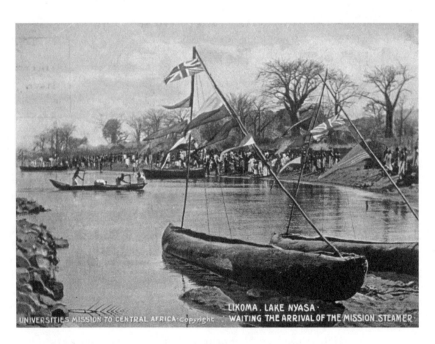

Figure 7.6. Awaiting the arrival of the mission steamer, Likoma.
(Source: USPG.)

of the UMCA's pioneer period. In time, the UMCA's hospitals generally featured separate wards for men, women, Africans, and Europeans, and a dispensary, outpatient department, and operating theater. No hospitals at new locations were established after the mid-1920s, although in 1936 the UMCA built a new hospital at Manda to replace the old one put up by the Berlin Mission.

EARLY MISSIONARY BIOMEDICINE

In its first year of operation (1903), Malindi Native Hospital took in forty-two inpatients, including two each "admitted" from the *Charles Janson* and the *Chauncy Maples*. One was a woman with severe yaws. Other diagnoses ranged from tertiary syphilis, acute and chronic ulceration of legs, and hookworm disease to scabies, septic wounds, and bronchitis. Many patients remained in the hospital for two to three months, while some with advanced ulcers stayed from six months to a year. During these long stays, even some Muslim adults might be persuaded to question their own faith and look more favorably on Christianity.

The record of activity at Malindi in 1903 also offers information on the work done at the dispensary (dawa), medical itineration in the villages, and local epidemiology. The dispensary recorded 3,240 attendances, or an average of 270 visits monthly by Africans. Sometimes the dispensary closed because the nurse was ill or she had been called to assist at another hospital, such as at Mponda's or Ft. Johnston. By 1910, Dr. Howard's last year as UMCA Medical Officer, the annual dawa attendances at Malindi had increased to 2,899. Thus on average nearly 300 visits occurred during each of the ten months the dawa was open.[6]

In 1903, another twenty-four people living in the outlying Muslim villages received treatment at home from the nurse and doctor stationed at Malindi Hospital (table 7.4). The twenty-four ill people, ten of whom are sampled in the table, received ninety-three visits from the nurse or doctor. This frequency of return visits to people at home suggests a high prevalence of people with foul-smelling,[7] chronic, and disabling tropical or other ulcers who were unable to walk to a dispensary. Social practices such as alcohol abuse and geophagy are also evident. UMCA staff viewed their village visits as opportunities to find slivers of opportunity in which to introduce their Christian message among the Islamized, skeptical, and often-hostile Yao people.

Also in 1903, the medical staff compiled a combined "Index of Diseases" based on records returned from Likoma, Kota Kota, and Malindi Hospitals.

Table 7.4   Patients visited and treated at home: From Malindi Hospital, 1903

Patient	Diagnosis and notes
1. ?	Tertiary syphilitic ulceration of arm and back. Periostitis.
2. Male	Ascites. Cause cirrhosis?
3. Female	Septic superficial dermatitis.
4. Female	Headache, dyspnaea.
5. Female	Pneumonia, pleurisy.
6. Female	Attempted suicide by hanging ("had been drinking all day and in evening quarreled with her husband").
7. Male	Abdominal growth, enlarged liver. Allegedly beaten earlier. Died.
8. Female child	Acute mania? Anemia, chorea? Regular earth eating. Died.
9. Male	Atheroma, chronic; edema of legs; nephritis.
10. Female	Parturition. Some uterine inertia.

Source: 145-DOM-10-4-6. MNA.

Overall, the 790 cases were divided among fourteen biomedical classes of diseases and conditions (table 7.5). Males accounted for 70 percent of all inpatients.[8]

In 1910, the mission recorded by name and ailment all persons, men, women, and children, who were inpatients in its three existing hospitals on January 1 (table 7.6). Only crude inferences can be made about the kinds and extent of the health problems then experienced by the tens of thousands of people for whom these hospitals were not accessible or available.

Undoubtedly, ulcers ranked among the most serious afflictions of those outside as well as inside the mission hospitals. The profile of 116 patients in Likoma, Kota Kota, and Malindi hospitals points to the preponderance (43 percent) of incapacitating, painful, and foul ulcerations. Most commonly found on the legs and feet, tropical and other ulcers can develop on virtually any body site. Many ulcers emerged after years of dormancy following the sufferer's experience with other infection(s) such as yaws, smallpox (the most common source of blindness), or the exotic jiggers. Poor nutrition increased the risks of complications from ulcers. If neglected, a new ulcer could progress to bone degeneration, gangrene, and amputation. The high proportion of "tertiary ulcer" diagnoses among inpatients suggests their widespread chronic progression.

The information in tables 7.5 and 7.6 suggests the biomedical baseline that provided a frame of reference for the early medical missionaries. An obvious and fundamental reality of the African-missionary frontier was that

Table 7.5 Index of inpatient diseases and classifications, Diocese of Likoma, 1903 (selected examples in rank order)

Disease/Ailment Classification

General Diseases (N = 168 cases)
  Tertiary syphilis, pyrexia (7 types), malaria, varicella, *chikuku*, yaws, pneumococcal sept., tubercular leprosy, typhoid.
Parasitic Diseases (N = 35)
  Ankylostomiasis, Bilharzia haematobia, Ascaris, *matakenya* (jiggers), snake-bite, cancer (stomach, pancreas), scorpion sting, scabies.
Alimentary System (N = 67)
  Spleen (enlarged), diarrheas, malnutrition (want of food, exhaustion), neglect, constipation, ascites, inguinal hernia, vomiting, stomatitis, abdominal tumor.
Respiratory System (N = 50)
  Pneumonia, bronchitis, cough, broncho-pneumonia, pleurisy, asthma, pigeon breast.
Circulatory System (N = 43)
  Anaemia (from hookworm and malaria), tachycardia, anaemia with debility, oedema, dilated heart, morbus cordis, atheroma, fainting, collapse.
Genito-Urinary System (N = 27)
  Mastitis, circumcision complications, Bright's disease, orchitis, epidymitis, parturition problems, cystitis (bilharzia and TB).
Nervous System (N = 54)
  Neuritis (leprous, beri beri, alcoholic), headache, epilepsy, hysteria (bewitched; tremors), convulsions, mania, shock, meningitis, chorea, infantile paralysis.
The Special Senses (N = 49)
  Diseases of the **ear** (N = 17): otorrhea, impetiginous eczema, acute oedema/abscess of mastoid gland, old otitis media w/deafness
  Diseases of the **eye** (N = 32): Conjunctivitis (incl. trachoma), corneal ulcer, proptosis (blindness from smallpox, syphilis), senile cataract, retinitis, ectropion.
Cutaneous System (N = 25)
  Septic dermatitis, scabies, eczema, tinea versicolor and circinata, herpes labialis
Bones and Joints (N = 115)
  Abscesses (various sites), inflamed glands (various sites), cellulitis (various sources), necroses, periostitis (syphilitic nodes), synovitis, osteitis depremans, gangrene, myalgia, arthritis (osteo-, septic).
Ulceration (N = 88)
  Tertiary syphilitic ulcer (N = 29), septic, chronic sloughing and septic (with complications from gangrene, warts, yaws, non-treatment), hidebound, tuberculosis.
Injuries (N = 64)
  Cuts (various sites), poisoning (mercurialism, earth eating), fractures (simple and compound), operations, contusions, burns, sprains, gunshot wounds.
Injuries from Wild Beasts (N = 8)
  Lion (3), leopard (2), crocodile (2), hippo (1).

Source: 145-DOM-10-4-6. MNA.

Table 7.6   UMCA native hospitals: Diagnoses of patients (N = 116) in hospital on January 1, 1910

Diagnosis	No. of Patients	Percentage
Ulceration	25	21.6
Tertiary syphilitic ulceration	25	21.6
Yaws	6	5.2
Anaemias (various origins)	5	4.3
Injuries (hoe, nail, gunpowder, etc.)	5	4.3
Malaria	5	4.3
Injury by wild animal (mauling by leopards and crocodile)	4	3.4
Rhinopharyngitis mutilans	3	2.6
Burns (feet of epileptic); arms and abdomen (baby boy)	2	1.7
Whooping cough	2	1.7
Pneumonia	1	0.8
Other (N = 1 each)	23	19.8

Necrosis of tibia, breast abscesses, gunshot wound, swollen knee joint, glossitis, swollen thyroid, cyst, marasmus, sloughing sores, *upele*, mammary growth, Whitlow, phthisis, asthma, chronic fever, fever and convulsions, tubercular thigh, severe abdominal pains, *mmatumbo*, elephantiasis w/ulceration ("patient wishes for amputation"), tick fever, circumcision complications, beriberi.

Source: 25-MAM-6-1-1. Malindi Native Hospitals: 1910. MNA.

both systems of healing were embedded in the respective cultures. The new biomedicine in Europe was still evolving, but rapidly gaining respect. In the early decades especially, whatever public health skills the missionaries had proved grossly inadequate to save the lives of many of their co-workers who died from malaria and blackwater fever. Indeed, the breakthroughs in bacteriology, parasitology, drugs, and tropical health were just emerging. Basic laboratory and surgery equipment and specimen analysis remained scarce or absent, especially in the early decades.

At the same time, many African societies had fairly well defined etiologies of disease that recognized both natural causation and contagion (Green 1998). However, the pan-African idea of human agency, or external forces, as a primary explanation for illness was probably the most deep-seated and striking feature of traditional cultures (Good 1987). As tables 7.5 and 7.6 suggest, the imported European etiology had few categories for the numerous African illnesses that indigenous peoples generally recognized as the healing province of traditional diviners, herbalists, and specialists. Western medicine had been slowly moving away from such a paradigm for more than a century. These two systems of mediating illness would be evaluated by the practical outcomes of treatment experienced by individuals.

By the 1890s, some Africans exposed to the new missionary medicine had already decided not to choose only one system and exclude the other. With the establishment of dispensaries and hospitals, a pluralist model of health-care began to evolve. Use of traditional and biomedicine, jointly or concurrently, expanded once people had witnessed the often dramatic effects of the "medicine of the needle," the healing of ulcers, or the cure of certain infectious diseases. In time, incremental pluralism became a significant component of African ethnomedical healing. Resort to imported and indigenous therapies remains in wide practice. This reality is profoundly relevant to addressing the vast unmet health-care needs of postcolonial African communities.

PLURALISM: OPPORTUNITIES FOR CHOOSING AMONG THERAPIES

In time, Africans who lived within walking or canoeing distance from a mission[9] could seek out at least three noncompulsory sources of care during illness. Foremost was the ubiquitous traditional system, epitomized by *asing'anga*, divination, and herbal remedies. Most missionaries detested *asing'anga* and their "pagan" rites, yet they remained in awe of their cultural and psychological hold on all African peoples. The UMCA worried openly about the competition it faced, and whether missionary healing and the principles of Christian living they sought to implant would prevail. Africans did not adapt to the new circumstances by abandoning their customary medico-religious institutions, and their selective use of biomedicine revealed that their own system was probably more open and flexible than missionary medicine. At a varying pace, according to their proximity relative to dispensaries and hospitals, religion, gender and other social factors, Africans began to seek out injections, and assistance with trauma and other needs. Not least, Africans began to benefit from the mandated compassion for patients the missionaries showed in their concept and practice of biomedicine.

A third alternative was to utilize elements from both systems. This last strategy turned out to be the most common, as medical facilities spread and larger numbers of people could gain access to them. It should be remembered that in the early stages of the medical missions era, only 1 or

2 percent of Africans lived within practical reach of a UMCA hospital or dispensary. Furthermore, in Malawi no government medical services were available to rural Africans (at least 95 percent of the total population) for the first thirty-five years of missions and colonization.

Today, there is no reasonable intellectual basis for assuming that missionary medicine could have fully replaced the indigenous systems. Many UMCA and other missionaries strongly and publicly condemned African practitioners (and their clients), with a view to stamping out what they saw as a pervasive evil and a stumbling block to the Christian life. In reality, African borrowings and adaptations of the outsiders' "health culture" proved highly pragmatic and instrumental. Change occurred mainly through a process of Africans adding on elements of missionary medicine, rather than simply subtracting or abandoning their own therapeutic traditions. Medical pluralism emerged as an essentially one-way process of selective, sometimes very gradual acceptance of techniques, such as surgery, available at mission dispensaries and hospitals. It was not necessary to understand the microbiology of an injection, or (eventually) how chloroform worked, to experience their potency. Unmet needs, natural curiosity, and a propensity towards belief in the power of the unseen proved strong motivators. Linden, who studied the work of the White Fathers southwest of Lake Malawi, observed that "the religious power of the dispensary lay in its medical technology; ... if the priest did not give an 'injection' he was [in African eyes] seen as failing in his religious duties to his flock" (Linden 1974, 60).

Medical pluralism thus grew in scope and complexity. Beginning at mission dispensaries, it became a defining feature of the medico-religious frontier in colonial and postcolonial Africa. Early patronage of a few dispensaries run by the Dutch Reformed Church Mission (DRCM) at Nkhoma demonstrates how quickly some Africans (mainly non-Muslims) responded to certain highly attractive elements of missionary medicine. In 1896, when the DRCM opened its first dispensary with no doctor on hand, about 200 people came in for assistance. By 1899, and the DRCM still without a doctor, some 12,500 people sought help at the dispensaries. This response removed any doubts about the need for a doctor (King and King 1991).

"Go Ask the Old Men": Tapping Personal and Institutional Memory

In 1989 and 1990, I asked four elderly at men at Malindi Mission to share with me their private and collective insights about how they, as colonial Africans, perceived and remembered the missionary medicine of the middle pioneer period.[10] In general, these short personal narratives by Archbishop

Chikokota, Shannon Bango, Chief Makwinja, and Chief Chiwaya offer insights that go beyond what is found in the UMCA's archives, which were of course compiled by Europeans. Each man had lived the greater part of his life in some connection with Malindi Mission, and as near as possible each man was asked to respond to the same set of questions. These oral histories remain unique and valuable. They are filtered through the wisdom of age together with the distorting effects of time. What they offer is a small, subjective window through which we can try to grasp how each elder constructs and interprets significant aspects of his own life in relation to the larger mission canvas (figs. 7.7 and 7.8).

Archdeacon Chikokota was born and baptized in Malindi in 1910. Brought up in the church, he was sent by the UMCA to Nigeria and other countries to study Islam. He said that his assignment was to become a specialist on Muslim affairs, and thereafter to assist the mission to better compete against Islam's powerful presence in the Malindi area and Malawi generally.

Describing Africans' responses to the missionaries' early medical efforts, Chikokota said people were "at first terrified of them," but acceptance grew over time and more people came in for treatment. The peoples' first impulse was to go to their chief and complain about the missionaries. Typically, the chief then went to the mission and told the Europeans that "these people are mine, not yours." Nevertheless, "the whites worked the chief hard" to gain his permission to do medical work. They would give the chief sweets, invite him for a cup of tea, or offer him a necklace—which was a very popular item with chiefs. The UMCA also gave gifts of cloth to the chiefs before establishing a clinic, hospital, or school. In this way they worked to convert the chief to Christianity. If the missionaries were successful, the rest of the chief's people usually followed his example.

Europeans treated abdominal pains, malaria, bilharzia, hookworm, relapsing fever, and tropical ulcers. Ulcers were endemic, and "almost everyone at the mission had bandages on his legs." Epidemics "came and went" during the colonial days. People suffered from plague, smallpox for a long time, chickenpox, dysentery ("bacilli"), and whooping cough. Cholera, which began in 1985–86, is still found all along the lakeshore. "People use the lake for a toilet."

Chikokota observed that "the early missionaries really worked hard at both prevention and cure." He recalled the Thursday masses at Malindi's St. Martin's Hospital and the special prayers for the sick offered outside under the trees. Offerings at church were used to help people in the hospital, especially the poorest folk. The Feast of St. Luke's Day was special for the hospital, blending Anglo-Catholic religious rituals with the social customs of

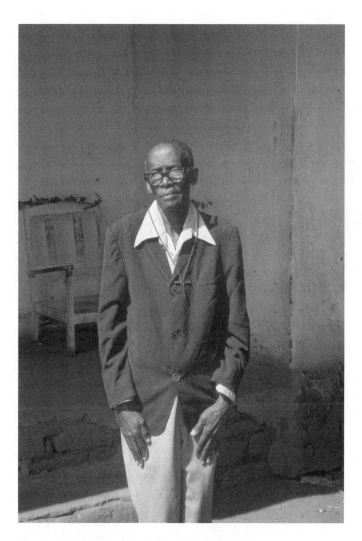

Figure 7.7. Archdeacon Chikokota, Malindi, 1989.
(Source: Author's photograph.)

the English middle and upper-middle classes. The priest conducted an open-air mass at the hospital and visited the sick. Ill people, especially the poor, received presents such as garments, blankets, sheets, and sometimes soap. Hospital visitation was followed by a party, where the priest and nurses sat together to drink tea. Today, said Chikokota, "most people go to the *sing'anga* in the village before going to the hospital."

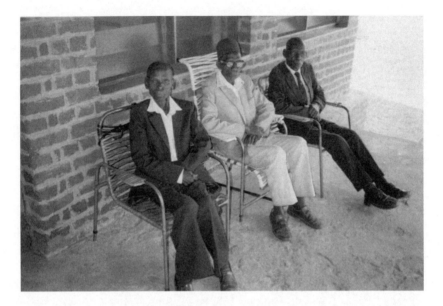

Figure 7.8. Shannon Bango, Chief Makwinja, and Chief Chiwaya, 1990.
(Source: Author's photograph.)

Rev. Stanley Mandala, Malindi's priest-in-charge in 1989, added that "three factors converted Africans to the use of missionary medicine." First, there was "propaganda" and "mass education"—teaching and communicating among the Christians; "they began to believe in it." Second, "whites were in power," and "fear of that power convinced many Africans to adopt their medicine." The whites also preached about the harmfulness of African medicine. Finally, "the money issue" played a role. Africans paid much money and goods in kind to *asing'anga* in comparison with the cost of Western medicines, which the early missionaries "gave freely."

Chief Chiwaya, a Yao born in 1912, said that his people were "taken" to Malindi by the missionaries when he was eight years old, and that "people felt safe there." He had become a village headman in 1939, worked as a court clerk in local government for twelve years, and was a sub-chief of Mangochi District. He recalled that in the beginning, going to the hospital was a frightening prospect for many people. The Muslim Yao feared that they would "be forced into baptism and Christianity." People paid for hospital treatment with eggs, flour, maize, and money, according to the sickness. In the early days, Africans who went to the hospital would always be asked if they were Christian. If Muslim, it was so recorded and they also received treatment.

This information was helpful in the event of a patient's death, when relatives were called. People came to the mission with a variety of ailments, such as headache, stomach problems, TB, whooping cough, pain in the body, and *nyamakazi* (Nyanja, "ulcer"). *Asing'anga*, on the other hand, treated a variety of conditions "including gonorrhea, abortions, and wizardry. They failed to treat malaria, spirits, and madness."

Reflecting on positive influences of the medical mission, Chiwaya offered that people were often cured, and they had come to accept the idea that "death is God's wish" [i.e., our lives are in God's hands alone]. At first, however, "the hospital was a strange thing: the people were still in darkness and did not understand that there was no harm in it." The medical work did help to improve disease prevention in the area because "people had been acting out of ignorance." Improvements included sanitation, the boiling of water, injections, and cleaning dishes, pots, and cups. People followed the chief, who started boiling his water in 1937.

Mr. Shannon Bango was born on Likoma Island in 1909 and came to Malindi in 1920. He was employed by the UMCA for over twenty years as an engineer on the *Chauncy Maples*, and took the name of its first European captain. Bango said that when the Europeans first arrived Africans found the sight of white people strange, and they "flocked to look at them." A white person was considered *chizyuka*, meaning (in Likoma Nyanja) "different," "not a real person," or "one who is a ghost and cannot talk." Yet "the Europeans could talk! Some whites could speak Swahili." Certain Africans "behaved courageously and would approach whites, communicating in Swahili or a sign language."

To encourage people to come to the hospital, the Europeans gave out collarless short-sleeve shirts made of a thick, white cotton material called Amerikani. They also gave away soap, salt, and sugar. Any person was treated. Africans did not have to submit to Christian prayers or ceremonies to receive treatment, although the whites did find ways to share the "good news of the Bible." In the early days, medical care was free; fees were introduced from about 1925. People were treated at the hospital even if they lacked the fees. "There were no invoices!" Payments, including such forms as eggs, fruit, maize, live chicken, and one tambala (penny), could be delayed until after a person recovered, as was the practice with traditional healers. As more people began to attend hospitals, some *asing'anga* began to cheat people, "charging them twenty-five tambola for quackery!"

Christian converts used European medicine more frequently than non-Christians did. Africans went to the hospital to be treated for ailments such as smallpox, measles, venereal diseases, toothache, and tropical ulcers. Bango recalled that he had been vaccinated against smallpox on board the *C.M.* in 1930, and soon thereafter experienced a mild case of the infection. People were brought onto the steamer for vaccination to prevent them from running away.

Bango believed that European medical skills ranked high among the UMCA's positive contributions to African society, along with education and craftwork such as carpentry and construction. He recalled that "Africans called all whites 'doctor'" if they had any association with the hospital. People were cured "much more often than was the case when they visited *asing'anga*. The missionary doctors' quick cure for tropical ulcers is a good example." On the other hand, Africans objected when they were "forced to dig latrines." They had been "used to defecating anywhere," and at first the latrines were unpopular. Such negative attitudes diminished when Africans began to see positive results from the use of latrines, protection of food, and so on. In other words, "they saw the connections between their behavior, way of life, and their health."

Africans, said Bango, took a "practical" approach to medical care. They would switch to European medicine if they were not cured by *asing'anga*, and vice versa. Today, even if hospital medicine is successful, many people go to a *sing'anga* to ask, "why me?"

Asked what Africans could teach the Europeans, Bango selected four specific themes: "African medicine, hospitality, singing," and a sense of "community life." An example of the latter is the custom of cooking food and taking it to a *mphala*, where all the men and women from each house in the village(s) gathered in two (gender) groups to eat communally.

Chief Makwinja, a Muslim and a headman, was born in 1920. He remembered that the missionaries might say that anyone putting on a [Muslim] *fez* "should not pass through the mission grounds." In the early days "Africans feared injections." They were also afraid of carbon tetrachloride, which was used for treating hookworm. Taken internally, it was bitter and produced nausea and pains in the neck and throat. Eventually, "injections came to be seen as one of the best therapies"—people could recognize the change in their physical health. Carbon tetrachloride reduced the swelling from hookworm disease; ulcers healed more readily than with traditional treatment; and when pit latrines came into use "it became shameful to see an adult going to the toilet in the bush."

Makwinja remembered that tó get people to come to the hospital for treatment the white nurses carried a gramophone with musical records into the villages. People gathered to listen and the nurses talked with them and gave free treatment and medicines for ulcers and other conditions such as scabies and malnutrition. Nurses sent messages to people in the villages informing them that they could get free items and schooling, and that their child could be evangelized, if they came in for treatment. They also distributed handouts such as "clothes, sweets, soap, and fish hooks." Getting the majority Muslim Yao to come in for treatment was more difficult. They were "ignorant" and thought they would be converted to Christianity, or that they would "be killed" at the mission. Such attitudes had begun to change by the 1950s. "Educated Africans" could then explain better than whites why nothing adverse happened if a Muslim went for hospital treatment.

The thing that impressed Makwinja the most about the missionaries was "their care for the people." In general, they would not report thefts to the police. Instead, they brought together the parties to a grievance so that they could settle their problems internally, through mediation. "Today," said Makwinja, "money is scarce in Malawi and people sometimes resort to stealing. For example, three of the accountants who worked in our local government offices have recently gone to prison. In contrast, recently an accountant employed by the Anglican church [Diocese of Southern Malawi, formerly UMCA] misappropriated Malawi *kwacha* 4,000. The church terminated his employment rather than having him tried and sent to jail."

It is noteworthy that these old men at Malindi emphasized the fact that the UMCA gave free medical treatment until the mid-1920s. Presumably, this policy resulted from an awareness of poverty and the desire not to lose potential Christians; yet affluence had certainly not arrived when a different policy was introduced. Accordingly, following a graduated scale "the patients, with the exception of the very poor, are expected to give something once a week, a little flour, some dried cereal such as rice, millet, or maize, perhaps a pumpkin or an egg. A well-to-do man gives the princely sum of one penny, this saves enquiries [about the outstanding balance] for a fortnight." A European nurse described the principle in 1934: "We are very emphatic on payment—the African should be taught to help himself, also his sick brethren" (*CA* 48 [1930]: 190).

IDEOLOGY, SOCIAL IMPERATIVES, AND MANAGEMENT OF MEDICAL RESOURCES: PRINCIPLES AND CONTRADICTIONS

Recruitment of Professional Staff and Conditions of Service

Any thoughts of further expanding the medical system collided with the diocese's perennially poor financial and recruitment prospects. Critical limitations included chronic shortages of funds, the already far-flung and thinly spread resources, and the disappointing results of its campaigns in Britain to attract professional medical staff. Appeals for doctors, in particular, fell on deaf ears and remained "to a great extent unanswered" (Dale 1925, 243).

In contrast, recruitment of UMCA nurses for Malawi was conducted through the Guild of St. Barnabas in England, and the Nurses' Guild pool apparently became a reliable source of nurses. "The great use made of, and responsibilities entrusted to, the nurses" thus became "a peculiarity of the medical organisation of the Universities' Missions" (242). In 1924, for example, the bishop stated from Likoma that nurses who came out to the mission field commonly found themselves managing all of the health-related functions on their own, without relief, for very long periods. Their responsibilities included the hospital, dispensary, procurement (drugs, food, other supplies), and custodial oversight, and they might be on call twenty-four hours. Nurses also had to manage the health problems of Europeans on the mission staff, and when possible consult with the doctor regarding their condition. Given these burdens, some nurses worked themselves to exhaustion and became so ill that they had to be sent back to England to recover. Nonetheless, the bishop informed UMCA constituencies at home that "we are splendidly staffed with nurses" (*CA* 42 [1924]: 122).

It is not surprising that the UMCA's medical staff in Malawi were prompted to compare their own unorthodox situation with the apparently more abundant resources at several other medical missions, most notably Livingstonia. Why, said Dr. Howard in 1907, "does not our church answer the call for another doctor? Why is it that our Presbyterian neighbors in the Livingstonia Mission have nine medical men on their staff while we have but one?" (*CA* 26 [1908]: 153).

The heavy dependency on nurses continued to grow, and only six were working when Dr. Howard left Malawi in 1910. In addition, the diocese had failed to recruit a replacement for Howard, who as noted earlier was obliged to relinquish his post when he married Kay Minter, a UMCA nurse. A year and a half passed before Dr. Wigan stepped into the breech.

The priests, doctors, and many of the nurses who carried out the UMCA's medical work were recruited mostly from Britain's middle classes. They were not permitted to begin service until age thirty, and could not join after age forty. For women, this age policy traded on the fact that most who had not married by the age of thirty would be unlikely to do so. By then a woman was typically viewed as "unsalable," and would probably remain a spinster.[11]

Nevertheless, the mission decided that, ceteris paribus, a woman was still "young" enough to commit herself and talents to the mission field.

Most of the men and women who applied for mission work were well educated, and nurses typically had been trained and certified at well-known hospitals in England. Many of the men had studied the classics and theology at Oxford and Cambridge, and valued the life of the mind. While no means test was formally required, especially for women, all English mission recruits, including medical staff, agreed to work without pay and to accept a life of frugal simplicity. The mission provided for a member's outfit, his or her passage to and from africa, and an annual allowance of £20. No one was expected to draw even this small sum unless it was really required. The "unique charm and attractiveness" of service in the UMCA, wrote E. M. Nelson, "was the knowledge that the self-oblation of each and all the members is absolute. No one can be the gainer by joining." Members with private means might even wish to "refund what the mission expends for them" (*CA* 19 [1901]: 26–27).

Use of personal funds to augment a missionary's resources was not condoned. Exceptions might be made to permit an occasional gift, for some special project such as a hospital ward. During their period of commitment the missionaries, all bachelors and spinsters from start to finish, would have no local source of savings for their retirement or other future needs. This stricture limited the field of applicants, favoring those who were financially independent. Thus for the clergy and other professional staff, ownership of property and an independent source of income in England or elsewhere were important considerations when they applied for a career with the mission. For Dr. Howard and Dr. Wigan, and several nurses and teachers, their mission service was virtually a lifelong career.[12]

By the mid-1920s, the diocese's only doctor had a crushing workload that encompassed nine hospitals with their dispensaries. There were freestanding dispensaries in five other places. By the 1920s, two segregated leprosy centers treated hundreds of residential and outpatients.

Between them, Dr. Robert Howard (1899–1910) and Dr. William C. Wigan (1911–47) provided nearly five decades of extraordinary medical service of incalculable value to the mission staff and to African populations in the lake basin. During the UMCA's nearly seventy-five years of hospital operations in Malawi, in only three of those years did the tours of two medical officers overlap even briefly (table 7.7).

As the mission expanded its mandate into a vast territory with relatively isolated stations and hospitals, distances, the steamers' unpredictability, and lake weather conspired to limit the doctor's supervisory visits to once every

Table 7.7   UMCA (Malawi) diocesan medical officers (in bold type) and other doctors

Name	Dates of service	Notes
Dr. (Bishop) John E. Hine	1889–91, 1893–94, 1894–99	Doctor first. Appointed Bishop of Likoma, 1896–1901.
Dr. Frederick A. Robinson	1894	Served few months only. Invalided to England. Hine covers while bishop.
Dr. Robert Howard	1899–1910	Broke celibacy rule by marrying UMCA nurse Kathleen Minter. Couple obliged to vacate positions and Nyasaland.
Dr. William C. Wigan	1911–47	Served longer than all other doctors combined. Nearly 71 yrs. old when retired from Nyasaland. Awarded M.B.E. for Africa service.
Dr. Kathleen Vost	1927–30	A second doctor (short term).
Dr. Trefusis	1937–47	A priest first, from 1914. Qualified as doctor by 1931. Intensive medical work 1942–47. Declined to succeed Dr. Wigan as M.O.
Dr. George Maclean	1948–55	Left diocese 1955, age 66.
Dr. Ursula Hay	1952–60	In charge of all medical work in Milo, Manda, and Liuli Hospitals, leprosy settlement, and dispensary in new Diocese of South West Tanganyika.
Dr. John Dingley	1955–57	Former head of TB Sanitorium in Sussex. Began as M.O. at age 65. Served 18 months.
Dr. Ian D. Findlay	1957–59	Accompanied by wife, a trained nurse. Short stay in diocese.
Dr. David Stevenson	1958–62	Overlapped Findlay for just over one month. Diocese's only doctor.

Table 7.7 *Continued*

Name	Dates of service	Notes
Dr. Robert Brown	1963–64	American. DMO in 1963. Left Nyasaland July 1964 for specialized training in neurosurgery.
Dr. R. H. Mumford	1962–64	Based at Likoma.
Dr. Andrew Johnson	1964	American GP, married with three children. Intended permanent service. Likwenu base.

Sources: *Central Africa;* Malawi National Archives; secondary sources, including Winspear 1956, Gelfand 1964, King and King 1991, and others mentioned in the text.

three or four months. Typically, full responsibility for the day-to-day running of the UMCA hospitals fell upon its British nursing sisters. Many of these single women had to manage a hospital alone or in pairs for many months at a time, and they also had full responsibility for the health of Europeans at the station.

Clever improvisation and adaptation of standard nursing practices in British hospitals was generally the rule in Nyasaland. Teaching Africans the imported, scientific principles of hygiene and disinfection—so instrumental to physical and spiritual healing as well as to maintaining personal and community health—could not be accomplished in a day. The visible and invisible presence of an African-European cultural frontier, and growing social contact, revealed a multitude of divergent and conflicting beliefs and practices related to health. For example, the imported (European) standard of inpatient care had patients stay in their beds during the day. Windows were kept open throughout the day and night for proper ventilation of hospital wards. In the early mission hospitals these policies conflicted with African social psychology and sociability. Instead of lying down all day, Africans preferred to vacate their "mats," or beds, for the outside environs, exercise, and the fresh air. Some even walked to the lake or river to bathe. A European visitor to the hospital was amazed to see that only 10 percent of patients stayed in bed during the day (Dale 1925).

To keep windows open after dark was to invite visitation by the *wafiti.* These fearful creatures had witches' natures and were often embodied in dangerous animals such as leopards. Eventually, a structural solution was found to accommodate these terribly real anxieties. The UMCA's hospitals were renovated, leaving large spaces for air flow between the roof and walls of the buildings. Windows could then be kept closed at night, and patients could not see out or be seen. This change at least partially neutralized the frightening powers of witchcraft, sorcery, and body snatchers lurking around at night. *Wafiti* practiced cannibalism. Local psychology held that these creatures could peer into and even enter a hospital ward to drag a person out into the night (*CA* 19 [1901]: 14–15; Dale 1925).

Accommodating inpatients' dread of the *wafiti* seems to have proved a simpler task for the mission doctor and nurses than teaching proper drug dosage and hygiene, convincing people of their need for surgery or European midwifery, or making appropriate use of medicines. It was one thing to reconfigure the mud, wattle and thatch, or bricks and mortar, of a cottage hospital. It was another to communicate in such a way that a patient did not mistake the liniment for his leg ulcer as something for him to drink; or to convince a mother that when her infant refused a powered medicine she could not help the child by taking it herself.

By 1928, the UMCA had two doctors and eighteen nurses in Central Africa. Ironically, this prompted then Bishop Cathrew to write that this growth was "really the big change in the diocese during the last sixteen years," not least because the European nurses related to Africans "more quickly than anyone else" (*CA* 46 [1928]: 103). Cathrew boasted that the medical staff was now "equal in numbers to that of the European clergy and considerably larger in nurses (though not of course in doctors) than the staff of any other mission or the government itself." The bishop neglected to mention that the resources for medical work in the diocese had for long been overextended relative to its resources; and he ignored the hardships, frustrations, and health problems this policy brought to the staff.

In 1926, Dr. Wigan had been the diocese's Medical Officer for fifteen years. At this time his official responsibilities had been extended to a region 160 miles south of Lake Malawi. There, beyond Blantyre, he treated both faithful and lapsed Christians in the European settler community. Travel between the mission headquarters at Likoma and Milo Hospital, situated in the northern reaches of the diocese, was slow and arduous. This itinerary required traveling for six days, "roughly 100 miles by lake and 70 [steeply inclined] by walking" (*CA* 44 [1926]: 16). Today, such demands on one's time and health, and the arduous schedule of hospital visitation and outreach, seem an unconscionable and intolerable burden. Even by the standards of the time, and the historical and spatial context, extraordinary feats were expected of the UMCA's medical staff.

Commitment, an unshakable sense of mandate and duty to proclaim God's kingdom to the "unconverted," and satisfactions gained through self-sacrifice were values that strongly influenced the behavior and vocational decisions of the mission's "medical man" and nurses. As the following discussion makes clear, the UMCA's medical staff and the peculiar constraints of its modus operandi were evidently held together by strength of character, belief, and values, usually in the absence of material resources. These factors grew more important as their work with inpatients, outpatients, and administration expanded.

Ultimately, the disproportionate workloads and responsibilities that fell on the medical staff fostered tolerance in them for managing with meager resources. This outlook had a price: the mission and medical staff could not realize many of their presumed objectives and goals. Great areas and many populations that had been targeted lay outside effective reach. That so few Africans were trained as medical assistants, nurses, and midwives is one of the more obvious strategic mistakes that limited the scope of public health activities in colonial times. This factor profoundly affected what the mission passed on as its legacy to a new generation of Africans at independence.

Central Africa, a journal to inform readers in Britain, and the *UMCA Annual Review,* carried repeated, often desperate pleas for new doctors. Critical vacancies for Medical Officers were created in 1909–10 and 1947 by the departures of Dr. Howard and Dr. Wigan, respectively. During their terms the UMCA was unable to honor the many public and private requests for a second doctor. With the two short-term exceptions of Dr. Kathleen Vost, who served with Dr. Wigan from 1927–30, and Father Dr. Trefusis in the mid-1940s, the many compelling pleas for a second doctor from the missionaries in Malawi fell on deaf ears. Virtually from the beginning, the doctor and nurses in the Nyasaland Diocese apparently received far less financial support from the UMCA's London headquarters than they required to carry out the mission's medical mandate. That they would have felt let down or angered by this situation is predictable. In his annual "Medical Officer's Report" for 1937, Dr. Wigan emphasized

> the inadequacy of our staff. The number of nurses which the diocese can afford is no more than adequate for the work; two doctors, one [Trefusis, a priest] tied to a station by non-medical work leaving only one to supervise

nine hospitals with 400 miles traveling between the most distant ones, are quite insufficient. A reference has been made in *Central Africa* to our need for a young medical man, but so far there is no sign of one coming in the near future. (*UMCA Ann. Rev.*, 1937, 103)

One year later, the Bishop of Nyasaland pleaded that we

most urgently need a second doctor to help Dr. Wigan in the exacting work of medical supervision.... He has been coping with this gigantic task single-handedly for over twenty five years with an energy that seems providentially to increase with the amount of work to be done, and he spends at least three quarters of the year up and down the diocese, only lodging occasionally for a few days in his house at Likoma. (*UMCA Ann. Rev.*, 1938, 95–96)

By 1946, when Wigan was seeking to retire and attend to serious family matters at home, medical understaffing in Malawi had sunk to "tragic" proportions (*UMCA Ann. Rev.*, 1946, 35). His frustrations now finally surfaced in print, leaving little guesswork about his feelings. The work he had been doing for thirty-five years, and the tremendous efforts of the British nurses had, in effect, been taken for granted and devalued by the mission's administrators. Writing in *Central Africa* primarily for a British readership, Wigan pleaded:

How long is this diocese of Nyasaland to be left with one doctor (perhaps none shortly) in nominal charge of nine or ten hospitals, with a distance of 400 miles between the northern and southern ones? For years I have asked for an assistant, recently I have asked for three to replace me; it seems a modest demand, but, I suppose for financial reasons, *Central Africa* asks [advertises] for two only. (*CA* 63 [1945]: 109)

Wigan further pointed out that they had no permanent doctor to support the large hospital and outpatient workload that had developed in the northern (Tanganyika) sector of the diocese. No government doctors were "anywhere near" Manda,[13] Liuli, or Milo—the latter sixty miles inland from the lake. Pointedly, he remarked that Liuli Hospital had recently "had a welcome visit from the S.M.O. Lindi, 400 miles away [at the Indian Ocean], the first visit for years" (ibid.) (fig. 7.9). Coincidentally, the neighboring UMCA Diocese of Northern Rhodesia was still waiting for its first-ever doctor at the end of World War II (*UMCA Ann. Rev.*, 1944, 14).

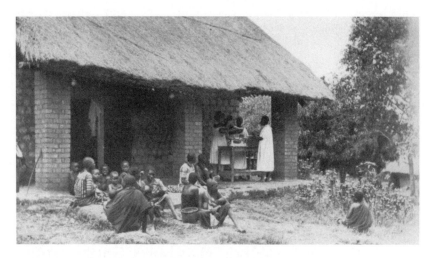

Figure 7.9. Baby Clinic, Liuli Hospital, Tanganyika.
(Source: Wilson (1936), facing p. 110. From the archives of the USPG.)

Whatever the UMCA accomplished in the name of African health, it was facilitated only through the dedication of its African dispensers/hospital assistants, and the sacrifices, even heroism, demonstrated by many of its British nursing sisters. Even though the nurses had "volunteered" for mission duty, it is not too rash to conclude that on many occasions, the UMCA superiors both in England and in Malawi had allowed the nurses' health, good will, ingenuity, and formidable skills to be exploited in the name of financial urgency.

Perspective on Recruitment and Understaffing

Why the UMCA in effect "institutionalized" its medical understaffing in Malawi is paradoxical if not ironic, because the healing component of its ministry was consistently celebrated in the organization's journals and papers. Part of the explanation must lie with the UMCA's hierarchical structure in Britain. Circumstantial evidence suggests that they were not sufficiently creative to attract and sustain a flow of new, committed subscribers. Apparently, endowment earnings were inadequate to support the extensive and ambitious infrastructure that the missionaries were striving to create in Central Africa.

In 1936, for example, the Diocese of Nyasaland received a total "vote" of £21,500 for its General Fund from its London headquarters. This included an allotment for maintaining the doctor and nurses and meeting some hospital expenses. The overall vote for Nyasaland was the largest among the four dioceses, and 24 percent higher than that for the Diocese of Zanzibar (the next highest). However, only 3 percent (£600) of the Nyasaland budget was for running its ten hospitals and dispensaries; 21 percent of the diocese's entire budget (£4,600) was earmarked for the *Chauncy Maples*. Zanzibar, with no steamers to operate, received £919 (nearly 6 percent of its vote) for its eleven hospitals and dispensaries. Thus, the Diocese of Nyasaland had to trade off its hospital funds for the upkeep of the *C.M.*, which required nearly eight times the amount allocated to its basic medical facilities.

There was also a separate contributory Hospital Fund to which friends of the mission were encouraged to make donations. In 1936, the total grant from this source to the UMCA's four dioceses tallied £2,275, of which Zanzibar was promsied £785, Nyasaland £700, Masasi £500, and Northern Rhodesia £240. This funding source was earmarked for drugs, dressings, and appliances. According to Dr. Robert Howard, up to 90 percent of this money might be spent early in the fiscal year (*CA* 55 [1937]: 215). My point here is not to second-guess and generalize about the allocations made in 1937. Rather, I wish to highlight the magnitude and distribution of resources relative to place, and the UMCA's potential access to resources given its connections in society and its role in the broader polity of religions in Britain.

Church auxiliaries in England, and later on the British Red Cross, provided important quantities of supplies such as bandages and blankets for the mission's hospitals and dispensaries. By the 1930s, grants from the protectorate government and the British Empire Leprosy Association provided some assistance for special programs. The Mothers' Union supported one and later two women workers from England. Individuals were solicited to commit to the mission's "Covenanted Subscriptions" for seven years (*CA*, vols. 49–55).

Dozens of subscribers supported the innovative "Mat Fund," initiated by Dr. Howard in 1903. A subscription of £3 provided one bed or mat, a blanket, and a patient's food for a year. When Dr. Wigan became the mission's Medical Officer in 1911, the Mat Fund still adequately provided for the number of patients in the four existing hospitals. By 1922, patient numbers in these places had increased, and two new hospitals had been added. However, the Mat Fund had become stagnant. Other income from church and individual donations, and special solicitations (e.g., on the BBC) for the General Fund also rarely yielded real increases for the medical sector. Consequently, after World War I, the mission limped and stumbled along from one annual accounting to the next. Dr. Wigan warned the readers of *Central Africa* that patients would have to be turned away unless income increased. On the other hand, he noted, in the "Mohammedan districts, where we are trying to get the people's confidence, less compulsion can be used in the matter of payment" (*CA* 40 [1922]: 137). How just, and Christian, he wondered, was a mission strategy that enforced payments by non-Muslim patients while Muslims received special considerations on political grounds?

During the mid-1920s to 1930, discourse within both mission and government medical services hints of a more "can do" attitude, and a slow but distinct awakening to the broader health needs of African populations. Occasionally the unexpected reinforced these progressive instincts. In 1926, the Nyasaland Diocese received a £300 grant from the UMCA's Hospital Fund in London. Said Dr. Wigan, it was "the first time that the hospital work has cost the diocese nothing, except the maintenance of the doctor and nurses" (*CA* 45 [1927]: 93). Looking ahead to 1927, he noted that several new grass roofs for hospitals would be needed, requiring slightly heavier expenditures. As usual, hopes of more sustained commitments were raised, but not realized.

Regardless of why the UMCA's budgetary problems persisted, the overall financial and development support coming from the London headquarters was stingy. Under these circumstances, those struggling to teach, evangelize, and heal the sick could resign, or muddle through, without symbolically or otherwise challenging the status quo. Penny-pinching became the perennial order of the day because the UMCA was weak at raising funds and expanding its base of support. Despite frequent pleadings in *Central Africa* for more support from the British faithful, strong-arm tactics in fund raising campaigns seemed inappropriate in matters of faith and conscience. People should respond as God moved them.

Capital funds for new buildings, infrastructure, and better equipment were usually scarce or nonexistent. In no sense was support proportional to or adequate for the scope of work that the medical staff ultimately staked out, with the encouragement of the UMCA's policy makers. Furthermore, in addition to Nyasaland, available funds had to be allocated among the UMCA's dioceses in Tanganyika and Northern Rhodesia.

As a member of the Conference of Missionary Societies of Great Britain and Ireland, the UMCA received shares of targeted funds raised in BBC radio appeals for medical missions undertaken in 1940, 1943, 1950–51, 1959, and 1962. In June 1940, 1,224 people responded to the BBC's call with £650.8.11. In 1942, a relatively successful wartime campaign in Britain to raise the UMCA's income from subscriptions, donations, and collections netted almost £6,000. Together with additional income from legacies and "covenant recoveries," enough funds were amassed to restore individual dioceses, in proportion to published expenditures, to their prewar levels (*CA* 62 [1944]: 25). By comparison, the UMCA had spent at least £12,000 for its medical work alone in the previous year. Nineteen years later, the UMCA's total spending on its medical work amounted to £31,250. Nevertheless, the BBC appeal for 1959 netted the mission a mere £562. These "home" fundraisers thus yielded puny amounts relative to the mission's needs.[14]

It is not that UMCA officers always sat on their hands. However, their strategies for raising general funds, recruiting more doctors, or filling a vacancy evidently produced mostly frustration. Good intentions aside, the record does not bear out that they vigorously pursued alternative approaches for wooing doctors or for supplementing operating and capital funds. Locally, the UMCA doctor and nurses were left to view with admiration and envy the relative abundance of doctors who served the Church of Scotland at any one time in Livingstonia and Blantyre. How could the Presbyterians do it? Certainly part of the explanation lay in the latter's Calvinist reformist and social activist traditions, and not least in their acceptance of missionary families in the mission field.

Two World Wars and the Depression deepened retrenchment and hampered flexibility. Half way through, the UMCA had only five doctors and forty nurses available to cover all its African work, which was spread across three colonies and four dioceses. In 1944, these individuals had responsibility for 38 hospitals and 1,033 inpatients. While numbers of patients grew after World War II, the number of hospitals dropped from 38 to 25 by 1959. The mission counted seven doctors and forty-nine European nurses. Thirty-three dispensaries, 281 African medical assistants, and sixteen leper clinics rounded out the UMCA medical establishment.[15]

In a number of places the material conditions under which the mission provided medical services were extremely poor and even hazardous to health. For example, at Milo Hospital and dispensary, the numbers of both in- and outpatients had reportedly doubled between 1925, when the UMCA took over the responsibilities of the German missionaries, and 1932. During this seven year period the UMCA made few changes to the physical infrastructure they had inherited. Originally cowsheds, these structures had become a perfect site for *O. moubata* infestation. Vectors of relapsing fever, these hardy ticks were spreading the disease at Milo among patients and others (*CA* 51 [1932]: 150, 233). Making long overdue changes, even in the face of resource scarcity, was most often a question of leadership. For example, twenty-five years later, when Dr. Ian Findlay arrived as Medical Officer

(1957–59), he discovered that the hospitals in the south of the diocese were in a deplorable state. As the bishop later reported, the doctor found them "thatched with straw and left them roofed with iron" (*UMCA Ann. Rev.*, 1958, 11).

In retrospect, it is evident that the available medical support was spread too thinly and unevenly, or not at all. Over the years the mission was permitted to stake out a huge, unwieldy diocese that comprised parts of Nyasaland, Portuguese East Africa, and southwestern Tanganyika. Resources had to be stretched to the limits of endurance—and sometimes the breaking point. Professional health-care training for Africans was brought along slowly. For example, a "Medical School" for African dressers opened at Malindi in 1952. Certainly there was considerable ambivalence among the European staff about turning over the highest-level responsibilities to Africans.

These unavoidable conclusions have major implications for interpreting the mission's achievements and failures in medicine and in raising living standards. During its sixty-plus years of medical service in Malawi, the UMCA's pattern was that of taking one step forward, and one or two underfunded steps backward. As if further evidence is needed, consider, for instance, the following scenarios. In 1949, the superintendent of the leprosy settlement near Liuli, Tanganyika, and his wife went on leave in August. Since they had no backup, for patients this meant sulphetrone treatment was postponed for the remainder of the year. At Mponda's Hospital, also in 1949, when the only nursing sister in charge left on leave at mid-year, there was no European (or African) nurse to replace her. Consequently, the hospital's female inpatient section closed and the antenatal work stopped (*UMCA Ann. Rev.*, 1950, 21).

Circumstantial evidence strongly suggests that the UMCA compromised its medical agenda and later its potential in public health through its doggedly conservative insistence that a married person was unacceptable for mission service. Perhaps the most blatant and harmful example of this policy was its application to the Howard–Minter marriage in 1910, which deprived the Nyasaland Diocese of critical medical and nursing talent.

This vow not to marry was a "Condition of Service," and remained largely in effect until the last European clergy and most other professional staff left Malawi around the time of independence (*CA* 74 [1956]: 183). The mission's celibacy policy, along with vows to accept a lifestyle of simplicity, and "full obedience to my bishop," was revisited again in an editorial published in *Central Africa* in 1951. Celibacy is, and should remain, said the UMCA's Duncan Armitage, a "hallmark of the UMCA." Whereas this promise may "seem strangely old-fashioned" by present standards, and run counter to young men's' demands that they be allowed to marry, it represented, Armitage continued,

> the secret of the Mission's power . . . Only the utter offering of self without restriction can be worthy to present to the crucified Lord. So UMCA expects of its missionaries a freedom of intention which will set the whole man at liberty for service wherever the call may be. . . . If we are to win Africa for Christ our own lives must bear Christ's stigmata; and part of that wounding may well be a call to the single state for some years, perhaps for life. (*CA* 69 [1951]: 3–4)

After Dr. Maclean's retirement in 1955 at age sixty-six, the mission was again unsuccessful in its efforts to recruit a Medical Officer to oversee the entire diocese (tables 7.3 and 7.7). Several retired doctors provided emergency, short-term filling-in service, but a successor was always "urgently needed, ASAP" (*CA* 74 [1956]: 183). Nonetheless, *Central Africa* editorialized: "There is no crisis in Nyasaland. The crisis is in England" (ibid.). In the 1950s, the years of the Central African Federation, a dire need for medical leadership presented the mission with an ultimatum: hire a married doctor or do without. Subsequently, Drs. Findlay, Brown, and Johnson, each of whom was married, provided short-term doctor services in the diocese between 1957 and 1964.

UMCA human relations policy was grounded in a powerful Anglo-Catholic ideology, legitimated through hierarchical traditions and practices (Thomson 1950, 107–8). The policy of excluding married persons from service was based on an assumption of marriage being incompatible with missionary work. Institutional and theological imperatives outweighed any benefits that married couples could offer. Marriage presumably interfered with one's ability to devote full effort and undivided attention to the primary tasks of evangelization, Christian teaching, and healing. Single missionaries could best remain focused in a life of piety and devotion to service. They would cost less to support, and not get distracted by the needs of European children running about the mission compound. In the historical record there is little evidence of, or even allusion to, how the latent sexual tensions and anxieties of a celibate psychological "landscape" shaped missionaries and life on mission compounds.

In Britain itself, Anglo-Catholics within the Church of England were outnumbered by low-church Protestants, including the Methodists, Presbyterians, Quakers, and the large body of Anglicans who looked to the Church Missionary Society. They had disassociated themselves from the Romanism of high-church Anglicanism, with its insistence on celibacy and practices centered on the institutions of clerical office, vestments, and ritualism.

Alternatively, factors working for the recruitment of spouses included their companionship and mutual support, which in theory would have improved the maintenance of health and enhanced longevity. Finally, if Western Christian ideals represented an instrumental bargain, might married missionary couples, particularly when they had produced children, not exemplify a family model that was socially and culturally whole and thus more comprehensible in African terms?

The profile above is reinforced by the experience of the Presbyterian Dr. Walter Elmslie, a pioneer Scottish medical missionary among the Ngoni people. Elmslie worked in Malawi from 1884 to 1924 and was a close friend of and collaborator with Dr. Robert Laws. He opened a dispensary for Africans in 1884 at Njuyu Mission, but could do nothing to prevent the serial deaths of his three European colleagues in just two years. In 1886 Elmslie married a woman from Scotland at Blantyre Mission and brought her to Njuyu. On arrival, the chief greeted him with "yesterday you were a boy, today you are a man and can speak." There can be little doubt that being married enhanced Elmslie's status among the Ngoni. In a later reflection, Elmslie stated that "matrimony has been more helpful to my work than celibacy" (King and King 1991, 73).

In contrast, the UMCA brooked no compromise on spouses until 1957, when a married doctor and nurse volunteered for a short-term stint in the diocese (table 7.7). Under duress, the mission was fortunate to acquire the couple's services. This event, and the example of Dr. Elmslie seventy years earlier, strengthens the following hypothesis: dogged adherence to celibacy was a self-defeating policy for the UMCA because it severely narrowed the field of available professional talent and interest in Britain. Furthermore, celibacy distanced the missionaries from Africans and in the long run probably diluted their influence.

Most men and women in the English middle classes married. Among those who did not marry, presumably only a fraction had medical and nursing backgrounds. This pool narrowed even more because most medical professionals would not choose to leave behind family, friends, or material comforts and other amenities, or risk their health, by going out to Malawi for sheer "adventure." Celibacy thus interfered with and undermined the UMCA's ability to attract, retain, and utilize the necessary numbers of doctors to nurses. While mission service was voluntary, celibacy deprived missionaries of basic human comforts, the benefits of cooperative spousal work and support, and the experience of parenting. Considering African social values, celibacy was not normal. Traditional religious beliefs about procreation and the soul made it next to impossible for Africans to identify with celibacy. It was strange and unnatural to them. Thus, it was not solely a question of celibacy narrowing the opportunities to recruit medical workers, teachers, and other professional and lay staff. In reality, the policy diminished the UMCA's strenuous efforts at spiritual and "whole-life" conversions of Africans.

UMCA DIOCESE OF MASASI, TANGANYIKA: "GODLY MEDICINE" COMPARED

In his analysis of the UMCA and "Godly Medicine" in southeast Tanzania, Ranger (1981) observes that the mission's vision, or Christian "theory," of medical work, had become a heady, self-confident mix of paternalism joined to scientific rationality and evangelicalism. However, he also asserts that the local African society exercised dynamic self-direction by filtering change and shaping its own responses to missionary medicine. Consequently, the missionaries were obliged to abandon their early "theories" that their medicine, writ broadly, could eliminate or at least neutralize the indigenous healing system(s).

Instead of "one or none," Africans in Tanganyika and elsewhere chose to fashion various configurations of medical pluralism (see, e.g., Janzen 1978; Good 1987). In Malawi, too, they selectively adopted those elements of missionary medicine that were complementary to the responsibilities entrusted to their own *asing'anga* and others involved in physical treatment and healing rituals. Once the missionaries arrived on the scene, rubbing out African traditional healing meant somehow eliminating the magico-religious system upon which it was grounded. The prognosis did not favor success. Of all African cultural beliefs and practices, religious institutions and behavior were the most resilient in the face of outside influence. Supplanting African core values with the foreign medical technology and system of values was not a path the missionaries found open.

Ranger's uses six "tests" to assess the UMCA's success at realizing its psychological therapeutic goals. These include the management of disease; the role of kin-based groups in therapy management; the challenges of alternative therapies and spiritual healing among African Christians; and the influence of African medical assistants and others who acquired some medical training. Ranger concludes that the missionaries had to reduce if not abandon their expectations that acceptance of their medicine would render "profound ideological transformations" in traditional African thought and practices (Ranger 1981, 261).

As revisionist medical history, Ranger's study reflects the significant shift underway by the 1970s towards giving greater attention to the African socio-political domain as a shaper of change. There are important findings that certainly find parallels in the Diocese of Nyasaland, including passive resistance to "biomedicalization." However, Ranger's assessment does not examine other "practical" issues such as celibacy, understaffing, and financial policy, and the intentional overextension (relative to resources) of medical services. These factors loomed large in the patterning of work, relationships, and accomplishment in Malawi, and their pertinence in the neighboring Masasi Diocese remains unclear. Certainly, the UMCA's institutional character suggests that socio-political forces akin to those in Malawi also affected the medical achievements of Masasi's missionaries.

To determine whether a broader, trans-territorial continuity of policy and medical outcomes existed across colonial and ecological boundaries, the Masasi Diocese archives must be read with a different set of questions in mind. There are strong hints that Masasi suffered from the same kinds of institutional malaise as plagued the UMCA medical missionaries in Malawi. In 1929, for example, *Central Africa*'s subscribers could read that "all our doctors and nurses are conquering them [African diseases such as leprosy] all one by one with a wonderful spirit, and Masasi at the moment is fighting desperately without a doctor at all!" (*CA* 47 [1929]: 179).

Under Dr. Robert Howard's guidance, by 1905 the Diocese of Nyasaland had begun to formulate a vision of medical ministry to Malawians. Strategic medical facilities had been erected at Likoma, Kota Kota, and Malindi, and a few skilled and dedicated British nurses had already demonstrated their commitment to caring for the sick. The *C.M.* had shown its worth as a transport vessel for the ill and injured gathered in from lakeside villages, and it carried the mission's doctors, nurses, and African dispensers to their assigned stations and patients. As the next chapter explains, before and after World War I further persistent and sometimes valiant institutional and personal efforts were made to build up a chain of hospitals and dispensaries on this early foundation. With much faith but little material support, the missionaries clung to the belief that they could reach far more souls with their Christian message, and keep more believers believing, with a larger system of medical and health services as their ally. Limited collaboration with the protectorate government in areas such as leprosy and immunization became institutionalized. By the 1930s, the UMCA, influenced by secular international trends, began to integrate welfare and community development concerns, particularly maternal and child health, into its Christian medical mandate.

NOTES

1. The report includes a brief profile of the health of mission workers at all land stations, and on the steamers, between 1885 and 1903.

2. In 1894 Laws moved the mission one hundred miles north to Khondowe (Livingstonia) on the Nyika Plateau. Dr. Howard, the UMCA's first full-time Medical Officer, did not arrive until 1899.

3. Medical and Surgical Report, Likoma, 1899 and 1900; Likoma Dispensary Record, 1899 (Notes on the Smallpox Epidemic and on Vaccination). 145-DOM-10-4-7. MNA.

4. Malindi Station Diary, 1908. 145-DOM-10-4-1. MNA.

5. Malindi Station Diaries, 1904–1905. 145-DOM-10-4-1. MNA.

6. Malindi Reports, 1910: Dawa Summary. 25-MAM-6-1-1. MNA. On average it was open 26 days per month, with 290 attendances.

7. This descriptive term is widely used in the various sources of UMCA medical history.

8. In certain years, statistics may have been kept for each dispensary (counting those at hospitals, thirteen had opened by 1924), but such accounting either remained in the locality or was not given priority for collection at Likoma. More comprehensive reports about dispensaries were prepared following World War I, particularly from 1922 to 1927. It is likely that some statistics remain hidden away or were inadvertently destroyed.

9. Or the relatively small number who could be physically and/or temporally positioned to get space on the Mission's steamer, the *C.M.*

10. The interviews (Malindi Orals, St. Martin's Hospital) were conducted with the assistance of the priests-in-charge at Malindi: Ven. Stanley Mandala (June 15, 1989) and Father Oneika (May 24, 1990). Mandala, who had lived at Likoma for many years, also contributed some of his reflections during the Chikokota interview.

11. I owe this point to my colleague, Dr. Thomas Howard, Department of History, Virginia Tech.

12. The combined records of women UMCA nurses and teachers still in service in Nyasaland at four time periods shows that in 1917, seven of twenty-one had served 11 to 16 years. In 1921, five of twenty-four women had worked for 17 to 20 years. Of thirty-two women on staff in 1927, three had already served respectively for 23, 25, and 26 years. In 1937, four women had service of between 17 and 25 years (*CA* 35 [1917]: ii; 39 [1921]: i; 45 [1927] ii; 55 [1937], ii).

13. Ironically, Manda station "headed the list of contributions to the Restoration Fund for bombed churches in England last year with the generous total of £15" (*CA* 64 [1946]: 72).

14. BBC Appeal for Medical Missions. UMCA, S.F. Series, SF 27 (1940–70). RHL.

15. Secretary General, UMCA, to Mr. Lovejoy, Conference of Missionary Societies in Great Britain and Ireland, July 23, 1959. RHL.

CHAPTER EIGHT

Gauging Change: African Health and Well-being

FOR THE MOMENT WE ARE CONCERNED WITH CHRIST'S
WORK FOR PEOPLE'S BODIES. IT IS IMPOSSIBLE TO THINK
OF THE GOSPEL AND OF OUR LORD'S LIFE APART FROM
THE SICK AND AFFLICTED.

Alice Simpkin (1926, 11)

I have characterized important ideas, opportunities, and challenges that influenced the UMCA's quest to create a mission field populated by African Christians and many more potential believers. A new medical system of European provenience for Africans was first perceived as desirable and, later, as necessary and instrumental, to achieve the mission's evangelistic and welfare goals in Malawi. It remains to answer the most compelling and significant questions raised so far in the study. Specifically, given the UMCA's imported technologies of steamer transport and Western-type scientific medicine, what obstacles did it face? And what was accomplished, after all, with Africans in terms of medical care and improved health status during the mission's tenure? On balance, what can be seen in terms of the positive gains of this imperial intervention? How might evidence of relative success be balanced against the consequences of significant failures of practice and policy, of omission or commission?

Numerous elements figured in the mission's ability to influence African health. These include:

• growth in numbers of patients, and patients' access to facilities;
• collaboration with government medical services and traditional healers;

- the special emphasis on leprosy;
- the cure vs. prevention debate;
- maternal and child welfare;
- public and environmental health;
- control and management of disease, including endemic problems and epidemics;
  - past and present profiles of disease and health indicators;
  - availability, uses, and effectiveness of Western drugs, surgery, and other technology; and
  - the UMCA's legacy, including preparation of Africans for medical practice and nursing.

I begin by examining two centers of influence in the UMCA scheme of medical services. First is that of hospitals, including patterns of use, dispensaries and outpatient trends, and the role of African dispensers. Second, I identify the forms and consequences of collaboration between the UMCA and the colonial government, with special regard to leprosy and drugs, and to the mission's contributions to the health of women and children.

Measuring changes in health based on available qualitative or quantifiable criteria is a formidable task. Pertinent historical records of health-related activities are often thin and uneven. Understanding health changes focused in time and place also demands an accounting of the role played by nonmedical factors, such as schools, gender, relative location, and quality of archival material. It cannot be overemphasized that the policies and developments, and successes or failures, of missionary medicine must be evaluated in their historical context.

A minimalist position might argue that any documented reduction of suffering, improvements in healing, or enhanced longevity attributable to the UMCA's medical work should be counted as a favorable outcome. While not without merit, this approach is likely to overlook or underplay evidence of limited or no positive outcomes, including instances in which the missionaries (whether due to policy, resources, or ignorance) may have inadvertently worsened African health status. A broadly postmodernist, deconstructionist approach would probably rely on a historical analysis and insist on the impossibility of reaching any generalizations apart from the writer's own. My approach does not build "a case" that is dependent on a single theoretical argument throughout, such as therapeutic landscapes, political ecology, gender, or innovation diffusion. Instead, I draw upon both critical and competing concepts when they appear to strengthen explanation.

INTERPRETING OUTPATIENT AND INPATIENT RECORDS

Evidently, keeping records of medical services was never among the UMCA's highest priorities. Investigation of the mission's archives on three continents revealed much missing data regarding outpatients and inpatients for the period 1890 to 1963. These incomplete hospital and dispensary statistics nevertheless do shed light on the evolution, utilization, and value of the mission's African medical and health services.[1]

The UMCA provided "services to the sick" within an ecclesiastical bureaucratic structure. Likoma Island, for decades the official residence of the bishop and the medical officer, was the distribution point for medical stores and site of the oldest hospital. Great distances separated Likoma from the other hospitals and most freestanding dispensaries. Any of these places could be cut off for months at a time if the steamers were down, or if the nurse or doctor was diverted elsewhere.

Supervision of all medical work depended heavily, at least in theory, on a British-qualified doctor. But the doctor's cyclical travel among the dispersed diocesan hospitals generally did not allow frequent visits to any one, with the possible exception of Likoma. In 1900, for example, the mission had succeeded in placing a nurse at each of its three stations, but an interval of three months punctuated the MO's visits to each place. Typically, the European nurses in charge depended on their own ingenuity and personal commitment to cope with the daily routine of patients and their families, itineration among villages, local disease outbreaks, and emergencies (*CA 28* [1910]: 40). A nurse was often stationed at one hospital for years.

Gradually, a small number of mission-trained African dispensers, or medical assistants, helped to increase services. Some had charge of a dispensary away from a hospital, such as those in Portuguese East Africa. Like the European nurses, dispensers also worked alone in remote places for lengthy periods, sometimes separated by great distances from supplies and professional consultation.

Unlike the government medical services, the UMCA's mandate did not require the missionaries to develop into a professionalized cadre with a constant eye to gathering better patient statistics. Remoteness and lack of assistance evidently took their toll on the systematic collection, analysis, and forwarding of data to headquarters at Likoma. Inevitably, some hospital and dispensary records have been lost or destroyed by such things as insects, mildew, and inattention.

In fact, the MO and head nurses often seemed more obliged to report detailed accounts of revenues and expenditures, as opposed to the numbers of people who sought and received treatments and follow-up care at a hospital or dispensary. For example, Dr. Wigan's Hospital Accounts and MO's Report for 1919–20 contains a detailed breakdown of the Diocesan Building Fund for each of the mission's four hospitals. Its focus is the annual revenues and expenses for inpatients and outpatients at each place. Reflecting on the immediate postwar climate, Wigan noted that "the work of the hospitals is in full swing once more" (*UMCA Ann. Rev.*, 1919–20, 44). Yet no count of patients who attended these hospitals and their dispensaries is provided. In 1920–21, reference is again primarily each facility's revenues and expenses. An annual tally of inpatients (943) and outpatients (97,000) is provided for the whole diocese, but there is no sorting out by hospital or dispensary. Such reporting methods complicate the possibilities for discerning spatial patterns of medical work carried out during the period of the study. In contrast, The MO's report for 1921–22 departs from the previous two years. It includes inpatient and outpatient totals for each hospital and dispensary in the diocese as well as financial accounts. But once again, in 1923, only "total inpatients" (1,005) and "outpatients" (130,536) data appear. The greatest blocks of time for which annual statistics are practically unavailable are as follows. Inpatients: 1909–20, 1931–37, 1946–49, and 1955–62; outpatients: 1898–1920, 1930–40, 1944–50, and 1955–62.

The size of the inpatient population at the start (1899) and end (1963) of UMCA record-keeping efforts is known. Likoma's total of 27 patients in 1899, when it was the only hospital, contrasts with its 3,526 patients who entered the six hospitals still open in 1963. Overall, the number of African patients who stayed in a UMCA hospital in 1963 was 130 times greater than in 1899. This progressive growth in inpatients over time is based on eleven "index" years and their yearly means. The averages compiled reflect hospital to inpatient ratios, and suggest a crude yardstick for measuring relative change over time. Although the scale is modest, a fairly steady pattern of hospital work and outreach to African villages is discernible (table 8.1).

Comparing inpatient expansion in the UMCA's hospitals against population growth to the end of the colonial era is hampered by the fact that most of the increases occurred at UMCA stations inside Portuguese East Africa and Tanganyika. Since the scales of administrative reporting units do not match, a valid comparison of population growth and inpatient expansion in the diocese is not feasible. What remains is to contrast the rate of population increase in Malawi as a whole from 1901 to 1966 with the rate of inpatient growth in the diocese. Thus in 1966 the protectorate's African population was 5.5 times greater than in 1901 (Nelson et al. 1975, 65, table 1). In contrast, UMCA hospital admissions in 1963 were over 130 times greater

Table 8.1   Growth in numbers of hospital patients, Diocese of Nyasaland, 1899–1963

Year	Inpatients	Mean per hospital	Hospitals
1899	27	n.a.	1
1902	88	44	2
1903	197	66	3
1907	459	153	3
1921	943	157	6
1922	1,005	144	7
1925	2,058	257	8
1927	2,640	330	8
1929	2,199[a]	275	8
1950	2,683	335	8
1953	1,993	399	5
1963	3,526	588	6

Source: Reports in *Central Africa*, the UMCA *Annual Report*, and the *Nyasaland Diocesan Chronicle*.
   [a] Includes 396 lepers.

than recorded in 1899. This assumes that population growth in the UMCA's mission field was roughly similar to that for the protectorate as a whole.

If nothing more, this crude comparison of two different measures suggests that inpatient admissions exceeded the population growth rate by a substantial margin. It also provides a yardstick of how "African" treatment grew more inclusive with the growing availability of the mission hospital system. On the other hand, these inpatient records reflect utilization. Alone, they cannot tell us the extent to which UMCA hospital admissions reflected medical needs in the African community.

GROWTH IN NUMBERS OF HOSPITAL PATIENTS

Steady growth of inpatients was not always predictable at the pioneer hospitals of Likoma, Kota Kota, and Malindi. At Likoma, the sphere of Christian work embraced thirty-three lakeside villages by 1897. Fed patients by the *C.M.* as well as those from the mainland, Likoma Hospital admitted 376 patients in 1909, but the total fell to 138 in 1915. This decline may reflect fewer patients due to the wartime commandeering of the *C.M.* Across the lake, Kota Kota admitted 106, 83, and 395 respectively in 1904, 1921, and 1927.

Likoma's African hospital accommodated 376 patients in 1909, but this level could not be sustained (CA 28 [1910]: 216). Comparable patient intake was not achieved again until the 1920s.[2] By 1911 inpatient totals dropped to 221, a decline of 40 percent (CA 30 [1912]: 258). The causes of this drop-off included the island's growing population, a decline in arable land, and accordingly both localized and island-wide food shortages. In 1910 the mission was forced to refuse admission to "any but the worst cases." At the same time, "a good many village cases—pneumonia, accidents, and minor things" resulted in frequent travel to patients' homes by European nurses. Called *Dona wa Dawa* by the Africans, the nurses were carried overland in machila chairs by porters. By this time also, increasing numbers of mothers were bringing their small babies to Likoma Hospital for treatment and advice (*CA* 28 [1910]: 238).

In 1911, Likoma regularly had forty to fifty inpatients at one time (near or at the maximum number of its sponsored "mats"), and at times exceeded seventy. Most patients originated on the mainland in Mozambique or Tanzania and thus came to the hospital by steamer. Many suffered from chronic illnesses, while others often presented life-threatening wounds received in attacks by crocodiles, leopards, or other wild animals. On average an inpatient remained in the hospital for seven or eight weeks. The precise length of stay depended partly upon the sailing dates of the *C.M.* (*CA* 30 [1912]: 258). At this time Archdeacon William Johnson was clearly enthused by what he saw as the growing acceptance of missionary medicine. On the mainland opposite Likoma, he said, "confidence is conquered all round. Where formerly they hid from the doctor, they now get canoes and paddle for hours against wind and current to come to the hospital—it is immense" (*CA* 29 [1911]: 5).

In 1909 Likoma's dispensary was "well equipped" and stocked with "all the necessary drugs . . . arranged most conveniently, solids, liquids, and tabloids and pills." A typical morning at the dispensary had the European nurses on the scene by 8:30. By then the dispensers had put out dressings and lotions and prepared hot water. People from local villages arrived first: "Most are mothers and babies, some poor little darlings with malaria, others with bad coughs, bad eyes. These mostly bring for payment an egg, little bundle of cassava roots, or in season native cucumbers or pumpkins which . . . flourish on the island" (*CA* 28 [1910]: 271). Such payments-in-kind, or *nchembe*, remained a norm for many years at hospitals and dispensaries (*UMCA Ann. Rev.*, 1926, 3).

For the missionaries, constant asking for *nchembe* in exchange for treatment was an unpleasant chore. "Really poor people" received medicine for free.

In the view of the mission medical staff, since patients had to pay good sums for services they received from African traditional healers, it should also be expected that they learn in the same way to value mission medicine. Indeed, it was the missionaries' "parental" responsibility to teach that "it is the duty of every Christian to give, and that it is becoming in a heathen to show a little gratitude." A European nurse at Likoma advocated that such lessons should be accompanied by the raising up of "self-supporting native hospitals" staffed by "trained African men and women" (*CA* 31 [1913]: 93–94).

Edward Nemeleyani and Raphael Mkoma, the most experienced African apprentices, arrived at their positions in Likoma Hospital by 9:30. By 10:15 young men and little boys came over from the mission school, many with small sores. At 11:00, the nurse observed, "the girls descend on us in numbers. None bring payment, but the teachers and workmen have got dawa tickets, which are available for six months at a cost of about 4 pence. Occasionally teeth are extracted by Edward or Raphael, who are adepts. By 12 noon the dispensary work is completed. What remains are just the various records to make in the books" (*CA* 28 (1910): 271–72).[3]

Across the lake at Kota Kota, the UMCA's largest station in Malawi, the evangelistic and medical hinterland had expanded to encompass an area of "about 170 miles in circumference" by 1909 (ibid., 209–10). The area is part of Malawi's Muslim heartland, and the UMCA set to work among the predominantly Muslim populations around Kota Kota, Mponda's station, and Malindi, along the south and western sides of the lake.

Designed and built by Dr. Howard, by the end of World War I Kota Kota's African hospital, originally a 17′ × 12′ reed structure, was providing sixty to eighty outpatient dressings daily. Occasionally daily attendance exceeded 250 (*CA* 37 [1919]: 183–84). Situated on the lakeside, Kota Kota's "dreadful" crocodile menace reportedly produced about one known death in the locality each week. Washing of clothes, water collection, and inshore fishing activities entailed great risk. The crocodiles could drown their victims, sever limbs, or cause massive puncture and tear wounds. Amputation, a procedure that was not always accepted, was often the only strategy against gangrene and certain death (*CA* 25 [1907]: 164).

Early in 1903, Kota Kota's nurse-in-charge recorded: "I have six patients in the native hospital right now." Such small inpatient populations could be very time-consuming, but they often also gave a missionary nurse opportunities to pursue her curiosity and ways to relieve boredom and loneliness. In her encounter with one not-too-sick Muslim patient—"the chief of Msumba, a dear old man, a gentleman entirely, with the charmingest of naive manners"—the nurse provided him with a cup of tea and fruit in exchange for shared conversation (*CA* 21 [1903]: 17). Encounters of this nature occurred sporadically in the early years of mission building, yet they gave encouragement to missionaries anxious to capitalize on any small signs that their efforts to Christianize African followers of Islam might some day succeed.

By 1909, inpatients drawn from the large Muslim stronghold around Kota Kota, on Lake Malawi's west coast, numbered at least one hundred annually. Data on inpatient admissions for the years leading up to and during World War I are sketchy. From 1921 to 1927 Likoma's average intake substantially increased to 413 patients, ranging from a low of 335 in 1923 to a high of 481 in 1923.[4]

Despite markedly uneven growth, by 1927 inpatient admissions at Kota Kota had reached 395. This expansion began with the hospital's initial intake of twenty-one patients during 1902, and increased to 174 inpatients in 1921. Thus by 1927 Kota Kota well exceeded the average intake of the mission's eight hospitals (table 8.1). Viewed from a broader perspective, however, in 1927 Kota Kota's average intake was only slightly above one new patient daily during the year. When all hospitals are considered, the average intake was less than one patient daily. By 1950, the average total and per diem admissions to UMCA hospitals were nearly identical with those for 1927. In 1952 the UMCA created the Diocese of South West Tanganyika and transferred three hospitals from the Diocese of Nyasaland (Milo, Manda, and Liuli) to this new unit.

Mponda's Hospital was situated near a junction of land and water routes at the southern tip of the lake, a part of Malawi's Muslim heartland. Opened in 1912, it experienced substantial growth through 1924, when it tallied over 600 inpatients. But competition from the nearby government hospital and other factors reduced attendees at the mission's facility. In 1963, just before Malawi's independence, Mponda's admitted only 373 patients.

As at Kota Kota and Mponda's, Malindi's predominantly Muslim population did not welcome hospital work with open arms. Inpatient admissions began in 1903, in small hospital buildings made of wattle and daub. After several months Malindi's resident nurse reported that the hospital "has been fairly full ever since its opening." Patients had come in from "villages distant one or two days' march," while the *Chauncy Maples* transported some others from lakeside villages (*CA* 22 [1904]: 206). Said the nurse:

> I do very little for them [patients]. In the morning I attend to their wants, and I look in and out during the day and do what is necessary. They fetch their own firewood, catch their own fish, cook their own food, and sweep

the house. Wednesday is also *posho* [maize flour] day, when I give each enough cloth and salt to buy food for the week. The hospital window overlooks the high road, and they intercept any rice, flour, or corn which passes. (All of which sounds very strange to our English notions of the functions of a hospital.)

At Malindi, the mission constructed new stone hospitals and a brick dispensary for Africans in 1908.[5] Patients began to come in from across the lake and distant hill villages. Yet the missionaries felt conflicted by African responses to their offerings of medical services. Writing in 1912, the Reverend R. Russell, a priest at Malindi, felt distressed upon witnessing

> many horrible cases of sickness which might be cured if properly attended to. And in most cases nothing can be done to help, the people absolutely refusing to have their sick carried to the Mission Hospital... owing to the fear instilled into their mind by the false teachers amongst them. The utter helplessness of some of these poor souls is too pitiable for words. (*CA* 30 [1912]: 144)

Simultaneously, teaching and preaching in the villages also met "with little response. In this district no great crowds gather round to hear the missionary (which is a picture usually set before English minds of the missionary preaching to the heathen). Fear, superstition, lust and vice claim these people body and soul" (ibid.).

Fear and mutual hostility sustained African resistance to the mission's medical work. UMCA missionaries openly preached their belief in the degraded character and inferiority of local Islam, calling it the "Dreaded Octopus." In return they garnered resentment and deeper mistrust. Nonetheless, writing again later in 1912, Rev. Russell commented optimistically on the mission's success in overcoming this mistrust:

> Mohammedan teachers put in circulation all kinds of stories as to the cruelty of the mission, and in consequence many poor folk suffered untold agonies, through starvation and neglect, when they might have had instant relief. Some natives risked the anger of Mohammedan teachers and headmen in the villages, and came to the hospitals, many of them being able to return home quite well. Opposition was now broken down, [however], and people sometimes brought their sick many days' journey across the mountains, knowing that they would never be refused admission to the hospitals. (176)

During the war years of 1917 to 1919, the mission was unable to supply a nurse for Malindi, and the closest was nine miles away. Under these conditions, an African dispenser who had been trained by UMCA nurses was given full responsibility for the station's hospitals and outpatient work (*CA* 37 [1919]: 184).

These statistics underscore the reality that, regardless of its vast medical service area, the UMCA's doctor, nurses, and dispensers could reach but a mere fraction of the population that obviously needed care. Inseparable from this situation was the fact that in most of the diocese the perpetually small medical staff found themselves increasingly swamped by their workload outside the hospital wards and operating rooms. The numbers and needs of outpatients, village visitations, and from the 1930s, the attendees at maternal and child care clinics, continued to grow in scope and complexity. The diocese's medical missionaries also had every legitimate reason to believe that their work was undervalued by the UMCA administrators and the church in England, and quite possibly as well by some of their local nonmedical colleagues who put greater stock in more direct approaches to Christian evangelization and education.

THE *CHAUNCY MAPLES*'S 'STATION': SICK TRANSPORT AND DISPENSARY

Arrival of the UMCA's new steamer in 1901 raised the missionaries' confidence about what they might accomplish in Malawi in the new century. The steamer symbolized many things, especially an unprecedented opportunity to expand and consolidate the mission's influence in the lake region. It was a means to empower the mission's fledging hospital system, providing as it did a conveyance and a safety-net for seriously ill mission workers and Africans. The *C.M.* also stirred feelings of nationalistic pride among the European mission workers—an understandable response from foreigners whose voluntary commitments obliged them to live in long-term relative isolation, thousands of miles from home.

Little time was wasted in getting the steamer into its medical transport mode. By 1902 the special sick bay had already proved "a great boon," and Dr. Howard started to see patients on board during his periodical rounds at Kota Kota, Malindi, and Likoma Hospitals (*CA* 21 [1903]: 143). Accommodations on board permitted the *C.M.* to transport a relatively large number of patients from the lakeside villages to one of the three hospitals then operating. On one voyage in 1903 "no less than ten patients (with two wives as extras) arrived at Likoma" (ibid.). This scene remained typical for many years, as the steamer became the primary means of moving patients from the lakeside and adjacent mountains in villages to the nearest UMCA hospital. By 1905, at least, most patients treated in Likoma Hospital had been collected from villages on the Portuguese mainland and landed by steamer (*CA* 24 [1906]: 147; also see "A Day on the *'Chauncy Maples,'*" *CA* 26 [1908]: 104–6). By 1910 at Kota Kota Hospital, two-thirds of the inpatients arrived by the steamer, while the other third came from the town and outlying villages (Mills 1911, 126, 128).

Two of the *C.M.'s* European crewmen did occasional dispensary work on board in between the MO's visits, but they kept no records.[6] Hopes were voiced that a trained African dispenser would be permanently stationed on the steamer. It was already impossible for one European doctor to meet the expressed needs for medical care in the mission's growing realm of accepted responsibility.

In September 1911, a nurse at Likoma reported that the *C.M.* had just brought in thirteen patients to the hospital. In another instance the steamer had transported "seventeen patients from the northern villages, nearly all suffering from deep chronic ulcers and in several cases the bone diseased, several children with these dreadful ulcers aged between three and eight" (*CA* 30 [1912]: 49).

Transporting ill people could be a mixed blessing, saving a few while possibly endangering many more. In 1903 a disease known by Africans as *Mtetekuwanga*, characterized by a generalized rash and glandular swelling and more severe than chickenpox (*varicella*), was present "both on the *C.J.* and *C.M.*" Little known at Likoma, it was thought to have been acquired at Malindi.[7] Also in 1903 several African masons arrived at Likoma aboard the *C.M.*, accompanied by an unspecified number of patients. Within five days two masons had developed pneumococcal-like meningitis infections they had acquired "on the journey down." Both died within the week. Another patient who had slept in the hospital developed a foul sloughing condition of the cheek. When she died five days later, "the hospital was thoroughly burnt out and whitewashed."[8]

Shortages of African staple foods on Likoma Island often proved a "great drawback" to accommodating patients in the local hospital. At one point in 1913, the hospital refused admission to patients aboard the *C.M.*, in contrast to Kota Kota, Malindi, and Mponda's hospitals, where food was usually more regularly available and inpatients thus managed more steadily (*CA* 32 [1914]: 100–4).

As for the smaller, aging *Charles Janson*, no one intended that it might be lost in the *C.M.'s* shadow. Rather, it would be used as an "emergency and despatch boat," working to unite lakeshore stations and "overcome to some extent that isolation which in cases of serious illness is one of the greatest dangers of Central Africa" (*CA* 21 [1903]: 143).

BELIEF AND BEHAVIOR: AFRICANS, MISSIONARIES, AND THE MEDICO-RELIGIOUS FRONTIER

Hospital stays benefited many Africans who suffered conditions such as traumas, deep ulcers, severe burns, fractures, anemias, typhoid, dysentery, childhood malaria, and difficulties of childbirth, including those who underwent major surgery. As a practical matter, dispensaries could reach much larger numbers of people more often, especially when located between hospitals instead of being part of one. In theory, if too little in practice, dispensaries enabled the caregivers to be more with the surrounding communities, addressing some of their acute, chronic, everyday health problems.

For the UMCA missionaries, however, providing European medical practitioners, building hospitals, and offering medicines and treatments for diseases with Western labels did not lead in a straight line to African acceptance or better health. Missionary medicine was essentially part of a distinct and still emerging therapy system based on a rapidly accumulating body of Western science. It was increasingly if not yet entirely centered on germ theory and the notion of specific etiology. Most importantly, in Malawi as elsewhere in tropical Africa, there was no possibility that it would be introduced into a void.

Strangeness, fear, and, where Islam was also rooted, religious animosities, generally meant that Africans did not immediately welcome the presence of a mission doctor or nurse. Such resistance was partly explained by a prevailing theory that African social norms produced apathy or even antipathy toward people with needs who were not part of one's own immediate or extended family. Similarly, it would be difficult to understand, or trust, the altruism of a relative stranger, particularly a white one. A mission observer at Kota Kota stated in 1911:

> The people were suspicious. It was incomprehensible to them that anyone not of their race or language or even colour should wish to help the sick, and frankly they did not believe it. In time, people grew less suspicious, and began to come in for the treatment of small sores and minor ailments, but no serious cases ventured near. The first Mohammedan patient would not come inside the modest little dispensary, but stood some distance off, and explained his illness through the mouth of his slaves, and they received

the medicine and conveyed it to their master, having first tasted it to be sure that it was not poison. (Mills 1911, 110)

After six years with the UMCA in Malawi, Dr. Howard had the opinion that mission medical work provided Africans with an object lesson. As a race, he said,

> they have intense natural affection. The love of a mother is as great as it is in England. But they have not natural sympathy. I do not think the African cares anything for his fellow man as such. If he is a member of his family, or of his tribe, yes, then he has duties towards him; but he has no sense of responsibility for his neighbor. (*CA* 24 [1906]: 201)

For example, observed Howard, "suppose a man on a journey falls sick in a village, the chances are that he will die there. He is a stranger; what claim has he on anyone in the village?" (ibid.).

Speaking in London to UMCA members and prospective medical recruits, Howard advised: "It is of no use going out to [Malawi] and thinking at first you will have grateful patients flocking to you. You have got to work slowly, gradually, and it is slow building up a practice in Africa" (ibid.). Recall that Dr. Howard's influence in UMCA circles had risen rapidly with his leadership on malaria control and other public health concerns.

Referring to nurses' work, Howard had come to believe that "the whole idea of helping the sick is Christian and utterly alien to the ordinary heathen conception" (*CA* 26 [1908]: 151).

To choose not to give or accept medical help from someone outside your immediate kin group was undoubtedly a reflection of the peoples' pervasive witchcraft beliefs and practices (*ufiti*) that were mediated by public opinion, traditional diviners, and other religious specialists. Human agency—the idea that some other person(s) is responsible for the bad things that happen to oneself or one's family—was a central pillar of African belief and practice. It embodied witchcraft's potent fear syndrome and social control mechanism. This deeply embedded sense that the harmful desires or actions of others explain why an individual or group has been made sick, or failed, or been injured was, and often still is, invoked in order to assign causes and blame for illness and misfortune. Enticed by fear, fatalism, and hysteria, in more extreme circumstances death was a possible real consequence of one's belief in bewitchment.

While the missionaries may have highlighted the pervasiveness of witchcraft to garner support for their evangelistic campaigns, there was evidentiary truth in their references to "the atmosphere of terror in which the native lives" (*CA* 28 [1910]: 173–74). Dr. Howard concluded that Africans' nearly universal use of charms and amulets, the poison ordeal, and belief in the reality of bewitchment showed that "heathenism teaches nothing except care for your own family" (175). He also believed that compassionate missionary medicine, if it stayed the course, was the antidote to such conditions.

Howard, the diocese's only doctor, wrote with a broad comparative perspective about the effects of witchcraft on African society and on missionary medicine. He also recorded details of indigenous medicines and treatments such as bleeding, cupping, counter irritation, massage, setting of broken bones and sprains, use of laxatives, and surgery, and referenced cases of witchcraft-associated conditions. Howard advised how important it was in African medical work to understand the "tremendous hold" of superstition and suspicion of others on patients' thoughts and behavior. He and others noted the widespread dread of body-snatchers (*afiti*) believed to work in and around mission hospitals at night. How difficult it was, he said, to fight such ideas "even among Christians," and how futile to argue with patients about them. Even in England some people had "a lingering belief in charms, and in Italy the idea of the evil eye is firmly rooted" (*CA* 24 [1906]: 253).

Early resistance to missionary medicine was common, and fears of it understandably tended to linger longer in more remote places. Furthermore, the UMCA had chosen to focus its efforts among predominantly matrilineal societies, such as the Nyanja and Yao peoples. As discussed further in chapter 9, their traditions called for specific consultations with several relatives of a sick or injured person prior to a treatment decision, a practice which often delayed or eliminated visits to a dispensary or hospital (*CA* 12 [1894]: 137–41).

Before World War I growing confidence in the imported medical practices was registered virtually everywhere in the diocese. This theme became a fairly steady drumbeat intended especially for UMCA benefactors and policy makers. By 1918, the UMCA reported that African belief in European medicine and treatment was "firmly established," forming "a very strong antidote to witch doctoring and the use of charms" (*CA* 37 [1919]: 183). Opportunities for all kinds of medical interventions had markedly increased; with more staff and funds the work could be greatly extended.

From the medical missionary's vantage point, the mission hospitals and dispensaries had a humanizing effect on the African people. Said "C.T.," a nurse whose outlook was widely shared in the mission, at the time:

> To care for the sick is not a general virtue among them. This is not
> intended to imply that there is not much real tenderness and care displayed
> frequently to sick members of their own families, and mothers being much

the same all the world over, the women show the same devotion to their ailing little ones as white ones do, though naturally they are not always wise in their treatment. But to help a sick person who has no direct claim on them, simply because he is a sick person, this does not occur to them. Indeed, it is often considered derogatory—the work of a slave. (CA 27 [1909]: 303)

However, missionary paternalism and maternalism projected confidence that humanitarian impulses could be tapped to advantage when Africans had an opportunity to stay in a mission hospital. According to nurse "C.T.," Africans, "always lovable," became even more so when they were sick. They called the nurses "*Amatee,* our mother, and . . . they are indeed as her children [and] behave almost always with wonderful decorum, [otherwise] one reading of the Riot Act is usually quite effective." "C.T." observed further:

Once there a patient realizes that the sick are considered quite important people, and that at least one white person, and one or two native assistants, make their well-being one of the chief objects of their life and work. It is not long before they begin to do little services for one each other—before they learn, to some extent, self-control, kindness, patience, and all this must make for righteousness. (303–4)

AFRICAN OUTPATIENTS: THE DISPENSERS AND DISPENSARIES

African Dispensers

In 1907, the mission's first trained dispensers, Edward Nemeleyani and Raphael Mkoma, began alternating month-long stints on the *C.M.* around the "Steamer Parish." Between them, they had already accumulated seventeen years training and experience in Likoma's dispensary under the tutelage of Dr. Howard and the mission nurses. Said Howard of the dispensers' first year of work on the *C.M.*: "They are really 'Medical officer.' They have to look after the crew and go ashore at each village to see the sick folk, and select patients for the hospitals. Even the European staff not infrequently come to them for treatment for minor ailments" (CA 26 [1908]: 301).

Without doubt, both men had "risen well" to their responsibilities, making major contributions to the growth of outpatient and hospital work. They grew more able to select those patients who could most benefit from treatment, and also increased the number of ill people who actually reached the mission's hospitals. They looked after the medical needs of both the crew and European staff, and went ashore at villages along the route to treat the sick and to identify people who needed hospitalization. The *C.M.'s* resident clergy also expressed satisfaction with their work, and the experiment was judged a success.

In the meantime, Edward Nemeleyani and Raphael Mkoma had to "put up with a good deal from the unsympathetic side" of African passengers on the steamer. While they proved "willing enough to benefit by their skill," many Africans evidently found little to admire in their fellows who dressed others' sores, dispensed medicines, and performed minor surgery (*CA* 26 [1908]: 301–2). Dr. Howard noted that most Africans did not "take" to such work and showed "a cordial dislike for anything at all nasty."

Systematic dispenser or dresser training did not begin at Likoma until 1912. During World War I, when the *C.M.* was in government service, five dispensers underwent training at Likoma (*CA* 34 [1916]: 82). It required about five years to "turn out" a dispenser. Women also gradually entered this training and proved themselves capable of high standards. Twenty-five dispensers trained at Likoma in 1919.[9]

To be eligible for consideration, a prospective dispenser had to be at least fifteen years old, a Christian, possess a "good general education," and rank "near the top of the school" prior to leaving it.[10] Some entered training as schoolboys, while others started the course as adults. Training included special lessons in elementary anatomy and physiology at St. Michael's College, and "ambulance lectures." Success was rewarded with increased clinical duties, and ultimately responsibility for a dispensary or hospital (*CA* 26 [1908]: 299). Practical and theoretical work was done at Likoma Hospital, and at an appropriate time in their training the dispensers received thermometers and a (prestigious) watch. Generally kind and patient, most trainees showed keen interest in the "theoretical work," but found the nursing and night-duty responsibilities "disagreeable."[11]

The mission trained far fewer dispensers than needed. Teenage boys often started in the dispensary as "bottle-washers" for 2 pence a week, but few stayed long enough to qualify as apprentices. Dr. Howard noted in 1908 that the process of training someone for medical work was "always tedious and often disappointing" because most had a distaste for "nasty" work. Also, access to dispensary stocks tempted some trainees to steal small bottles or boxes in which they put their snuff, as well as pieces of linen and calico "which could clothe a small brother" (ibid.). Some patients would come when the supervising nurse was away and ask to be given medicine without paying for it.

Dr. Howard made an ethnic distinction regarding recruitment. He observed that during his first eight years with the mission, no Yaos completed dispenser training. Of them, he said: "The sight of operations seems too much for them. This is all the more strange since they are naturally a race of hunters and raiders, with no tender feelings toward their slaves or captives" (300). Newly certified dispensers thus often found themselves posted to a smaller station, especially in Yaoland, where the mission desired that they help proselytize the Muslim Yaos. However, since the UMCA's pay scale for dispensers was typically inferior to what other missions such as Presbyterians, or the government, offered for similar training, it was often difficult for the Anglicans to hold onto their investments.

Recruitment of dispensers remained a problem into the 1920s. In a speech on "the work of healing" in Malawi at the UMCA's sixtieth anniversary convocation in London, Canon Dennis Victor asserted that Africans continued to show little enthusiasm for doing anything for people outside their families, or at best "possibly someone in his own village" (*CA* 41 (1923): 181).

Over the years the mission's African dispensers made immeasurable contributions to its medical work. At one hospital, presumably Likoma in 1920, the dispensers reportedly examined over 1,000 specimens in one six-month period, especially for bilharzia and hookworm (King and King 1991, 135). In 1930, one dispenser reportedly managed 25,000 outpatient attendances and also made many visits to the sick in outlying villages. With the aid of a small microscope, he spared a priest from a dangerous relapse of tick-borne fever by taking timely blood slides and sending them to the doctor at Likoma (ibid).[12] Regarding the dispensers, Alice Simpkin remarked in 1926 that

> no people in the Mission . . . work harder, the nurses could not get on at all without them. They prepare the operating theatre, visit in the villages, help with evangelistic work. Our head man, Edward, is very good at diagnosis; and his courtesy and bedside manner are equal to those of any physician in Harley Street. (Simpkin 1926, 56–57)

The task of getting medical care to people who could benefit from it was often frustrating, even when dispensers' own work stations and homes were relatively near the populations they served. Carrying a small biscuit-tin of dressings, they also frequently left their regular posts to visit mission outstations. As often as not, people away from the mission feared the new medicine and often believed they would be poisoned. In 1915, for example, Mponda's dispensers had gone out for an entire day, but came back "having seen only a very few who were ready to trust them" (*CA* 34 [1916]: 68).

By World War I both European and African staff used bicycles extensively to reach outstations in the lake plains near Mponda's. Carrying a flask and sandwiches, they could "save much time, energy and expense" (67). The UMCA recognized that the dispensers' strategic value stretched far beyond their medical, laboratory, and interpersonal skills. Indeed, their special status gave them ample opportunities to help break down public and private "prejudice" toward evangelical work. As they worked for the "relief of sickness and misery," they were also collaborators in "Christ's battle in Africa," helping lead "the fight against superstition and witchcraft" and "winning over the Mohammedan" (*CA* 44 [1926]: 50).

Dispensaries

Providing dispensary services to large numbers of dispersed people was an uphill struggle for several reasons. First of all, the UMCA's huge territory and resource constraints ensured that the number of dispensaries was inadequate to the task of reaching the populations who could benefit from the services. Of the thirteen dispensaries established between 1890 and 1925, nine were physically part of a hospital station and thus served the same villages around it. Over half of these dispensaries did not open until after World War I. Until the war ended, the only freestanding dispensaries opened were Unangu (1893) and Msumba (1906) in Portuguese East Africa (fig. 4.9).

Msumba developed into one of the mission's higher-volume dispensaries. In 1923 a veteran nurse observed that it "had more than justified its existence. Both Selwyn and Paul [dispensers] have done excellent work there. A nurse from Likoma has visited them quarterly, and each time she was besieged with requests for injections for yaws and other diseases" (*CA* 42 [1924]: 132–33).

Eventually, the mission added male and female wards at Msumba, and in 1934 the MO reported that inpatients had increased 50 percent. Most patients had their own food brought to them by family members, which helped the mission to balance this expense. At Mponda's, in- and outpatient work had also grown substantially, and women reportedly displayed noticeably greater trust in the medical services. Credit for these advances was attributed to "the medicine of the needle," which was "a means of bringing many Mohammedans to the hospitals" (*UMCA Ann. Rev.*, 1934, 121–22). By 1938, over 350 outstations had been established within UMCA parishes, but these overwhelmingly emphasized evangelical and teaching activities. A dispenser or nurse could reach only a relative handful on a regular basis.

Second, Africans might be *treated* at a mission facility. Yet, when people returned to their daily living patterns—featuring well-established patterns of ecological and cultural relationships including daily or periodic movement within zones with diverse health risks—the effects of medical treatment could soon be nullified by the normal conditions of peoples' lives. Back in the village, the potential for hookworm infection, malaria, and other fecal-oral and vectored infections remained as great as ever.[13]

Truly maladaptive customs and community standards that harmed health could not be eliminated overnight, or perhaps even in a generation. Reoccurrence of ill-health was often the rule rather than the exception. The fact that Africans seemed to generally accept these circumstances of their habitat and lives reinforced the missionary sense that disease and poor health were often a sign of sin and backwardness. A faithful, consistent Christian lifestyle was, finally, the only true path to higher health standards for Africans. Not surprisingly, the missionaries seemed to put greatest energy into concerns that were, health-wise, comparatively benign, such as trying to protect virginity, and to eradicate polygyny, "lewd" dancing, and other sexual misdeeds. A large effort was also made to inculcate English domestic skills and comportment in African women and girls.[14] Meanwhile, the concept and practice of "community and public health" remained opaque, at best, until the mid-1930s and the post–World War II era.

At the very least, dispensaries offered users temporary respite from suffering. In many instances, treatment led to stabilization and healing. Such success was not lost on the local family and its social extensions, and thus the use of dispensary services gradually increased. A baby's gastroenteritis could be relieved, a cough stopped, an oozing leg ulcer dressed, or a dog-bite wound cleaned with antiseptic, sutured, and bandaged. Yaws reacted dramatically, even miraculously, to injections of the arsenicals. Local anesthetics deadened pain, and vaccine could immunize against smallpox. In 1909, a "rampant" smallpox epidemic swept through the area at south end of the lake. A government smallpox quarantine camp with over three hundred cases was set up near Malindi mission station. The government also initiated payment of a small fee to persons who provided notice of witnessing someone with smallpox (*CA* 27 [1909]: 208). Meanwhile, the mission was "doing all the vaccinating we can," which included "all [50] of our own children" in boarding school (ibid., 22). On Likoma in the central lake region, the mission vaccinated 3,178 people and sustained only one smallpox case (93).

Though it was toxic, the use of carbon tetrachloride (beginning 1920) produced positive results against hookworm. Applications of gentian-violet could slow certain bacterial and fungal infections. Any of these procedures, which were carried out by a European nurse or one of the African assistants, could greatly benefit a patient. An admonition along the way from the nurse or dispenser to wash hands, dig a latrine, or boil water could, in time, expand the benefits of dispensary attendance. Chances of such messages being acted upon improved if the patient was young and in school. Dispensary measures might slow the spread of an infectious disease such as smallpox by primitive (at the time) efforts to increase "herd immunity." This might be obtained by vaccinating a proportion of the population situated outward from a sentinel smallpox case, sufficient to stop its transmission.

As noted, a critical constraint on the effectiveness of the curative, service-point approach within the UMCA's dispensaries was that patients returned to their communities and accustomed habits after treatment. There, poor sanitary practices and hygiene, ignorance, and other predisposing conditions persisted, little influenced by the dispensary-hospital system. This evidently produced a broad recycling of the same cohorts of outpatients, accounting for the fact that the total population of individual outpatients was only a fraction of total annual admissions. Records for 1944 through 1963 suggest that the average annual ratio of patients to outpatient visits was around 1 : 10 (table 8.2). As outpatient admissions grew over time, record-keeping customs generally did not provide for a distinction between new patients and those making a repeat visit in a given year. Records also offer little insight into seasonal variations, and thus their comparative health implications, in dispensary and hospital attendance.

A comprehensive, annual record of outpatients for all UMCA dispensaries is not available for any year before 1922.[15] The most complete reports available for individual dispensaries show annual attendance across the diocese for the years 1922 through 1927. *Total outpatient attendance* (the sum of individuals receiving treatment times the number of visits they made) at all dispensaries is available for the years shown in table 8.2.

By 1923–24, the financial and manpower strains of World War I in Britain had begun to ebb somewhat. By 1925, the protectorate's Medical Department expanded its dispensaries to 78, and outpatient attendances grew three times from 1922 to 1926. Vague, embryonic notions of "welfare" and "development" began to emerge for the first time in the discourse of empire, as reflected in Britain's Colonial Development Act of 1929 (Beck 1981).[16] Unfortunately, the global depression was just around the corner. It soon produced a drastic downsizing of vision and resources for the expansion of economic and social welfare activities, in both the metropoles and colonies. Just a few years later, World War II would further hammer away at development aspirations among Africans and sympathetic colonial officials.

Table 8.2 Outpatients: UMCA dispensaries (selected years)

Year	Total attendance	No. of outpatients
1909	29,943	—
1921	97,000	—
1922	103,305	—
1923	130,536	—
1924	150,700	—
1925	216,827	—
1926	200,508	—
1927	224,690	—
1929	187,022	—
1941	316,464	—
1944	895,000[a]	87,000
1950	310,255	23,999
1951	320,904	24,622
1954	223,105	19,469
1963	394,843	52,000

Source: MNA; *Central Africa*.

[a] Figure for all UMCA Dioceses: Nyasaland, Tanzania, N. Rhodesia. See *Central Africa* 62 (1944): 6. Mission statistics at this time for all dioceses included 5 doctors and 40 nurses to staff 38 hospitals which averaged 1,033 inpatients.

Records for fourteen years between 1921 and 1963 show nearly three million outpatient attendances across the diocese, or about 250,000 annually. Growth in attendance exceeded three times from 1909 to 1921, four times between 1921 between 1993, and thirteen times from 1909 to 1963. During the UMCA's last five years in Malawi, with its control of medical services rapidly winding down, outpatient attendances grew by one-quarter to more than 310,000. The conservative attendance to outpatient ratio shown in tables 8.2 and 8.3, when applied to the years from 1921 to 1963, suggests that UMCA medical services reached a total of about 25,000 individual Africans during a typical year (applying the 1 : 10 ratio of patient : attendances). This modest figure yields slightly less than 2,000 outpatients for each of the mission's dispensaries.

Finally, the geographic distribution of clinic activity for 1963, together with ratios of patients-to-attendances, is shown in table 8.3. Results are mixed, and the distribution of visits by patients and gender cannot be known. However, no significant change in the patient : attendances ratio (1 : 10) is apparent for 1963 over previous years.

Table 8.3 UMCA outpatient activity in 1963: A sentinel year

Dispensary	Outpatients	Attendances	Ratio, O to A (rounded)
Mponda's	7,555	91,556	12
Likoma	4,121	72,528	18
Mkope Hill	5,043	67,444	13
Kota Kota	5,328	43,513	8
Likwenu	6,785	38,067	6
Malindi	3,248	32,932	10
Cididi	3,496	28,296	8
Matope	2,162	10,387	5
Totals	37,738	384,723	10

Source: Diocese of Malawi (Nyasaland), Med. Dept. Ann. Rep., 1963. MNA.
   Table excludes returns for Chizimulu Island dispensary, incorrectly listed in above report as having 14,562 outpatients and 10,120 attendances.

Several factors contribute to the visitation pattern. Resistant and repeat cases are numerous. More than a few patients would have made mistakes with their self-administered medications and follow-up procedures on arrival back in the village. Chronic, "needy" repeaters also figure in a tally of this kind. Further, circumstances suggest that European and African medical staff did not actively discourage repeated visits by a patient. After all, these were moments for encouraging a potential convert, and strengthening him or her in the faith.

MISSION MEDICINE AND COLONIAL GOVERNMENT

In Malawi, the various missions provided virtually all medical and education services for Africans from 1893 until the end of World War I (Gelfand 1964). No secondary schools opened until 1940, nearly fifty years after the protectorate's establishment (King and King 1991, 132). As in most of the British Empire, the colonial medical authorities waited until the 1920s and 1930s to begin to develop even a limited framework of basic curative services. Until about 1930, British colonial policy in the protectorate relied on a few "tools of empire"—the missions and highly localized public health measures—to try to fill the void. Instrumental measures might help to slow, prevent, and control epidemics of plague, smallpox, and cerebro-spinal meningitis, or dysentery. They might reduce morbidity and mortality levels within the tiny segments of population deemed essential to maintaining colonial law and order.

In the early decades these targeted groups for medical attention included European administrators; European, African, and South Asian troops and police in towns and military camps; ancillary African employees of the administration; and some migrant mineworkers. Total expenditure by the protectorate on European and African medical services in 1909–10 barely exceeded £8,000. A large percentage of this sum went to pay the salaries of European doctors and nurses attending European patients in segregated hospitals.[17] As late as 1935, the protectorate Medical Department in Chikwawa District reported that government dispensers and headmen were not reliable sources of case and mortality information regarding a then ongoing dysentery epidemic. Instead, "it is most of the Missions and their teachers that report the proper number I expect."[18] This small example serves a larger point about the administration's often guarded dependence on missions in education and public health.

Another public health example graphically illustrates the arrogant disregard of necessity and commonsense by colonial officials in Britain and Malawi. In 1934, conditions in Zomba Township, the protectorate's administrative center, which also housed the Medical and Sanitary Department, revealed just how little the colonial authorities had done to protect even their own British officers. A laboratory was opened there in 1930, and in 1934 the stools of African cooks, house servants, and others turned up rife with *E. coli* and *E. histolytica*. By then, years of neglect, including failure to install sewers and piped water, had led to the fouling of government compounds and houses. Writing to the Director of Medical Services (DMS), the protectorate's Sanitary Superintendent stated:

> The spread of infection is largely, if not totally, due to flies. Zomba has *for the past forty years* been used as disposal ground of night soil and refuse from the houses they occupy. In many cases it is impossible to find space within a compound in which pits have not already been dug, filled in, and re-opened. The condition is so bad that, in certain cases, the houses are rendered uninhabitable. This is so with regard to the houses of Dunn, Rossiter, Paddick, and Scott where it is impossible to find room for disposal in the garden ground attached to the house.[19]

Not surprisingly, from 1931 to 1934, fifty-eight Europeans were hospitalized with amoebic dysentery in Zomba. That such conditions existed indicates that the colonial authorities, while harping on the need for Africans to build latrines and desist from fouling the bush, set a poor example in their own behavior. After all, had not Britain's own "Sanitary Revolution" begun eighty years earlier?

Before 1911, the protectorate medical establishment comprised a Principal Medical Officer (PMO) and nine Medical Officers (MO), assisted by three to four Asian Sub-Assistant Surgeons. They staffed stations at Zomba (the first station with a "proper" hospital [1896]), Fort Johnston, and Blantyre, each of which had separate European and African hospitals. Government dispensaries also existed at Port Herald and Karonga, over five hundred miles apart in the far south and north of the country, respectively. Early annual reports indicate staffing was so short that "any routine medical work in the Lake districts, which comprise a large part of the Protectorate, was precluded."[20] In 1914 the three existing hospitals accounted for sixty-two beds, while Port Herald (4) and Karonga (2) dispensaries had six others. At this time the country had approximately one million African inhabitants.

During the 1914–18 War, seven of the twelve government doctors and several mission doctors (the UMCA's Dr. Wigan included) were drafted into the army, primarily for duty in Tanganyika. The war could never have been fought on either side without the conscription of huge numbers of porters. Nyasaland's Field Force included 169,000 African Carriers, whose primary responsibility was to carry supplies to the front. Seven carrier hospitals were set up, each one run by a doctor, employing over one hundred medical dressers (King and King 1991, 147).

After World War I, stations with government MOs increased from five to seven, and "the district bordering on the lake received more attention."[21] Nonetheless, medical reports in the early years after the war underscored the effects of severe financial constraints. The drug shortage was drastic, and it was reported "most of the hospitals remain half empty" (King and King 1991, 108). World War II further set back development aspirations among Africans and sympathetic colonial officials.

By 1929, the government had added a European Health (Sanitary) officer, a sanitary superintendent, and sixteen African Sanitary Inspectors. The number of European nurses grew to sixteen up from five in 1912. Protectorate staff had theoretical responsibility for an African population said to exceed 1.36 million, as well as 1,655 Europeans and 1,117 Asians. The government's infrastructure also included 12 African hospitals, 87 rural dispensaries (cf. 6 in 1912), and 170 hospital beds, or roughly 1 bed:8,000 people. Inpatients numbered 3,821.[22]

Given its daunting inadequacies, the Medical Department recognized that it was "merely in embryo." There had been "little progress" up to 1929, which the department saw as a watershed year.[23] In 1930, based on recommendations of the Shircore Report,[24] the Medical Department received a significant boost in the form of a grant exceeding £75,000 from Britain's Colonial Development Committee. It was used to construct twelve new African hospitals by 1934, as well as thirty-six rural dispensaries, three maternity and infant welfare clinics, and staff housing.[25] While modest, such measures suggest a government awakening to the realization that it needed to pursue a more effective role in addressing African health needs. Unfortunately, few of the seeds planted in the 1930s actually germinated. Depression and retrenchment, war in Europe, and the failure of the colonizers to treat health as a development priority undermined any pretense of sustainable progress.

Neither the Colonial Office in London nor British officers in Malawi perceived it as their business to *enable* African societies to become healthier. In 1919 the Medical Department's health budget was about one-thirteenth of total government expenditure. By 1929 the allotment had grown in small increments to almost one-eleventh, or the princely sum of £34,655, of the total available government monies.[26] From 1929 onward, whatever notable accomplishments might be documented represented mere holding actions, particularly in view of African population growth.

By 1940, the Colonial Development Advisory Committee admitted that the Development of Act of 1929 had done little to advance the interests of colonial peoples. Development planning was not a priority, and the Colonial Office, ever reliant on its "pay-as-you-go" policy, "dared not risk new enterprises without a reservoir of accumulated surpluses in the various colonial territories" (Beck 1981, 3).

A Memorandum from the Conference of Missionary Societies in Great Britain and Ireland to the Secretary of State for the Colonies in 1941 criticized the government for the generally poor state of public health in Britain's colonies and protectorates. In medicine and public health, noted the Memorandum, there had

> not been the same planned cooperation as in education. Indeed in some countries an opposite tendency can be detected and we think it is time to say that if Government had made it their policy to co-operate with Missions in the development of health services as they have in education, much more would have been accomplished and at less cost, and some serious mistakes would have been avoided. We would urge that machinery

similar to that which has been evolved for education should be adopted for all matters of health—both in the Colonial Office and by Advisory Boards in the Colonies and Protectorates. For the health departments cannot alone undertake the vast problems of preventive medicine, nor overcome the scourges of tuberculosis, leprosy, and sleeping sickness, nor build up a healthy people through a right dietary. Many missions have their own fully trained medical and nursing services and can help in this matter as efficiently as they can in education.[27]

The Memorandum goes on to point out:

> The training of female nurses in Government Hospitals has not on the whole been a success; in some parts the nurses' quarters are a disgrace and no decent girl will go to be trained. In our opinion work of this sort, for the present, should be done in co-operation with the Churches. [Regarding] medical assistants, [they] were being trained in various centres long before the Government medical schools were founded, and there is much training still going on, e.g., the Universities Mission to Central Africa. Nurses, of varying standard it is true, have been a universal output. In their training character has not been neglected. . . . Moreover, it should not be forgotten what great use has been made of the widespread organization of the Church throughout Africa to teach popular hygiene in the communities in which it is set.[28]

Since this is the "missions" view, one could call it self-serving; yet the overall evidence validates the views expressed.

Some government officials recognized the sacrifices and contributions of medical missions, but others maintained ambivalence and suspicion about them. A wider cooperation remained feasible only in theory. Ironically, these officials also believed that it was a government prerogative to provide medical services. Regardless of the thirty-odd years in which missions had been the only providers, once government did get involved it sought to minimize if not eliminate mission involvement in health policy-making.

Thus, for rural Africans in the colonies, even rudimentary government medical services remained absolutely unavailable for at least a generation after the initial missionary commitments. In this light, skepticism of the argument that Western medicine achieved its greatest importance in imperial ideology and practice from 1880–1930 seems warranted (see Arnold 1988). In truth, limited government initiatives in basic health services did not arrive until the 1920s, and maternal and child welfare did not surface until the 1930s. This pattern was repeated in other territories. In Kenya, for example, if Africans wished to have the benefits of dispensaries, health centers, and maternity facilities, they had to tax their own communities to pay for them (Good 1987).

LEPROSY: COLLABORATION OF MISSIONS AND GOVERNMENT MEDICAL SERVICES

It is against this background that the UMCA and other missions entered into limited collaboration with the government medical services, primarily through grants-in-aid. Practically all formal arrangements focused on special-purpose interventions, notably leprosy and maternal and child welfare. There were also small-scale collaborations to aid some blind Africans. Certain missions, including the UMCA, also later received annual "in lieu of fees" stipends from the government to partially offset unrecoverable fees for medical services. The Medical Department also supplied or occasionally sold the missions drugs for treating yaws (in some areas a large percentage of people with leprosy also suffered from yaws) (*CA* 40 [1922]: 203), bilharzia, and for hookworm campaigns. In 1926, for example, the missionaries received free Hydnocreol oil (Hydnocarpus tree) for injecting into lepers, and free carbon tetrachloride for treating hookworm.[29]

Leprosy was widespread in the protectorate, with some districts having an "alarming prevalency."[30] Although the Medical Department recognized the need to address the disease, as usual, it lacked the resources and manpower to plan and carry out the social experimentation and voluminous required injections. Government strategy was to encourage selected missions, including the UMCA, to strengthen their commitments to leprosy treatment via grants-in-aid. The UMCA had started small programs for lepers as early as Dr. Howard's tenure as MO in the years before World War I (see *CA* 27 [1909]: 213–14, and 28 [1910]: 2). Apart from the small cash subsidies, this secular-religious division of labor allowed the government to take itself off the hook. Presumably, Medical Department personnel could focus on other problems since they did not have much on-the-ground involvement with lepers. For their part, the missions were anxious to remain on good terms with the Medical Department. The UMCA, at least, viewed this collaboration as another means to demonstrate its value to the overall colonial enterprise. As late as 1925, the UMCA was believed to be the only agency that had made any attempt to deal with leprosy.[31]

Meanwhile, the Medical Department remained ambivalent about the leprosy emphasis and its ancient associations with religious societies. It was also defensive about suggestions that it was lax in its own responsibilities to lepers. Responding to a British Empire Leprosy Association (BELRA) official in London immediately after that organization's site visit to Malawi, the Director of Medical and Sanitary Services quite correctly and ably countered criticism of his department's apparent position:

> Though true in the past I do not think that Government can fairly be accused on "doing nothing for lepers" seeing that it supplies Missions with all drugs they require, and treats Lepers at all Government stations where there is a Government Medical Officer or Sub-Assistant Surgeon, 15 in number.... It should also be mentioned that Leprosy is not by any means the only or even the most important of the diseases with which this Department has to contend, seeing that trypanosomiasis is prevalent in very large areas, Plague is endemic in certain parts, and upwards of 100% of the inhabitants are infected with Ankylostomiasis, to mention only a few of our problems.[32]

The UMCA was the first mission in Malawi to work with lepers. It established special leprosy settlements and treatment centers at Likoma, near Malindi, and Likwenu. Before World War I, German authorities in Tanganyika, aided by native police, had rounded up lepers living along the coast of Lake Malawi and herded them into a settlement on remote and previously uninhabited Lundu Island (*CA* 27 [1909]: 213–14). The UMCA formally inherited Lundu's people after the war. Archdeacon Johnson, usually traveling alone, visited Lundu to preach to its quarantined residents. Situated two miles from the Tanganyika shore, it required an often hazardous canoe journey from Liuli of three to four hours.

In 1921 the Lundu camp contained 128 lepers, existing in horrible conditions. Occasionally a nurse and doctor came over on the *C.M.* with dressings. Dr. Wigan observed that most residents lived "in one village of miserable little huts all crowded together into a small space" (213). A large proportion of them also suffered from yaws, which added to their misery and made their leprous ulcers harder to treat.

Wigan recognized that "a time of financial drought is a bad time to be starting fresh work, but an opportunity (long wished for) has come to us of helping these people, who, for the good of the community, are compulsorily removed from the homes." However, he seemed determined to find a way to "clear the island of the disease" by a combining a new annual grant for medical work on Lundu from the Tanganyika government (£20), and sheer faith in the UMCA's ultimate resourcefulness (*CA* 40 [1922]: 203–4). In 1929 the UMCA moved all patients from Lundu to Mngehe on the Tanganyika mainland, a few miles from its Liuli station. For Dr. Wigan, the addition of a second nurse at Liuli meant that at last it was possible, "with reasonable efficiency, [to] look after the hospital and manage the two leper colonies and leper outpatients" (*CA* 48 [1930]: 211).

In 1924–25, the UMCA treated 199 lepers with 3,808 injections of "Moogrol," an extract of the Asian chaulmoogra oil. This treatment apparently proved ineffective, and few patients stayed with it (King and King 1991). The arrival of supplies of Hydnocarpus oil from Calcutta in 1926 offered an alternative that was "probably better than Chaulmoogrol."[33] It was like a golden syrup, and in cool weather it was necessary to warm it in order to inject it. Patients reportedly accepted the extremely painful, large-needle injections with stoicism, and afterwards vigorously massaged the sites "with a bloodstained gray swab" (ibid., 81–82, quoting a European nurse at the UMCA's leper center at Likwenu [Malosa] in the 1940s). In 1927 the protectorate's Agriculture Department began to plant Hydnocarpus trees with a view to producing the oil locally.[34]

At the isolated Maingande peninsula settlement on Likoma, the mission nurse and her assistants visited the resident patients three times weekly. They dressed sores and gave injections in "cheerfully" outstretched arms. They socialized, listened to patients' stories, and offered teaching and prayers. Typically, the team stayed until after evening prayers and hymns. To the nurse's eyes and ears these leprosy patients were "happy and contented [although] each one has a pathetic story; there are husbands forsaken by wives, and vice versa, because of the heavy burden they have to bear" (Simpkin 1926, 46–47). A priest also visited regularly (some lepers became baptized Christians), often accompanied by an African teacher. Nurse Simpkin remarked on how the patients loved to be read to and "ask for the Gospel." Such visits very often ended with the patients receiving "a distribution of tobacco" (47–48).

Other missions that grew active in leprosy treatment in Malawi included the Catholic White Fathers (two main centers), the Scottish Presbyterians (five), and the Seventh Day Adventists (two). Additional advice and financial support over the next several decades came from the British Empire Leprosy Relief Association (BELRA), whose Secretary visited the country in 1927. After his tour he reckoned that with an energetic effort "there should be little leprosy left in Nyasaland in twenty years, perhaps less."[35] The Medical Department guessed that the protectorate then had around 6,000 lepers[36] (or about one in every 215 Africans), while the UMCA's Dr. Wigan estimated leprosy prevalence in the protectorate at four people in every thousand, or 1 : 250 people (*CA* 45 [1927]: 154).

BELRA estimated that the whole Empire had at least 300,000 people with leprosy.[37]

While no one could challenge the notion that lepers deserved help, the government recognized that missions had their own historical, biblical, and spiritual reasons for developing leprosy as a focus. Consequently, missions with leprosy "mandates" had relatively fewer resources to devote to other health concerns that affected more people. Maintaining close oversight of the missions' current uses of grants-in-aid work would enable the government to keep the missions on their toes and exercise some control over future grants. The first leprosy grants and free drugs were authorized in 1927: the UMCA received £300, the Church of Scotland £200, and the White Fathers and Seventh Day Adventists £100 each. In addition, the Medical Department agreed to pay the salary of a hospital assistant and orderly at each leprosy center.[38] By 1943 the government made grants to mission leper settlements at the rate of £4 per 1,000 patients per day, along with free issue of drugs used.[39]

An early example of government's exercise of its oversight powers arose in 1927, when the Medical Department challenged the UMCA's allocation of resources for the leprosy settlement at Maingande on Likoma based on its relative location. This settlement, it pointed out, "serves Portuguese Territory and by virtue of its geographical position can do little for Nyasaland."[40] Three years later, of the patients under treatment at Likoma, twenty-six were Portuguese subjects, only two British. Dr. Sanderson, Medical Department Director, put Dr. Wigan on notice that he was aware of the situation, and that he was "holding up the cheque in respect of the Likoma settlement until I hear from you."[41] In response, Wigan noted that the previous Medical Director and he had held the same view on the matter, namely, that the UMCA was attempting to meet a need regardless of whose colonial subjects they might be. Islanders and mainlanders, he pointed out, were "mostly related" through families and social interactions. Thus, there was some danger of the disease spreading to others. Taking the high ground, Wigan wrote that "I shall of course miss the grant and shall probably have to reduce our numbers as soon as we can do so."[42]

Likwenu mission, south of Lake Malawi, eventually became the UMCA's largest leprosy treatment center. In 1926, the protectorate donated three hundred acres of land situated near the station for the purpose. Here lepers could build their houses, have convenient access to water, and re-create quasi "villages," often along ethnic lines. Thus "the leprosy settlement was a place where a new identity and new community could be forged" (Vaughan 1991, 83).

By 1927, about fifty-two patients had moved into the settlement at Lik-wenu, where they could take advantage of a new concept in case management that featured "no restrictions, no quarantine, and no isolation" (*CA* 46 [1928]: 9). Customarily, Africans segregated lepers from the rest of the population. However, by the mid-1920s the government began to discourage this practice. The old coercive or segregated model was a source of discomfort for both the missions and government, and unsuccessful, because Africans who might benefit from treatment would instead hide themselves among their own people.

By 1927, the Director of Medical and Sanitary Services stated that "it is now definitely accepted as a basic principle that compulsory segregation is not only undesirable but actively harmful. [However], lepers who are in an infective state should be segregated as long as they remain a danger to their families and the community."[43] Rejecting caution, the director believed there was "no doubt that all lepers can in time be made non-infective, even if it is still in doubt whether all can be permanently cured" (Beck 1981, 3).

Alternatively, allowing lepers freedom, including visits by family and friends, meant that they willingly came in for treatment and then stayed in the settlement. Food brought by their relatives helped the mission financially (*CA* 46 [1928]: 9). From the mission's perspective, many of the patients soon experienced "marked improvement." While "fingers and toes" could not be put back, said Dr. Wigan, "sores have healed up and many cases patients have improved in weight . . . and cheerfulness" (10).

Government-mission collaboration on leprosy continued during the remaining thirty-five years of colonial rule. Fluctuations in grants and enthusiasm occurred, reflecting the financial climate and occasional tinkering with policy. In 1929, leprosy treatment was available from six missions (UMCA, Seventh Day Adventist, Dutch Reformed Church, Free Chuch of Scotland, Church of Scotland, and White Fathers). Together they operated ten leprosy centers, three of them run by the UMCA. The total government grant-in-aid was £962 for all centers, and another £200 for drugs.[44] Outpatients attending UMCA centers reportedly numbered 236, yet the government recorded only 188 for all missions. Treatment regimens at this time included multiple, painful injections of Moogrol or Hydnocreol oil. At the UMCA centers in 1929, the 632 patients received 29,491 injections, or 47 per patient (*CA* 48 [1930]: 214).

Malamulo (SDA), in the lower Shiré River region, was the largest leprosarium in the country by 1933. Drugs issued for use included variously Hydnocreol (gaining favor), Alepol, Moogrol and Chaulmoogra, as well as trichloracetic acid, and potassium iodide.[45] By 1934 the missions had opened twelve leprosy treatment centers. The protectorate Medical Department was forced to admit that its £900 grant to missions, plus only £100 for both hookworm and leprosy drugs, "no longer covers needs."[46] At the same time, the government recognized that the number of leprosy patients was increasing rather than decreasing. It was doubted "whether, without properly qualified staff, any real headway is being made."[47] This was echoed a few years later by the DMS, who remarked that "despite valiant Mission efforts, leprosy is not on the wane."[48]

By the late 1930s, the government was taking a tougher attitude towards mission subsidies and also staking out its professional and "turf" positions. It conceded that the missions were "pioneers of medical work and still continue to perform very valuable services," while it alleged that their overall work revealed much variation in quality and quantity. Government subsidies should be restricted for the use of trained European staff, not for less well-trained African student-staff in training. To qualify for a subsidy, missions would have to conform to Medical Department standards "with staff to the scale required." Medical missions "should be open to inspection by government MOs and Medical Headquarters given authority to reduce government payments if approved standards are not maintained."[49]

A new, centralized approach to leprosy was entertained in 1940. The Medical Director proposed that the government invite mission societies to "provide for and maintain" three leper institutions, along lines recommended by Dr. E. Muir, Secretary of BELRA, during his recent tour of Nyasaland. Lepromatous patients formed a surprisingly high 61 percent of the Nyasaland cases seen at that time. He noted the small annual cost to the government (£900) for the care of some six hundred lepers, who were primarily males. Efficiency in these places varied with the availability of skilled medical supervision. Such work needed a larger scale of operation to justify a full-time doctor and two nurses or layworkers. This could be accomplished by increasing the number of patients at a center to four to five hundred or "by combining a moderate sized settlement with preventative work." Whereas Nyasaland's situation called for at least two regional centers, "unfortunately the care of lepers is divided among nine comparatively small units, which, with one exception, are without medical supervision and most of which are of the nature of asylums and of little value towards the control of leprosy."[50]

Muir named the mission centers of Malamulo (SDA) in the Southern Province and Mua (White Fathers) as examples of places that could be further developed. An alternative would be a new government-operated scheme at

Salima.[51] He made no mention of the UMCA among the options, although Likwenu had been the first stop on his itinerary. Leprosy's highest prevalence seemed to occur in the southern lakeshore regions. In Dr. Wigan's opinion, the Malindi district was "about the worst in Nyasaland for leprosy" (*CA* 57 [1939]: 106). However, the mission's efforts to maintain a leper colony at Malindi, with some thirty highly infective, nodular cases in residence, were undermined by inadequate finances and staff. It also encountered great difficulty in preventing members of the colony from mixing with the general population. The facility was closed in 1939.

Muir's ideas proved attractive enough to the Medical Department to cause it to stiffen its attitude toward the operation of the mission "asylums," at least temporarily. However, with the outbreak of World War II, the Medical Department was hard put to keep the existing leprosy programs in operation. Drug losses were serious, especially Hydnocarpus oil imported from Calcutta. This caused relapses among leper patients who had progressed with regular injections. A lack of dressings led to the banana leaf "coming back into its own as a bandage" (*UMCA Ann. Rev.*, 1942, 22). It had previously been used in maternity cases during World War I, along with other local materials including kapok (for dressings) and raw castor oil (King and King 1991, 130). For their part, the missions did not choose to follow up the government's invitation to participate in a reorganization of their leprosy work.

In 1944, the UMCA received government grants of £104 and £150 for its share of leprosy work in Malawi and Tanganyika, respectively. Total all-purpose grants to the missions in 1946 amounted to £8,819. Of this amount, leprosy centers received £1,500, while all maternal and child welfare centers received only £1,050. The remaining £6,269 represented the value of drugs supplied for free treatment, including venereal diseases.[52] The leprosy vote to all missions remained again at £1,500 in 1947. A specific formula for grants was announced in 1950. A mission center would receive "9d per day per leper receiving accommodation, food and treatment in institutions with special accommodations for lepers, or 3d if lepers are not fed."[53] In 1950, the UMCA's share was £222 plus drugs. This increased to £301 in 1951, together with supplies of the new sulphone drugs.[54]

The UMCA's Medical Financial Report for 1953 recorded the "usual" government subsidy. While it is difficult to judge need, amounts on hand in the Likoma (£527) and government (£406) Leprosy Funds, respectively, did not suggest bankruptcy. When in 1953 the government gave only half the usual grants, at the end of the year the Likoma and government funds held £535 and £93, respectively. The latter fund had been depleted by a transfer of £301 to Likwenu, where fully 90 percent of the UMCA's leprosy expenditure was concentrated.[55]

With the inauguration of the Central African Federation (CAF) in 1954, Malawi's Medical Department became a federal agency. Funds and drugs for medical and health services, including leprosy, grew considerably, including the budgets for missions with qualified staffs. Yet new funds could not compensate for the mistrust the CAF's birthing process had created in both government and mission personnel. Morale was low, and the UMCA was sensitive to the "need to be careful not to lose control of our own policy."[56] Under the CAF, the number of European doctors and home-generated funds required by the missions began to shrink. Older doctors on the government staff in Malawi received an ultimatum to transfer to the federal service (and risk being reassigned) or resign, by 1959. Understandably, few Malawian staff wanted to transfer. Others health professionals thought twice about working for an African government in a soon-to-be independent Malawi. Meanwhile, trust between European administrators and Africans further deteriorated as a result of botched efforts with smallpox and polio campaigns, along with failed World Health Organization (WHO) schemes to assess TB and spray Anopheles mosquitoes (King and King 1991).

In 1949, Malawi's missions accommodated 942 inpatients and 436 outpatients with leprosy. With the development of oral sulphone drugs in 1941, new hope for a cure emerged on the horizon. But another ten years passed before their use began in Malawi. And despite the ability of sulphones to arrest infection in a large proportion of leprosy patients, and occasionally possibly curing someone in the early stage of the disease, many new cases continued to emerge. By 1957, it was evident from around the world that sulphones were "not the final goal of chemotherapy."[57] And in Malawi, the reservoir of infectives still seemed vast.

Dramatic success with leprosy control did not occur until after Malawi's independence and the availability of more effective drugs administered in combination doses. The government-subsidized work of the missions was essentially a good-faith effort that helped to highlight the extent of this seemingly intractable and multifaceted disease. Few people were cured, but over the years improved living conditions and diets, human compassion, and palliative care eased the suffering of many.

Church-based work continued after independence, including nine treatment centers at first under UMCA auspices. In 1963 the UMCA received 1,024 leprosy outpatients. Their 35,277 attendances reflect three visits per patient each month. Inpatients numbered 116, with an average stay of 333 days each. Likwenu remained the most prominent leprosy settlement, accounting for two-thirds of all outpatients and nearly 80 percent of all inpatients.[58]

In 1965, BELRA started a home-based control project that placed 4,000 people under treatment with sulphones by 1966. By 1970, the project had 11,000 registered and 220 cured patients, and encompassed all of Malawi. The most satisfying results emerged with the addition in 1983 of the powerful antibiotic Rifampicin to the therapeutic regimes (King and King 1991). Given orally, this drug kills leprosy bacilli quickly, and patients who take it may be considered minimal health risks within a few days (Miller and Keane 1987). Case rates dropped from 38.3 per 100,000 in 1978 to 13.7 in 1987. By 1981 the numbers cured drew even with 2,000 new cases. In 1988, for the first time, new cases fell below 1,000 (King and King 1991). Most Malawians above six years old have been exposed to the leprosy bacillus, and a majority acquire full immunity. In 1994 the World Health Organization certified that leprosy had been eradicated from Malawi. Unfortunately, the government allegedly then cut the budget for leprosy control, and the disease resurfaced in persons with extremely advanced cases only six years later.[59]

HEALTH OF WOMEN AND CHILDREN

After two laborious decades spent in building up its hospital and dispensary medical services, the UMCA lacked a policy with which to guide its efforts among the most vulnerable groups in African society. At this time there was a growing sense within the mission that improving the health and souls of pregnant women, women in labor, newborns, and children under five was essential to Christianizing and "saving" African societies from was perceived as their inherent baseness. Many missionaries had come to believe that their responsibilities must also include efforts to strengthen Africans against the evils of the secular colonial society. Influenced from Europe, the ranks of missions and secular social agencies also began to respond to an emerging age of medical professionalization. UMCA missionaries worried about medical work shifting away from its "evangelising force," and "getting swamped by the increasing 'professionalization' of our hospitals" (CA 65 [1947]: 78).

Similarly, there was a developing sense of medicine's strategic connections to social welfare through public health. Such currents suggested that the quality of attention received by women and children would be a litmus test of the legitimacy of missionary and government intervention in the very foundations of African life. Would European doctors, nurses, and administrators working in the colonies ignore the progressive impulses influencing standards of professional practice at home? After World War I there was a growing consensus that without systematic attention to the special needs of these groups, African communities would become retrograde. Poverty, uneducated mothers, and horrendously high infant mortality ensured that African societies would achieve neither their own aspirations, nor satisfy the economic demands of the colonial system.

Religion, Sexuality and Fertility

Childbirth and its biological enablers, virility and fertility, are deeply embedded in the wider moral, spiritual, and symbolic aspects of African life. In these descent-based societies (primarily matrilineal in Malawi), reproduction and childbearing were essential, potent signs of wholeness and success for entire lineages as well as individuals and families. For women, especially, infertility was feared, and its presence a terrible scourge. Social constructions of reality tended to mask male sterility, placing the onus on the woman. In some African societies, a woman might "overcome" barrenness through social adoptions arranged, for example, between a woman, a fertile co-wife, and their husband.

For men and women without children, death signified their gradual annihilation from the memories of living kin and the unborn. Their spiritual connectedness to venerated ancestors became tenuous. Without offspring, there was no succeeding generation to look after their familial estate on earth, or in the next world. In these and other ways, reproduction was at the heart of African religions. In contrast, the reproductive mores and values of UMCA missionaries proved doubly foreign to African sensibilities. As celibates, they went out of their way to ensure that they would have no biological heirs of their own to claim. Indeed, given the cultural constraints, it is curious that the UMCA and Malawi's Roman Catholic missionaries (White Fathers and White Sisters) managed to attract any men or women into ordained roles. The presence of a cultural and moral frontier could not have been clearer.

European missionaries often became preoccupied with African sexuality and reproduction. Expressions of male virility, fertility dances and ceremonies, polygynous marriage (*mitala*), and "fornication"—reinforced through myths, fantasy, and occasional direct observation—absorbed a large share of the missionaries' psychic energy.[60] In time, the UMCA reported that those districts in which they had experienced most success in Christianizing the populations also had many children. In comparison, the still non-Christian and predominantly Muslim districts, such as the southeast coast of Lake Malawi, allegedly had lower numbers of children born. The mission believed that these demographic differences attributed to Muslims could be traced to higher rates of polygyny, venereal disease, easy divorce, and the "many irregular unions" (*CA* 40 [1922]: 6).

All Africans who entered the UMCA's domain underwent constant, close monitoring of their personal behavior by the missionaries. The latter strove to indoctrinate the idea that Christianity required a certain manner of life, not simply a form of consent to doctrine. Like most non-Africans, many Africans must have found it difficult to meet or rationalize such standards. They fell in and out of grace, particularly for "sins of the flesh." Once out, they had to submit to discipline as the price of regaining access to church participation. The following five cases, drawn from the mission records at Mponda's station, illustrate the missionaries' reactions to perceived wrongful behavior of African Christians.[61]

Aidan Barnaba Kastasi, a schoolboy at Mponda's, had been baptized in 1908 and confirmed as an Anglican Christian in 1909. His English patrons worshipped at St. Aidan's, Gateshead. Kastasi, whose occupation was described as that of "server" in his school, was considered a "very unsatisfactory" student and Christian. He was "always breaking out of the dormitory and going to dances." His larger offenses began in 1913, when he brought a prostitute to the station and tried to hide her in the mission's school for girls. As punishment, he was twice disciplined and barred from Communion by the mission. A few months later, in October 1913, Kastasi married Florie Kalhabeni [presumably in a "village" or non-church wedding]. He was restored to Communion at Christmas in 1913. The following year Kastasi went to work at "Gatoma Estate," leaving Florie behind with his relatives. In 1915 he was reported as still absent, but working hundreds of miles away in Chinde, Mozambique (at the mouth of the Zambezi), in a boarding house owned by the African Lakes Corporation. He returned to Mponda's in 1915. In February 1916 Kastasi was an employee of "Mponda's surgery." Shortly thereafter he was found "living with another woman" named Beda, from Kasungu in central Malawi. He was "disciplined" for another six months. In July 1917, he had separated from Florie, presumably left Mponda's, and "married Beda." One of the UMCA missionaries then "squared" (shared his concerns) with Kastasi's father about his behavior. In March 1918, Kastasi returned to Mponda's and started living again with Florie, denying "all knowledge of Beda." As the missionary who wrote put it, "I expect he means ruining both" women.

Charles Dimu was also a pupil in the UMCA's school at Mponda's, and "boy" to Padre C. Ker. A missionary described him as "a quiet, steady boy, and a good servant, not brilliant, but regular at school." He had run away from the school and "was training to be a Muhammadan teacher, but was rescued by Padre Jenkins." Charles later made a verbal commitment to Christianity and was "given the Cross" at Easter 1907. He was baptized in 1909 and confirmed at the end of that year. He became "engaged to a village girl" and then broke it off. In May 1911, he proposed to another local woman, Helen (?) Angambusye. The couple was "married in church on All Saints' Day 1911." (Thereafter, the name "Angambusye" does not appear in the mission log.) Two months after his marriage Dimu was "convicted of adultery and made to pay up." He was also obliged to spend three months with the local catechumens. In December, 1912, the mission recorded that he was "now steady." By August 1913, Dimu had "married another woman, *mitala* qua village [a polygynous arrangement]," and also had "apparently attached numerous other women." In March 1914 he was away, working at Gatoma Estate, and had not returned to Mponda's as of February 1915. The mission noted that "should he return, it should be quite clear that he has separated from the other women. Then he should have at least six months' discipline." Dimu did return in August 1915, and denied his non-Christian marriage. He was also reported to be "living all right with Helen now," and had been required to study with the catechumens until February 1916. In March 1916 Dimu was "restored to church," although, said the recording missionary, "I have no doubt he lived wrong himself and was purveying women to his European master at Fort J[ohnston]."[62] Dimu was charged with "another adultery" in May 1917, and died at Mkamba Bay, Malawi, in January 1919.

Emily Faith, baptized in 1912, was granddaughter of one of the old Christians at Mponda's village. In clipped style, the mission record notes that she experienced a sexual form of initiation: "She was danced April 1913, possibly by force. Restored and seems really anxious to go straight." A child, John Leslie, was born to Emily in 1913. In April 1915 it was recorded that her husband, "John H. had forsaken her & 'married' another."

Mission workman Manfred Tiputib was baptized on Christmas Eve 1913, and confirmed in April 1914. According to the mission recorder, he had a puzzling lifestyle: "I can't quite make out why he is not married, but such seems to be really the case. A bit given to drink. There are unpleasant rumours that he is mixed up with ufiti [witchcraft], but it is a charge that is quite impossible to sift. I think he is really keen, but doubt if he quite realizes that Christianity ought to mean a manner of life, not merely a form of consent to doctrine." In March 1915, Tiputib "married a heathen who comes to class in a desultory manner." In February 1916 the mission charged him with "adultery with Margaret," and gave him "six months' discipline."

Jonathan Samama was baptized in 1903. He had taken a "heathen" village wife in an unconsecrated marriage. The UMCA's recorder noted that she became blind, "so he put her away, I believe after making provision." He then took another wife, also a non-Christian. At the time of writing Samama was "self ex-communicated, judged by the Bishop to be under sentence of lesser ex-communication."

As the cases above amply demonstrate, once Africans showed more than a passing interest in the potential advantages of church membership, the mission subjected their lives to intense, perhaps even suffocating, scrutiny, especially regarding all things related to sexuality.

Traditional African midwives, typically older women, obviously served as key mediating figures in the reproductive process. Missionaries perceived them as secretive, superstitious, and unclean. Midwives provoked fear and loathing, not least because they exercised a powerful influence over beliefs about fertility and mother-infant roles. As Vaughan emphasizes, they were "the locus of the reproduction of many strongly-held beliefs." Furthermore, early missionary accounts contrast the "'darkness' of the African birthing hut . . . against the candles and white sheets of the maternity ward. Elder women who assisted in childbirth came to symbolize for these missionaries the immensity of the evil they were opposing in their work" (Vaughan 1991, 67). If Christianity was to flourish, the missionaries would have to neutralize the midwives' social and moral influence.

Given its ancient and central role in indigenous life, traditional mid-wifery remained the primary mode of delivery throughout the colonial era in Malawi. While European nurses eventually taught the elements of British birthing techniques to dozens of Malawian women, they were too new and too few in number to promote widespread changes in the behavior of most pregnant Malawian women.

Infant and Child Mortality

Mission responses to maternal and child welfare issues reflected international currents of change in public health. Dr. Wigan observed in 1933 that the mission's new focus had "claimed a considerable concern and interest in the Medical World in the last 5 or 10 years." Losing babies, he said, was a very serious thing among the African people, who still showed so much superstition and fear. It was through infant welfare centers that the UMCA could do the necessary work of caring for babies and checking their weekly progress; arresting sickness in the early stages and by preventive measures; providing simple talks for mothers on baby and self-care; and winning their confidence (*CA* 51 [1933]: 233). That such services could benefit the women and children was beyond question. With large numbers of living children the ideal, women spent much of their lives in serial pregnancy.[63]

From a missionary perspective, indigenous success in maternal and child health was greatly compromised by "gross carelessness" with babies and ignorance of hygiene. Few girls attended school, and the middle-aged and elderly women who served as midwives generally had little or no formal education.

In 1903, during house visits on the western side of the lake among Ngoni-land Christians, Dr. Laws and other Free Church of Scotland missionaries discovered in one district that 180 of 230, or 75 percent, of children born to church members had died. In a second district, 42 of 79 (53 percent) had died. At the Free Church station at Embangweni, 150 mothers surveyed by Dr. Agnes Fraser in 1924 reported that they had borne 611 children, and that 309 had died. Another infant mortality survey, undertaken by a physician among fathers in Karonga district in 1932, found that the under-six death rate exceeded 40 percent (King and King 1991, 166). In fact, at that time there was still little scientific knowledge of the average infant mortality rate (IMR) anywhere in Malawi. Bishop Cathrew asserted that infant mortality in the UMCA's sphere was a "terrible average 75 percent" (*CA* 46 [1928]: 105, and 51 [1933]: 233).

Government concern about Malawi's apparent demographic crisis emerged after the 1921 African census determined that the estimated population was 1,199,934 (Kuczynski 1949, 2:532.). Available information suggested a declining population compared to the 1901–11 period. Dr. Wigan spoke of the likelihood of a much greater decrease during the 1920s, given the pro-tectorate's "enormous" infant mortality and the interplay of malaria and famine (*CA* 40 [1922]: 91). Meanwhile, there was the little mentioned but ever-present migration of labor and its dimly understood interconnections to family structure and welfare, including infant and child health.

In 1925 a government order was issued through the DMS to various Medical Officers. Their charge was to conduct qualitative field studies to determine factors that affected local birthrates and infant and child mor-tality. Many of these reports were prepared by Sub-Assistant Surgeons, primarily Sikhs seconded from India. Original reports of risk factors for infant mortality in five districts, beginning with UMCA localities at the south end of the lake, paint a remarkably grim picture of infant survival prospects:[64]

> Syphilis is, I should think, the most important. . . . General unsanitary conditions and habits [body cleanliness, excreta disposal, etc.]. . . . Malaria must cause some deaths. . . . Bronchitis and bronco-pneumonia are common causes. (Ft. Johnston [incl. Malindi, Mponda's], Jan. 16, 1925. Medical Officer to DMS, Zomba)

> Scarcity of milk. . . . Immaturity and ignorance of the mother. . . . Early marriage. . . . Custom of marrying 10–12 girls at a time without looking after their children and unable to feed them. . . . Lack of education. . . . Hereditary tendencies. . . . People live in unsanitary conditions. . . . Improper feeding. I have seen mothers giving solid food to v. young infants. . . . Other causes such as illegitimacy, quack midwives, and congenital defects. . . . [Male infants] most susceptible to cold and unsanitary conditions—catch bronchitis pneumonia. This is especially favoured by native habit of keeping infants without any clothing. . . . Debility at birth, measles and tetanus also play greater part in it. (Ft. Manning, Jan. 22, 1926. Sub-Assistant Surgeon, M.D., to DMS, Zomba)

> Immaturity. . . . Bad feeding. . . . Ignorance and carelessness on the part of parents. . . . Abnormally dry, hot summers and cold winters, which gives rise to diarrhea and respiratory infections. (Dowa, Jan. 18, 1926. Sub-Assistant Surgeon to DMS, Zomba)

> About 15 percent of infantile deaths are due to cold, diarrhea, and *longlonwe*, a native disease that starts at root of umbilical cord. . . . [Customs]: They don't give bath to the baby after birth, nor [do] they cover it. . . . After one or two days they push some porridge in its mouth. (Port Herald, Jan. 15, 1926. Sub-Assistant Surgeon to DMS, Zomba)

> Habit of nursing mothers giving their infants all sorts of utterly unsuitable food. . . . The widespread native witchcraft superstition tends to enhance the influence of the native doctor and to belittle the usefulness of the government medical service. . . . Diseases tentatively placed in the following order: (1) malaria, (2) intestinal diseases, (3) pulmonary. 1 and 2 vary in incidence according to local geographical and climatic conditions. (Dedza, Dec. 10, 1925. Medical Officer)

> [Summary of findings]: Infantile mortality is undoubtedly very high all over the country. . . . Natural causes do not appear to play a part in infantile mortality. . . . Habits and customs do play an important part in

increasing mortality. . . . Early feeding of totally unsuitable food causes dyspepsia and intestinal troubles. . . . Native superstitions encourage Native medicine and belittle European medicine. . . . It is a common practice of all medical men to have infants brought to them as a last resource after native medicine has failed and when it is too late to save them. Is not known to what extent if any the practice of destroying twins, deformed babies, and bastard or half-caste babies is carried out. . . . Diseases cause a still heavier infantile mortality. The common causes are malaria, diarrhea, dysentery, bronchitis, pneumonia, and infection of the umbilical cord just after birth. (Zomba, DMS to Superintendent of Census, Jan. 25, 1926)

The preceding commentaries from medical personnel in the field provide strong clues about infants' survival odds. In his regular annual report for 1926 the DMS concluded from census returns that total fertility was 6.3 children per mother and that forty-four out of a hundred children born alive "fail to become adults."[65]

In many African societies, social practices had not favored the survival of "abnormal" infants, particularly when their presence might be seen to stress local resources, or when their physical appearance could frighten adults and bring accusations of witchcraft. Alice Simpkin, a long-tenured nurse at Likoma, said in 1926 that it was "only lately that twins and weaklings have been allowed to live" (Simpkin 1926, 52). It was customary to kill a Likoma child who cut its upper rather than lower teeth first. Also, little was done for an orphaned baby if no relative was available to feed it.

Later on, Kuczynski's widely cited survey of colonial demography criticized Malawi's colonial medical officials for their fanciful and inappropriate speculation about infant and child mortality statistics. His survey also found little if anything positive to report about the general health of the country's peoples in the 1920s and 1930s: "They are born, live and die under the most insanitary conditions, they are despite the benefits of education and 'Pax Britannica' on the whole very poor and are ignorant even of the most elementary principles of hygiene" (Kuczynski 1949, 2:623).

While access to mission and government maternity facilities was life-giving and sustaining to some, child mortality in colonial Malawi remained very high everywhere. At remote Mua, a White Fathers-White Sisters mission situated near the southwest coast of Lake Malawi, 2,237 live births were registered in the first fifteen years after World War I. Of these children, 808 died before the age of two years (36 percent), 132 between two and five years (6 percent), and 53 between five and fifteen years (2.5 percent). Comparable data for nearby Ntakataka Mission, operated by the same Catholic orders, show only slightly lower rates of total mortality. This station recorded 3,160 live births during the same period: 695 children died by age two (22 percent); 166 died between ages two and five (5 percent); and 142 between ages five and fifteen (4.5 pecent), or thus 32 per cent mortality from birth to age fifteen. An analysis of these statistics emphasized that "with such mortality amongst Christians who had access to some medical facilities, and in most cases enough education to use them, child mortality amongst the general population along the lakeshore can be imagined" (Linden 1974).

At the International Conference on African Children in 1931, it was suggested that average IMRs in eastern Africa, including Malawi, "was 50 percent. or even higher," with the range from 82 percent in the "worst districts" to occasionally as low as 20 percent in a few others. In Lord Hailey's survey of British Tropical African Colonies (1937) the rate in the "Nyasaland selected area" was 154.6 per 1,000 (*UMCA Ann. Rev.*, 1941, 5). While unacceptably high even for the time, these rates appear much too low when compared with the post-independence era. By the 1990s, reportedly one third of Malawian children still died before reaching the age of five (King and King 1991, 167). If accurate, this observation suggests that few gains have been made in child mortality since the 1930s.

Credible statistics on women's childbearing in Malawi came only after educational opportunities for girls expanded, and time and experience had lessened the strangeness and cultural distance between women and those asking intrusive demographic questions. As late as 1933, the Medical Officer at Ft. Johnston (a heavily Muslim district) reported that he had been "unable to obtain satisfactory and reliable information as to facts or figures on . . . infant mortality." No child welfare work had been started in the district. At Mponda's Mission Hospital nearby, the UMCA's sister-in-charge assisted him to question several mothers at their child welfare clinic. Yet

> I found . . . that even there where they have been attending for many months—some for years—the mothers were most unwilling to give any history connected with their child-bearing, and rather resented being questioned; stillbirths and miscarriages were rarely admitted. Moreover, they seemed to have no idea either of the cause of, or age of death of any children who had died in infancy or childhood. I am of the opinion that the figures obtained would be quite valueless from a statistical point of view.[66]

As in most African societies, infants in Malawi generally received at least two years of on-demand breast-feeding. However, the supplemental foods they ingested such as *phala,* a thin, gradually thickened maize gruel, and sweet beer, did not win praise from colonial-era medical observers, who saw them as unsuitable and unnecessary for infants. It was claimed that this poor diet, and direct feeding from unsanitary adult hands, were "largely responsible for the high infantile mortality from enteritis."[67] At the beginning of World War II, the nurturing of most infants and children in the Diocese of Nyasaland was done in an environment that posed severe challenges to their survival, including the usual diseases associated with unsanitary surroundings, insect vectors, malnutrition, and ignorance of hygiene and child welfare practices (*UMCA Ann. Rev.*, 1941, 5).

OPENING MATERNITY SERVICES

Weakening the control of village birth attendants was not something that would be accomplished quickly. One of the first European-supervised African maternity cases in Malawi occurred in 1890 in Ngoniland. This was an extraordinary occurrence, since African "childbirth was handled almost entirely by traditional birth attendants in the villages." Women who had not given birth themselves were generally considered too young and ritually unacceptable to serve as midwives. Participation of European professional staff in African deliveries remained "an uncommon medical event for another half century," at least (King and King 1991, 164).[68] The fact that European mission nurses had no children must have been one factor in their slow acceptance as authority figures.

In Africa generally, pregnant African women—and society at large—did not interpret their condition as unusual or risky. Whereas European women of this period could be expected to deliver and stay in bed for two weeks,[69] an African woman might return to her gardens within a day or two after she delivered.[70]

In Malawi, the Dutch Reformed Church Mission (DRCM) hospital at Mvera evidently was the first place to attract substantial numbers of pregnant women for delivery. In 1910, Dr. William Murray reportedly had "many maternity patients," and he prepared the first formally trained African midwife in the country (ibid.). In *What We Do in Nyasaland*, the UMCA's Mills (1911) makes no reference to maternity work, which is also true of Gelfand's (1964) *Lakeside Pioneers*, a well-known "socio-medical study" of Malawi to 1920. After World War I, which brought greater exposure to outside ideas, attitudes began to change. A slow trickle of African women began to avail themselves of obstetrics and the unequivocally higher hygienic standards of European maternity practice.

The UMCA developed maternity facilities at Kota Kota (thirty beds and two out-clinics), Likoma, Mponda's, and Malindi Hospitals starting in the late 1920s. In time, midwifery schools and courses were opened at several locations under the auspices of the DRMC (1928 at Mlanda), Scots (1932, 1933 at Blantyre and Bandawe), and belatedly, the UMCA's St. Anne's Midwifery School at Kota Kota (1941 and 1947), where each week at least seven babies were born. This school started up with five students, all married, and all literate except a keen, much older woman. The two staff included St. Anne's European nurse and an experienced African hospital assistant from Kota Kota (*UMCA Ann. Rev.*, 1941, 6; and 1947, 19).

By the 1940s, African antipathy toward the idea of young unmarried women serving as midwives and nurses had begun to decrease. This was of course viewed in a highly positive light since it promised increased African staff and set an example that might further isolate the village midwives. In 1953, six of seven students passed the government certificate examination and received recognition in a capping ceremony at Kota Kota. Following a tea party and speeches, African drumming commenced, lasting until well after dark. "We took our leave when the drumming began," one of the two English nurses said, and they danced "until well after dark" (*CA* 72 [1954]: 129–30).[71]

By 1928, after thirty-five years of British rule, the government, too, finally got into the business of training midwives. Its first action was to facilitate the offerings of rural welfare and maternity services by the Jeanes Institute in the countryside around Zomba. Participation was miserable, and after eight years the institute averaged only two "confinements" per month. This poor showing was blamed on the fears and taboos of uneducated women, as well as insufficient propaganda and time to demonstrate results (King and King 1991, 165, citing the 1936 *Jeanes Report*).

By 1930, Malawi's low health standards finally caught the attention of Downing Street. In London, the Colonial Office viewed "with very grave concern" rumors that the protectorate's population was variously stationary or declining. Local authorities received instructions to intervene with measures to promote African population growth and raise its generally poor physique to an acceptable standard. Such action was "demanded by consideration both of their welfare and of their economic prosperity," a statement that reveals the intense concern of colonial officials, and planters, about the implications of an inadequate labor supply in the colonial economy. The protectorate's DMS was directed to furnish relevant demographic information, as well as provide "details of all customs in Nyasaland that may relate to health" such as female circumcision.[72] More than health was at issue here, as London wished to avoid a repeat of the disastrous bungling of African affairs then occurring in central Kenya.[73]

To alter these unfavorable circumstances it was seen as necessary to develop a greater emphasis on maternal and child welfare. By the late 1930s, confidential dispatches from the Secretary of State for the Colonies and the Colonial Advisory Medical Committee indicate that the protectorate government was under strong pressure to get results. Meeting on March 24, 1937, the protectorate's Native Welfare Committee unanimously agreed that more effort should go into training native midwives and health visitors for rural districts. The DMS recommended to the government that much of the proposed expansion in this area could be handled most economically by the Jeanes Centre, which embraced "every aspect of rural welfare," rather than the African Hospital in Zomba.[74]

Such shifting of loads was the only realistic alternative for a Medical Department that seemed, comparatively, at least, as starved for resources as the UMCA. Waste of available resources exacerbated this situation. In his report for 1937, the DMS pointedly noted that Zomba was the only place in Malawi with more than one government doctor (MO) and with European nurses. Only three African hospitals had any clerical assistance, two of which were overburdened with increased work caused by the medical examination of laborers headed for South Africa. Furthermore, the protectorate had no European sanitary inspectors outside Blantyre and Zomba, nor health sisters or lady doctors in its employ.[75]

Colonial Development Loan funds enabled the Medical Department to undertake a number of initiatives in the 1930s, including maternal and child welfare work and training of African Sanitary Inspectors, Laboratory Assistants, dispensers, and nurses.[76] Within a few years the Medical Department opened several infant welfare clinics, but in 1933 those at Ft. Johnston and Port Herald lacked staff and lay unused. It was generally recognized that "no real progress in public health can be anticipated until the women are educated in the management and care of their children."[77]

Small government grants-in-aid were started in 1930 "with a view to encouraging missions to undertake this work." Even the Portuguese administration gave a grant to the UMCA, which financed a new maternity hospital at Msumba inside P.E.A territory (*UMCA Ann. Rev.*, 1937, 102). Several missions including the UMCA also received protectorate grants for maternal and child welfare. In 1943 these subsidies amounted to £350 annually per mission, contingent on an understanding that a European midwife be posted to the designated center. In the following year the government offered per capita grants of £20 to approved missions that would train and post African midwives for government service.[78]

As with leprosy, small grants for maternal and child welfare became a regular fixture of the government-mission collaboration until the end of the colonial era. The extra funds enabled the missions to sustain a somewhat higher level of service in this key preventive area than was possible with mission funds alone. Missions could also reinforce awareness of the legitimate, essential functions they provided the colonial state. For its part, government delegated responsibility to a surrogate agency, receiving comparatively splendid returns on its small investment. It could thus claim some success at discharging its minimal responsibilities and, through the quid pro quo, maintain some control over mission agendas.

Still, some in government remained all too aware that collaboration might deliver the trump card to the missions. In 1938, for example, publication of the Sir Robert Bell Commission Report drew a strong "turf" response from the protectorate's DMS. Bell Recommendation No. 49 asserted that maternity and child welfare clinics should be left to missions, with financial assistance from government. Bell, the DMS responded, failed to appreciate the importance of government responsibility for maternal and child welfare work. "The future life of any state," the DMS instructed, "is dependent on the ante-natal and post-natal well-being of its child population." Rapid development of such services, he claimed, was occurring in many British African colonies, and by Union Miniere in the Belgian Congo. On a recent tour of Malawi the DMS had visited several mission centers active in this kind of work. He pointed out that while the African staff proved themselves quite busy and enthusiastic, there were too few of them and many seemed unqualified to teach others. Moreover, the only place where midwives could be effectively trained was the joint CSM/Government school in Blantyre. The protectorate's largest town government, he said, must not evade its responsibilities. While the DMS did not want to "belittle the beginning made by missions," it must be appreciated that "what they are doing is only a beginning and the government control and direction will be necessary if they are to develop satisfactorily. Mission centres will, however, touch only the fringe of the population."[79]

These defensive official comments, made just before World War II, reflect a brazen disregard of the government's own history of minimal or noninvolvement in African health services. They discount the colonial government's long dependency on the missions, and its continuing inability to do more than scratch the surface of the protectorate's basic needs for preventive and curative health service. Personal ambivalence and suspicions about missionaries, including their motives and qualifications generally, helped shape the attitudes of some government officers.

King and King (1991, 165) assert that the real turning point in maternity services was "the advent of obstetric surgery" in the mid-1930s, notably after the arrival of two Scottish surgeons who were posted at the government hospitals in Ft. Johnston and Zomba. Taking on numerous cases of abnormal midwifery, including Caesarian sections, they demonstrated that the lives of more women and infants could be spared through their procedures. When word of these results started to spread, maternity patients reportedly began to come to these two hospitals by the hundreds. In 1943, some 2,000 women delivered in government hospitals, and their numbers doubled during the next year. By 1951, confinements in government facilities had risen to 9,804 (ibid). This nearly 500 percent growth of hospital deliveries in only eight years was almost certainly related to the spread of information among mothers about increased infant survival rates, as well as growing access to maternity facilities.[80]

In the mission sphere, use of maternity services was distinguished by marked place-to-place variations. In 1927, all eight UMCA hospitals counted only fifty-three maternity cases, fifty of which occurred at Mponda's. Dr. Wigan took great encouragement from this particular accomplishment, considering Islam's hold on the people of Mponda's district (*CA* 45 [1927]: 94; Medical Officer's Report, *UMCA Ann. Rev.*, 1927). From 1930, the mission opened several maternal and child welfare clinics, and more mothers began to break with the custom of village birth. Whereas twenty years earlier European-style midwifery had been a "rare thing, by the early 1930s it had begun to experience marked growth" (*UMCA Ann. Rev.*, 1933, 103; *CA* 52 [1934]: 103).

In her analysis of this growing shift in birthing culture and politics, Vaughan (1991) argues that the UMCA missionaries celebrated the new births under their auspices as a kind of rescue operation. In Msalabani, Tanganyika, for instance, UMCA sisters assisted African Christians to construct a special "House of Birth." This place was consecrated on the feast day of the Nativity of the Virgin Mary in 1931. In Vaughan's interpretation of UMCA thinking, pregnant Christian and non-Christian women would increasingly choose "House" deliveries once they experienced or learned about the improved survival rates of both babies and mothers. If successful, this strategy would help to remove women from the powerful clutches of the "heathen grandmothers" who attended village births, who silently collaborated with practitioners of "witchcraft" and superstition.

The missionaries aimed to influence women to reject traditional midwives, who worked with diviners to transmit a backward and pernicious culture symbolized by the ubiquitous and "disgusting" amulets and "protective" charms fastened around the African child's waist and neck, or in the hair. A "mission baby," Vaughan accurately observed, was much more rarely stillborn or injured than in the village delivery system. It stood to gain a head start in life over village babies, with greater opportunities to fulfill the mission's criteria for discipline and good character. The child's mother would also be more likely to attend the mission's infant and child welfare clinics, thus creating more possibilities to expose the child and herself to good moral and health influences (ibid., 67).[81] As Vaughan asserts, " 'mission babies' were symbolic of a much larger missionary programme—the battle against the evils of pagan society" (68). As the following discussion indicates, efforts by the UMCA and other missions to guide mothers and children into their welfare clinics proved to be one of their most notable achievements in health.

MATERNAL AND CHILD WELFARE

Demonstration of life-saving obstetrical skills was not the only, or major, factor that convinced some African women to start delivering in a hospital setting. Health reports reflect major changes in the UMCA's thinking and acting on these issues. Key elements of public health philosophy in Britain had also begun to filter in, including ante- and postnatal care, and maternal and infant welfare clinics. This "new 'welfarism' " infused colonial policy during the 1930s and 1940s. It contributed to a more secularized discourse and practice regarding maternal and child health (ibid., 67). Growing from and complementing this trend was the institutionalization of grants-in-aid by a colonial government that had become more aware of the appalling health conditions under which Malawi's women and children lived and died.

Whereas progressive UMCA doctors[82] and nurses supported public health initiatives, the main impulses for broadening the concept of medical services came from outside. They include the influence of the public health movement in Britain and Europe, the International Conference on African Children (1931), and direct instructions from the Colonial Office to protectorate officials to halt Malawi's still-declining population. This last factor reflected concerns about the manpower needs of both European settlers and the protectorate itself. In response to these forces the government began to coopt missions to train African midwives and build facilities that offered maternal and child health (MCH) services.

The mission's approach to public health included the introduction of the Mothers' Union (MU). An imported British model, the MU was an agency of intentional culture change. Underwritten by the MU in Britain, it eventually had four staff in the UMCA dioceses, including one in Malawi. Mothers'

Union staff were highly trained, professional women whose primary responsibility was to train African women in hygiene. Their qualifications often included preparation as a teacher or evangelist. They worked "side by side" with the mission in Africa and in England (*CA* 57 [1939]: 249). Their formal assignment with the mission was to "uphold the sanctity of Christian marriage; awaken in all mothers a sense of their great responsibility in the training of their children; and organize in every place a band of mothers who will unite in prayer and seek by their own example to lead their families in purity and holiness of life" (*CA* 60 [1942]: 78).

In time, the local Mothers' Union trained Africans in British methods of visiting the sick, the poor, and the elderly, all of whom it was believed "have had little done for them in African tribal life." According to mission sources in 1942, European MU workers found that getting the African women to carry on with the work in their absence was "one of the most difficult tasks." In particular, visiting the sick was complicated by the persistent "mutual fear" that people generally had of one another. If an ill person's condition worsened after such a visit, the visitor would typically be blamed (ibid).

With their lives changed spiritually through the church and MU, African women could "create a Christian public opinion . . . to protest against heathen and superstitious practices" (*CA* 57 [1939]: 250). A primary target was Malawi's primarily matrilineal descent societies, in which fathers had little real responsibility or control over their own children. Fathers in positions of authority below that of their wives, and thus in homelife, directly conflicted with the UMCA's doctrine on Christian living. In 1949, a long-delayed Fathers' Union was initiated at Likoma, Liuli, and other places with a view to preparing men to act as "leaders of their fellows" in the villages (*CA* 68 [1950]: 160).

From the late 1920s, UMCA staff began to look for more opportunities to engage Africans about infant welfare and hygiene (*CA* 49 [1931]: 126). St. Anne's Hospital at Kota Kota recorded relatively quick advances on this front, although it must be remembered that the overwhelming majority of African women continued to deliver their babies in village confines. In 1930, the hospital had "fourteen ante-natal cases, twelve confinements . . . and 125 babies on the books." By the following year, with 3,254 attendance's at its baby clinic, St. Anne's became the UMCA's leading center for antenatal and child welfare work. A small round ward had also been built for maternity (*CA* 50 [1932]: 106). In 1942, with "260 babies born and 350 ante-natal cases," students in the midwifery school had no lack of "sufficient 'material' for their studies" (*UMCA Ann. Rev.*, 1942, 22).

In the interest of more uniform standards, a protectorate ordinance creating a Midwives Board was enacted in 1947. It covered both government and mission training schools, such as St. Anne's, and mandated certificates for women who attended a recognized training school who passed a common exam (*CA* 71 [1953]: 84).

UMCA staff naturally took great satisfaction in observing a gradual breakdown of African prejudice toward the mission's maternal and child welfare programs. This was no small task, especially in difficult cases where obstetrical instruments and chloroform might be required ("Nyasaland Diaries, A Notable Advance," *CA* 67 [1949]). In 1949, after mission staff had spent decades lamenting Muslim hatred and insolence, came the report that "Christian, heathen, and Muhammadan women have their babies in the hospital and many a life is saved in abnormal cases" (ibid., 27).

Postgraduate training in "district midwifery" was introduced at Kota Kota in 1949. It was initially designed for recently qualified midwives who staffed a health center situated in a densely populated area near the mission (*UMCA Ann. Rev.*, 1949, 21). Finally, almost fifty years after Kota Kota's founding, a Senior African Midwife was placed in charge of an outstation maternity clinic, situated in a Muslim village. Villagers built the clinic and staff houses, and looked after the well-being of the Christian midwives "in every way." Said the Bishop of Nyasaland, it was ironically "strange and sad" that Christians in an adjacent village, whose church the midwives attended, had shown little interest in supporting a clinic themselves (*CA* 69 [1951]: 29). Two welfare clinics near Kota Kota also opened in the early 1950s, with each center linked to more than thirty villages (*CA* 71 [1953]: 84).

Even in some of the most remote, poorly accessible UMCA stations, such as Milo in the Livingstone Mountains, attendance by mothers with children ages two weeks to two years was reportedly "very good" by 1932. The resident English nurse reported that "the Baby Clinic is my hope. It is a kind of Mothers' Union and Baby Clinic combined," where the babies are "weighed and remarked upon and the mothers are taught about their responsibilities as mothers" (*CA* 51 [1933]: 255). Nevertheless, for many people the mission compound remained a place of overwhelming strangeness. Those who did enter often ran away again out of fear.

At Likoma Hospital, where they experienced "many deaths in childbirth," the twenty deliveries and fourteen antenatal cases handled in 1933 reflected Mothers' Union work and the associated baby clinic. Said Dr. Wigan, it demonstrated "the need for us to push the antenatal work." Hookworm and syphilis were of particular concern because they appeared to be "the most common causes of miscarriages and labor difficulties." More people with hookworm were coming in than ever before.[83]

Also in 1933 an enterprising nurse at Mponda's began treating bad cases of hookworm with local fish livers, and with "considerable success," noted Dr. Wigan. That same year UMCA nurses also initiated contacts with local midwives in some of the station's outlying villages, teaching them "something of our methods." Progress toward better sanitation and hygiene lagged, not least in Southwest Tanganyika. Concerted efforts were underway in local antenatal clinics to help treat and reduce the prevalence of hookworm infection. This parasite was a major cause of death in childbearing, and most pregnant women needed treatment.[84]

While narrative evidence suggests that women joined the Mothers' Union in modest but growing numbers, evidence of actual numbers is scarce. A second European MU worker did not materialize in the diocese until 1954. When eleven new members at Mponda's (five with their first babies) were inducted in May 1955, members from the older MU at Malindi traveled about twelve miles to stand behind them ("acting like sponsors") (*CA* 73 [1955]: 219).

African acceptance of Western causes of infant illness and death was an ongoing, but never complete, process (Ranger 1981). This remains true today, especially regarding explanation of infant illness and death. Mission schools and hospitals aimed to facilitate the spread of ideas into and beyond their near hinterlands, thereby making inroads into small but widening segments of African society. Direct and indirect exposure to new ideas gradually enhanced maternal and child welfare before, during, and after birth. For instance, when school children later became parents, some would pass on their new skills and values to the next generation. School children also had opportunities to influence unschooled parents and peers about such things as hygiene, boiling water, nutrition, and child health.

By the late 1940s, maternal and child welfare work had become, with the schools, the UMCA's most important means of contributing to African health and welfare. In a related measure in 1945, the mission introduced lunches for all children in its schools.[85] This belated strategy benefited the small minority able to attend the UMCA schools. A sense of urgency over the call for prevention was not unique to the Anglicans. Writing to Governor Hall in 1934, Dr. Murray of the Dutch Reformed Church Mission revealed that he too had been caught up in the "preventive" work of infant welfare, prenatal clinics, and training of native midwives. Such activities, he said, had "even greater importance than Hospital help."[86]

Table 8.4   Maternal and child health: Activity in UMCA facilities, 1949

	Births	Antenatal cases	Antenatal attendances/ home visits	Infant welfare cases	Infant welfare attendances
Kota Kota	330	554	3,632	238	3,049
Mponda's	38	81	1,485	77	1,687
Likoma	28	141	898	82	962
Likwenu	11	49	238	68	247
Malindi	3	43	240	43	704
Msumba	33	60	383	61	761
Liuli	25	37	308	35	473
Manda	3	41	214	58	978
Milo	14	52	214	51	1,082
Total	485	1,078	7,612	713	9,943

Source: Diocese of Nyasaland, Med. Dept. Ann. Rep., 1949. Table 1. M3-1-80. MNA.

Eventually, virtually every UMCA station provided antenatal services, and 485 babies were delivered under mission care in 1949. Due in large measure to the mission's policy of concentrating resources at Kota Kota, this station accounted for over two-thirds of all hospital births. Likwenu, Malindi, Msumba, Liuli, Manda, Milo, and even Mponda's managed only a small fraction of Kota Kota's volume, reflecting mission policies that produced a skewed geographic focus in these activities (table 8.4).

Mkope Hill Hospital was at the opposite end of the spectrum from Kota Kota. Remotely situated in an agriculturally marginal area near the south end of Lake Malawi, it remained a destitute relative of Kota Kota throughout the colonial era. In 1949 it reported 20,204 outpatients, who made 98,268 visits. Although three people had surgery under anesthesia, Mkope Hill recorded no inpatients and no woman gave birth there. Only 25 women came to the hospital for antenatal checks, while the staff made 135 village visits for general and maternity cases.[87]

Infant welfare centers recorded over seven hundred babies and nearly ten thousand attendances at UMCA clinics in 1949. Throughout the 1950s, mission medical workers continued to contest and define African cultural practices associated with babies and young children. At Likwenu, for example, young African babies remained "most attractive," with "chubby little bodies with silky curls," until they reached six months old. Many mothers reportedly then ruined their appearance by "plastering the head with filthy sticky black medicine, and by tying on lots of dirty charms" around the neck.[88]

In 1949, the mission's infant clinics examined 2,745 babies, and over 1,000 women attended the mission's antenatal clinics an average of 7.5 times each (table 8.4). Curiously, in 1950 hospital births increased by 7 percent, yet antenatal and infant welfare attendances decreased by 21 and 32 percent, respectively (*CA* 69 [1951]: 197). Nevertheless, as the 1963 data show, this comparison of 1949 and 1950 does not diminish the fact that a solid base of maternal and child health services was emerging.

During certain weeks at Likoma in 1955 (the year the island first received electric light) the clinic examined over 140 babies. Virtually all of them had anemia. Clinic staff addressed the problem by having "the mothers come with bottles and take away a week's supply of iron tonic."[89] In 1959, many of the mothers and babies at the Welfare Clinic had come over from the Portuguese mainland in dugout canoes, across six miles of open water.[90]

By 1963, Kota Kota's share of hospital births and baby clinic enrollees had declined to 43 percent and 16 percent, respectively. Kota Kota's proportion of mothers receiving UMCA antenatal care also declined, from about one-half in 1949 to one-third in 1963. These changes provided evidence that opportunities to access these mission services had spread geographically to other places in the diocese.

Overall, 2,585 women made 19,028 antenatal visits (7.4 average) to the mission's facilities in 1963.[91] Corresponding increases from 1949 to 1963 were thus well beyond the doubling mark. The pattern reveals the growing use of maternal and child health services and also some leveling out across the various UMCA stations. Some of this expansion may have been facilitated by allocation of additional resources received during the otherwise disastrous years of the CAF.

However, the most important factor in maternal and child health was ongoing secular change involving the accommodation of new forces and values in Malawi's societies during the last twenty-five years of the colonial era. The remoteness of so many places had also become a bit less so by independence. People in both the villages and towns experienced ever-increasing exposure to outside influences through education, communications media, and the experiences of migrant laborers. For better or worse, these influences had softened many prejudices and feelings of strangeness surrounding both Western missionary and secular medical initiatives. Still, it must not be overlooked that the social geography of this process was markedly uneven. Unfortunately, a half-century later, the scandal of poverty embedded in

Malawi's political economy means that access to best practices in maternal and child health remain at grossly unacceptable levels.

There is no doubt that the direction and quality of change in maternal and child health in colonial Malawi was positive, even though sustained improvement developed slowly. Practically speaking, most Africans remained either on the fringes or beyond the reach of progressive maternal and child health services, whether mission- or government-based. Kota Kota provides an example of this pattern. Whereas absolute attendance levels at its baby clinic rose from 3,254 in 1931 to 5,867 in 1963, this growth of 80 percent over 32 years (2.5 percent on an annual basis) was quite low, especially considering the increased human fertility in the protectorate over the same period. At Malawi's independence, the reality was that a large majority of African mothers still delivered their babies into the hands of village midwives, and had few or no contacts with ante-or postnatal services. On the other hand, by 1963 a new breed of "village midwives" who had been trained by the UMCA at Liuli Hospital ran maternity services for the lakeshore villages around Liuli (*UMCA Ann. Rev.*, 1963, 36).

HEALTH CLUBS: VALUING PREVENTION FIRST

In 1949, the Medical Report for Nyasaland Diocese offered an ambitious and bold new vision for health care. It was the work of Dr. George Maclean, a doctor who had come out of retirement to succeed Dr. Wigan. Soon after his arrival Maclean recognized that the mission was presiding over a public health crisis. There were tens of thousands of people with urgent health needs. It was not to denigrate or discount what had already been accomplished with the old ways; but Maclean insisted that it was now obligatory for the UMCA step forward and implement principles of public and community health.

Maclean's plan aimed to create "family health and welfare services" at every station, emphasizing preventive and developmental aspects of health "perhaps more than curative" work. Once the system was adopted widely, "the average station" would serve "approximately a thousand families." The idealistic goal was to "build up nuclei of healthy communities at different centres" by promoting "sound beliefs and practices regarding personal, family and community health, and by eliminating, as far as practicable, all communicable diseases and preventable psychoneuroses; and by providing services for midwifery, for incipient ill-health and for injuries." Families would receive annual inspections for parasitic diseases and anaemias, and treatment of current ailments by a qualified nurse. Maternal and child welfare, and "confidential premarital examinations and advice," would be cornerstones of this policy. Financial support for these station "health clubs" would come largely from the families involved, based on the principle that as far as possible every locality should be "self-supporting."[92]

Maclean presented his proposal quite directly, indicating that it was, then and there, to be implemented as the diocese's new medical policy. While idealistic in terms of available resources, the plan was more advanced and grounded in principles of modern public health than anything previously proposed by the mission. It was both revolutionary and a logical attempt to pull together and connect a variety of smaller-scale, sectoral activities and ideas that some UMCA medical workers had expressed interest in over the years. The idea of contributory "Health Clubs" also received encouragement from the government side, including a hint that some small direct support might be possible.

Maclean recognized that 1950 was not the best time to begin such a venture, but nevertheless moved it forward. Unprecedented drought and a stinging famine that disorganized family budgets, "most acutely the maize-eating south," had ravaged the diocese: "Everywhere food, its presence or absence, and means of obtaining it, was the dominant preoccupation of people's minds and actions" (*UMCA Ann. Rev.*, 1949, 13).

To initiate the scheme, participating families at Likoma were sorted according to "healthier families" in grade A, "medium" families" in B, and "the poorest in health and those who demanded the most attention" in C. The subscription rate was regressive, so that Grade C families paid the highest rate. Anyone taking "undue advantage" of the facilities was bumped to a lower grade. Africans who did not join were to be "made conscious of their responsibilities" and made to pay something toward the treatment of disease.[93]

Health Clubs did form at Likoma, Liuli (*CA* 71 [1953]: 193–94), and a few other places. Liuli's Health Club, said Maclean in 1951, "if not active has continued, and a few more enrolled." At the end of that year Liuli had about forty families and one hundred single members. There was thus little indication that the clubs could be expected to facilitate dramatic changes in public health in this poor country before independence.[94] Health clubs may have been a good idea whose implementation was undermined, among other factors, by a poorly conceived payment scheme. Maclean apparently wanted to use the example of families in better health as an incentive to those in poorer condition. Somehow, the certain disincentives of poverty, fewer resources, and lack of empowerment to "move up" got lost in the idealism.

A few final observations connect the realities of plans, resources, and potential consequences. Certainly the UMCA did not depend on consistently modern, up-to-date facilities in its strivings to achieve good health results in African communities. That progress was made in maternal and child health, and to a lesser extent in other areas, is indisputable. Nevertheless, dreadfully outmoded facilities and concepts impaired the mission's efforts to meet spiraling needs. In 1924, Dr. Wigan called Likwenu Hospital "the most up-to-date hospital in the diocese" (*CA* 42 [1924]: 256). Curiously, in 1954 this hospital still had no running water. Supplies had to be drawn from a nearby river with steep banks. The operating theater was a tiny, multipurpose room. Since the doctor visited only two or three times a year for a few days, Likwenu's European nursing sister and African dressers operated on tropical ulcers and other conditions during the year. Sterilization was done on a wood fire ("just as aseptic as in an English hospital but . . . far more trouble"), and firewood had to be found in the forest and head-carried to the hospital. Yet with lost irony, Likwenu's European health workers recorded that most of their patients came from a "very backward" tribe. They lived in mud huts, slept on the floor, and were subject to powerful "old grannies [who] hinder progress."[95]

Malindi's condition, apart from its beautiful lakeside setting, was similar. In the late 1950s this hospital had little to recommend it in terms of facilities. An all-African staff had run it for many years, without capital or repair funds. Said a visiting doctor, it is

> a very humble affair. Three barnlike buildings; two, the outpatient clinic and the women's ward, are fortunate in possessing a cement floor, but the men's ward is just earth which is most undesirable when one realises that this means it can never be scrubbed or even washed down. . . . Alas, the equipment is wretched, rickety native beds, with only occasional blankets, sheets, and counter-panes.

Malindi's saving grace was Swinny Mtiesa, the unheralded, extraordinarily talented African man who served as its Senior Medical Assistant.[96]

With or without Health Clubs, women, children, and men in settlements up and down the lake basin were still better off by the 1960s because of the mission's twenty years of effort to build up maternal and child welfare services. Prospects for raising family health standards had brightened, although it was still mostly just a good idea. Curative work remained the overwhelming activity of the mission's hospitals and dispensaries, particularly as African trust in European medicine was continuing to spread (*CA* 73 [1955]: 234–39).

A small but growing proportion of women regularly received antenatal examinations, gave birth in the hands of trained midwives and under improved hygienic standards, and took their babies and young children to clinics. A health frontier with profound demographic significance had been breached and its population exposed to life-enhancing measures.

NOTES

1. Some records from the early years were so badly damaged that they were unusable. Destruction of paper records, particularly the oldest, by insects or inadvertently by people through ignorance, are significant factors. In some places the nurse or medical assistant at a dispensary may have collected certain information that was neither reported nor published as part of the mission's records. In some cases the staff's workloads, illness, or the "making do" adjustments forced on the mission in times of great stress, such as World War I (Dr. Wigan was seconded by the local British forces) and World War II, reduced the time given to record keeping. In several years the Medical Officer's Annual Medical Report (published in *Central Africa*, the *UMCA Annual Review*, or the *Nyasaland Diocesan Chronicle*) amounts to a few simple paragraphs containing minimal if any statistics on outpatients or inpatients. For at least nine years, only the annual "Total Attendance" at all dispensaries is available.

2. Data on inpatient admissions during World War I are scarce. Likoma's postwar average intake from 1921 through 1927 was 413 patients, ranging from a high of 431 (1921) to a low of 335 (1923). Diocese of Nyasaland, *Letter to Members and Friends, Advent* [published annually] (Likoma: Universities' Mission Press, 1918–27). File UMCA, D8 (X). Diocese of Nyasaland. Pamphlets. RHL.

3. A UMCA writer noted in this source that it was "rather misleading" to say so much country was worked because large parts of it remained untouched by mission influence.

4. Diocese of Nyasaland, *Letter to Members and Friends*.

5. Malindi Station Diary, 1908. 145-DOM-10-4-1. MNA.

6. Malindi Station Diary. Medical Work: *Chauncy Maples*. 145-DOM-10-4-6. MNA.

7. Malindi Station Diary, 1903. 145-DOM-10-4-6. MNA. At Zomba, important archival materials on the medical work in 1903, including the *C.M.*, Malindi, and Mponda's, have been badly damaged or destroyed by insects and rot.

8. Ibid.

9. Ibid.

10. The descriptions "dawa boy" or "dispensary boy," regardless of an individual's age, continued in use by the UMCA for many years.

11. Hospitals in Nyasaland Diocese, UMCA A3: 127–36. RHL

12. The number of patients the dispenser reportedly "managed" seems exaggerated, since it requires him to have seen an average of sixty-nine patients daily, Monday through Sunday, throughout the year.

13. For a useful model of risk zones, see Roundy 1987.

14. Mponda's Station Record Book, 1917–21 and 1929–31. 145-DOM-2-4-1 and 145-2-4-2. MNA.

15. Earlier, individual reports include Malindi (1903: 3,240 cases; 1911: ≈3,000 cases); Likoma (1909: 26,943 cases in first *quarter* of year, partly in response to drought and localized nutritional distress; and 1918: 41,200); and Msumba and Liuli (1921: each ≈7,500).

16. Beck asserts that although the idea of development was espoused in the context of Britain's own unemployment and manufacturing crises of the 1920s, in the 1930s "the concept of development had shifted toward the inclusion of the African in colonial society, a factor not considered before 1920" (1981, 3). Evidence with which to refute this argument is at least as plentiful as any to support it. Much hinges on the meaning of "inclusion." In the case of Malawi, labor policies and the exclusion of Africans from any meaningful say in the creation of the ill-fated Central African Federation do not support such an interpretation.

17. Vaughan 1991, 127, citing Nyasaland Protectorate, *Blue Book*, 1910.

18. Med. Dept., Chikwawa, to Director of Medical and Sanitary Services (hereafter, DMS), Zomba, Nov. 11, 1935. Medical Dept., M2-5-9. MNA.

19. Medical Dept., Survey of Stools of Native Servants Employed in Zomba Township, May 31, 1934. M2-5-9. MNA.

20. Nyasaland Protectorate, Med. Dept. Ann. Rep., 1937. Mimeograph, not paginated. M3-1-10. MNA.

21. Ibid.

22. Ibid.

23. Ibid.

24. Dr. Owen Shircore had been Government Pathologist in Nyasaland.

25. Nyasaland Protectorate, Med. Dept. Ann. Rep., 1937. M3-1-7. MNA.

26. Memorandum by DMS [c. 1929]. M2-14-1. MNA.

27. Conf. of Missionary Societies in Great Britain and Ireland to Lord Lloyd, Secretary of State for the Colonies. A memorandum Inspired by a Statement of Policy on Colonial Development and Welfare, CMD.6175. 15 pp. N.d. M2-24-45. File date Sept. 14, 1941. MNA.

28. Ibid.

29. Nyasaland Protectorate, Med. Dept. Ann. Rep., 1926. M3-1-7. MNA.

30. District Resident, Liwonde, to Principal Medical Officer, Zomba, Feb. 17, 1925. M2-5-12. MNA.

31. Provincial Commissioner, Southern Province, to Principal Medical Officer, Zomba, February 23, 1925. M2-5-12. MNA.

32. Acting DMS, Nyasaland, to Dr. R. G. Cochrane, BELRA, May 28, 1927. M2-5-12. 202/24. MNA.

33. Chaulmoogra is one of several southeast Asian trees of the genus *Taraktogenous*, family *Bixaceae*, and genus *Hydnocarpus*, family *Flacourtiaceae*. The seeds yield buttery oils that have been used for centuries as a germicides to treat leprosy, administered both internally (orally, or by injection, beginning in the 1920s) and externally to reduce bacteria and the severity of lesions. Relief of certain symptoms was often obtained. And expectations were raised when there were signs that leprosy's progress had been arrested. But there is little evidence that anyone was ever completely cured by these oils. As the text indicates, in common usage Chaulmoogra and Hydnocarpus tend to be used interchangeably

34. DMS to Chief Secretary, Zomba, April 11, 1927. M2-5-12. MNA.

35. Vice Presidents and Committee, BELRA, to Governor Sir C. C. Bowring, May 19, 1927. M2-5-12. MNA.

36. Act. Chief Secretary, Zomba, to Act. DMS, May 25, 1927. M2-5-12. 202/24. MNA. The author calculated the ratio based on a total estimated Protectorate African population of 1,290,885 for 1926. See Kuczynski 1949, 2:532.

37. BELRA to Governor, May 19, 1927. M2-5-12. MNA.

38. DMS Zomba, to Secretary, BELRA, London, Oct. 4, 1927. M2-5-12. MNA.

39. Chief Secretary, Zomba, to DMS, Zomba: Grants in Aid: Government to Missions. Nov. 18, 1943. M2-24-46. MNA.

40. DMS to Chief Secretary, Nyasaland, June 9, 1927. M2-5-13. MNA.

41. DMS to Dr. W. C. Wigan, July 17, 1930. M2-5-13. MNA.

42. Dr. W. C. Wigan, UMCA, to Dr. Sanderson, DMS, August 10, 1930. M2-5-13. MNA.

43. DMS, Zomba, to Chief Secretary, Zomba, May 25, 1927. M2-5-12. MNA

44. Memorandum, DMS (c. 1929). M2-14-1. MNA.

45. Potassium iodide was used to dissolve granulomatous tissue.

46. Nyasaland Protectorate, Med. Dept. Ann. Rep., 1934. M3-1-7. MNA.

47. Nyasaland Protectorate, Med. Dept. Ann. Rep., 1935, 22–23. M3-1-8. MNA.

48. Nyasaland Protectorate, Med. Dept. Ann. Rep., 1937. M3-1-10. MNA.

49. Medical and Health Services of Nyasaland, 1938, 41. Mimeograph. M3-4-4. MNA.

50. Dr. E. Muir, M.D., Secretary of BELRA. Report Submitted Following His Tour in Nyasaland Over the Period 2nd to the 15th June, 1939, 10–11. M2-5-13. MNA.

51. District Resident, Liwonde, to Principal Medical Officer, Zomba, Feb. 17, 1925. M2-5-12. MNA.

52. Mission Hospitals, by DMS, Zomba, September 1947. M2-24-45. MNA.

53. Mission Medical Facilities, 1952 and 1957–60. PCN1-26-13. MNA.

54. Medical Financial Report for 1952. UMCA 1/12/1. MNA.

55. Medical Financial Report for 1953, 1954. UMCA 1/12/1. MNA.

56. *UMCA Ann. Rev.,* 1954: Medical Report, 20.

57. "Treatment of Leprosy by Sulphone Drugs: Checking the Disease," reprinted from the *Times* (London) in *CA* 75 [1957]: 223–25.

58. Diocese of Malawi (Nyasaland), Med. Dept. Ann. Rep., 1963, p. 15. Hospital Statistics, 1963. MNA.

59. Afrolnews, "Budget Cuts Responsible for Leprosy in Malawi," www.afrol.com/countries/malawi/headlines2001/02_15.html; and "Leprosy Resurfaces in Malawi," http://allafrica.com/stories/200102160015.html.

60. The missionaries believed that "heathen customs" had an even stronger grip on girls and women than on men; and "a girl is often forced, through sheer terror and the threats of her mother and aunts, to take part in the [fertility] rites that her Christian teacher has taught her to know to be wholly evil." Thus girls' education was seen as the key to much-needed change in village society. It would inculcate a generation of girls "in the ideas that belong to a pure Christian home" (*CA* 21 [1903]: 47).

61. The following five cases all appear in Diocese of Southern Malawi. Mponda's Station—Record of Christians, October 1909–November 1920. MNA.

62. Linden (1974, 170) reports that in colonial Malawi African women frequently became "sexual objects for planters and the occasional colonial official."

63. Little information exists concerning the effectiveness of the traditional postpartum taboo on pregnancy patterns, and in particular how this custom affected the health of mothers and children.

64. M2-24-7. MNA. File I.D. for all reports in this section on infant mortality factors. It bears emphasis that these observations are impressionistic and are not supported by statistical surveys.

65. Nyasaland Protectorate, Med. Dept. Ann. Rep., 1926. M2-1-3. MNA.

66. Medical Officer, Ft. Johnston to DMS, Sept. 23, 1933. M2-24-7. MNA.

67. Kuczynski 1949, 2:629, citing Medical Report 1937, Appendix IV, The Native Welfare Report on Nutrition, p. 6.

68. The case cited was in response to a summons to Dr. George Steele, a Scot, to attend a case of complicated labor.

69. Headrick (1994) characterizes the general situation.

70. In 1978, Violet Kimani, a Kenyan colleague of the author, told how her mother had, in the case of at least one child, given birth in the morning and had returned to work in her garden in the afternoon.

71. Of course, for the nurses to join the Africans in their celebration would have been almost unthinkable—decidedly un-English, bad form, and risqué.

72. Passfield, Downing Street, to [presumably] DMS, Zomba, March 8, 1930. M2-14-1. MNA.

73. There, the decision of Presbyterian missionaries to force the Kikuyu and related peoples to choose between female circumcision or church membership was simultaneously yielding widespread defiance, destabilization, and African nationalism. See Good 2000.

74. DMS, Zomba, to Chief Secretary, Zomba, Training of Africans, Part B, April 5, 1937. M2-15-1. MNA.

75. Nyasaland Protectorate, Med. Dept. Ann. Rep., 1937. M3-1-10. MNA.

76. DMS, Zomba, to Chief Secretary, Zomba, Training of African Personnel of the Medical Department, Jan. 23, 1937, pp. 1–2. M2-15-1. MNA.

77. Nyasaland Protectorate, Med. Dept. Ann. Rep., 1933. M3-1-6. MNA.

78. Chief Secretary, Zomba, to DMS, Zomba, Grants-in-Aid: Government to Missions, Nov. 18, 1943. M2-24-46. MNA.

79. DMS, Zomba, to Chief Secretary, Zomba, re: Sir Robert Bell Report Recommendation 49. Maternity and Child Welfare Clinics Should be Left to Missions, with Financial Assistance from Government. Nov. 11, 1938. 29-11-38. S1-348-34. MNA. Of course, tension between the colonial medical dept. officials and missionaries was not preordained, especially when interests were served. In correspondence between the government MO for Kota Kota and the DMS, the local officer noted that he was "strongly in favour of the U.M.C.A. taking over [the local Government] Child Welfare Clinic," and further, that "they are at present doing splendid work with very poor facilities." This was "an opportunity of doing incalculable good." MO, Kota Kota, to DMS, Zomba, July 16, 1935. M2-12-2. MNA.

80. Data on survival rates were not found.

81. Vaughan's primary source is CA 49 (1931): 7–8. While the discussion is primarily about UMCA/Anglican attitudes and practices, she does not specifically refer here to the Diocese of Nyasaland.

82. E.g., Dr. George Maclean in the late 1940s.

83. Dr. W . C. Wigan to Dr. Williams, DMS, Zomba, September 1936. M2-5-10. MNA.

84. Ibid.

85. MO's Report, *UMCA Ann. Rev.*, 1945. RHL.

86. W. H. Murray, Supt. DRC Mission, to Gov. K. L. Hall, Nyasaland, Aug. 15, 1934. S1-348-34. MNA.

87. MO, Ft. Johnston, to DMS, Zomba, Annual Report from UMCA Mission. Appendix. Feb. 28, 1950. M3-1-80. MNA.

88. Typed notecards on health and education. Likwenu Hospital. Joan Knowles, c. 1955. UMCA Archives: UX 92A, Diocese of Nyasaland. RHL.

89. Likoma Hospital. Moyra Askew, June 1955. Source as in n. 88.

90. Likoma Hospital. P. M. Jennings, Aug. 1959. Source as in n. 88.

91. Diocese of Malawi (Nyasaland), Med. Dept. Ann. Rep., 1963, Hospital Statistics. MNA.

92. Diocese of Nyasaland, Med. Dept. Ann. Rep., 1949, Appendix 2. M3-1-80. MNA. Also *CA* 68 (1950): 189–92.

93. DMS, Zomba, to P.C., North Province, re: Proposed 'Health Club' to be established by the UMCA on Likoma Island, Jan. 12, 1952. PCN1-26-13. MNA.

94. In a letter to the D.C., Nkata Bay, Aug. 28, 1952, Dr. Maclean stated that the club subscription rate was 6d. per head. Members would receive free treatment at Likoma, as before, except for relapsing fever, amoebic dysentery, and cases requiring more than two month's attention during the year (e.g., TB). All members were expected to cooperate in public health efforts, esp. bilharzia control, and maintain a satisfactory standard of sanitation in their villages. Expectant and nursing mothers would receive free treatment for nine months before and after confinement whether club members or not. Everyone would receive free treatment for VD. PCN1-26-13. MNA.

95. Notecards on health and education. Likwenu Hospital. Joan Knowles, 1954.

96. See citation above in note 88. Malindi Hospital. Dr. John Dingley, c. 1957. RHL.

CHAPTER NINE

Treatment and Control: Limits and Contradictions of Science and Missionary Medicine

TIME IS THE GREAT PHYSICIAN.

B. Disraeli, *Henrietta Temple*, book 6, chap. 9

DISEASE: THROUGH THE BIOMEDICAL LENS

UMCA missionaries faced difficult challenges to their own health, apart from any aspirations they had to reduce the high levels of morbidity in the African community. When we add to this the limitations imposed by the mission's conservative institutions and modus operandi, it is clear that they faced astounding odds against changing the basic conditions of African health. For several decades, policies remained focused on curative help for needy individuals, who also received intensive Christian propaganda. Apart from smallpox, there was little interest in adopting secular developments in public health until the late 1920s and 1930s. This attitude was of course not peculiar to the UMCA. Yet when ideas about community approaches to health care and prevention did begin to seep into the mission's ranks, support for change was not unanimous. Some missionaries believed that such commitments would dilute evangelistic efforts and thus distort the true missionary mandate.

In truth, prayer was a staple of missionary life, and many prayed often and hard. Faith in answered prayer sustained hope in the possibilities of divine intervention. Yet there can be little doubt that some missionaries were conflicted by the realization that they could do little to promote, and would never witness, a significant transformation of the material conditions that defined the African communities they served. Faith, the "romance" of serving a foreign mission, and human transformation did not always produce elegant results. Time transcended everything, but in health matters it served as "the great physician" only to fortunate individuals or small clusters of people here and there; waiting did not bring healing to whole populations. Over time Africans had been quite successful at adapting to, and certainly accepting, levels of illness and suffering that had come to be viewed as unnecessary and untenable in Western societies. Certainly, in God's unfathomable time scheme, seventy-five years was an imperfect measure of what was needed to solve the deep-seated cultural, environmental, and political challenges on the African health frontier.

On the other hand, what was accomplished by a handful of isolated missionaries may be better appreciated when their experience and record are compared against the results of health interventions promoted by the WHO, World Bank, and other well-heeled international, bilateral, and nongovernmental agencies. Despite the huge success of smallpox eradication by 1979, and wobbly progress in selected areas of child health such as immunizations, highly publicized intersectoral goals including malaria control, sustainable community-based health/"Health for All," and HIV/AIDS amelioration in Africa and elsewhere have met with failure or at best marginal success. Poverty, poor interagency coordination, and bilateral/international policies that support systemic corruption at the national and local levels, especially, deserve much responsibility for these outcomes. Fossilized thinking in the powerful local and international allopathic sector is also responsible for misguiding and squandering health resources. Another limiting factor has been the slowness of biomedical professionals to "think outside the box"—to consider *whole* communities with their intimate connections to their changing environments, and to the preexisting system of traditional practitioners and other elements of today's medical pluralism.

UMCA archives reveal mission medical workers' persistent frustrations with the awful debilitating and killing power of disease. Eventually, many missionaries realized the strong connections between poverty and disease, and how they thwarted African social development. To a limited degree, the new and improved drugs that trickled out to Central Africa from Europe strengthened the mission's biomedical capabilities. Yet, the old diseases such as tropical ulcer, hookworm, and leprosy did not go away. "New" diseases such as TB, syphilis, and malnutrition spread widely in response to the social upheavals and mobility fostered by colonial policies and actions. Indeed, it is hard to imagine how the protectorate government, for its part, could take credit for any measures that substantially advanced the health or general well-being of Malawian peoples.[1]

Several views drawn at intervals from the *UMCA Annual Review*, 1926 to 1963, reflect the UMCA's uphill struggle to produce any long-lasting changes in the configuration of social, political, and environmental forces that shaped the diocese's disease profile:

1926: Yaws, syphilis, and hookworm are rife [at Milo Hospital] and about sixty per cent of our treatment for these diseases has been in Tanganyika Territory, leprosy too seems more common there than in Nyasaland. (*UMCA Ann. Rev.*, 1926, 2)

1941: The field that is open to medical endeavor is so vast that anything the Mission can do will no more than touch the fringe. There is always a good deal of illness among the children [Milo], and many turn to a witchdoctor to ask his help. (1942, 21)

1942: Foremost among [the causes of disease] we may place malnutrition, bad housing, and low wages. (1942, 25)

1943: Much of the curative work done in our hospitals in diseases such as ankylostomiasis and malaria is almost immediately undone by the patient's return after care to the same infected conditions at home which originally caused the disease, and therefore it is probably only as matter of time before he will be back again reinfected. (1943, 34)

1949: The health of the general population in the diocese was adversely affected by the prolonged drought, and also, in the case of children, by a widespread outbreak of whooping cough. (1949, 21)

1963 (the eve of independence): The old scourges remain. Malaria, hookworm, conjunctivitis and ulcers seem to be the most persistent; tuberculosis, dysentery, and bilharzia come next. In recent years much has been done to cure leprosy, especially if it is caught in the early stages. Yet leprosy seems to increase, perhaps because more cases are brought to light. (1963, 37–38)

Fragmentary UMCA reports of African health problems emerged by 1894. They were extremely sketchy and limited to Likoma Island. Dr. Robinson, who was the missionaries' physician for just a few months before he became ill and was sent back to England, ranked digestive disorders first. Mainly women and children were afflicted, and they cured easily after two or three applications of "the drops." "Weeping eyes," with "very melancholy looks," ranked second. Ulcers (*vilonda*) that needed cleaning and dressing, and fever (malaria) followed third and fourth, respectively, among known maladies (*CA* 12 [1894]: 138). Since fear of cutting into the body was widespread among Africans, surgical solutions to needful cases remained rare, particularly in the early years of contact.

As hospitals and dispensaries spread and more Africans took advantage of the UMCA's health services, a better outline of the most notorious endemic diseases emerged. In most places chronic tropical ulcers, yaws, malaria, hookworm, schistosomiasis, pneumonia, tuberculosis, and dysentery headed the list. Although endemic, these diseases, with the exception of falciparum malaria in children, generally did not cause death on their own. Instead, they tended to infect bodies concurrently in various combinations. A man, woman, or child harboring two to five different infections at once was commonplace. Since infections debilitated people, their immune system was subjected to great stress, thereby greatly complicating the task of staying alive. For instance, a child with hookworm disease, and thus by definition anemic, was far less likely to withstand an attack of cerebral malaria. A malnourished child infected with epidemic measles had to fight a disease synergism that greatly reduced her chances for survival. Time-wise, the UMCA's European and African medical workers focused their efforts on helping people cope with these often cyclical endemic diseases.

Epidemic, lethal diseases including influenza, smallpox, relapsing fever, cerebro-spinal meningitis, measles, and sleeping sickness only added to the insults. Primarily infectious, communicable, and intermittent, these potentially devastating and fearsome diseases could not be predicted before an outbreak had already started in one or more places. Colonial Malawi experienced recurrent outbreaks of these diseases, and panic and social disruption often accompanied their spread. Numerous "new" factors also contributed to such outbreaks, such as changes in population mobility (relapsing fever), long-distance migration and urbanization (TB), increased population density, crowding and poverty (cerebro-spinal meningitis), and ecological disruption leading to increased human-vector contact (human sleeping sickness).

Trends in Patterns of Endemic and Epidemic Diseases

Tropical ulcers crippled and debilitated, and yielded uneasily, if at all, to traditional medical treatments or to missionary methods (see chap. 7). Most began in childhood, although few individuals received early treatment. No discernible difference in incidence by sex was evident. As the lesions grew older, they enlarged to three inches or more, even eating into bone, particularly on the lower part of the leg. In the worst progressions people became lame, and were forced to spend much of their lives inside a dark hut. Old ulcers might become gangrenous. A former mission doctor in Kenya said that they characteristically turned malignant, with the limb in question requiring amputation if the cancer did not respond to local incisions.[2]

Dr. Robert Howard graphically portrays ulcer sufferers of long-standing who, "unable to walk . . . crawl down to the lake to wash and soak off the dry leaves which form the only dressing for their sores; they apply a fresh lot of leaves, with the object of keeping away the flies which torment them." Many could be helped and learn "to get about on crutches," which "never occurred to the native mind" (*CA* 22 [1904]: 141).

Some people had suffered with an ulcer five years or more at the time of first admission to a UMCA hospital (ibid.). Evidence suggests that susceptibility to and prevalence of tropical ulcer varied geographically, with strong suspicions of causal links to poor diet, undernutrition, and elevation. For example, in 1906, Dr. Howard commented on "the remarkable absence of ulcers" at Mtonya station in Portuguese East Africa. This place was situated at an altitude of almost 4,000 feet, which gave it less tropical and more "hill station" qualities. In this somewhat cooler place the "natives seemed a healthy lot" (*CA* 24 [1906]: 14). However, conditions surrounding Milo Hospital in Tanganyika seemed to counter the validity of the environmental theory of reduced disease. Whereas Milo was situated at an elevation of 7,000 feet, UMCA records reveal (but do not explain) that the people there experienced "ubiquitous ulcer" (*UMCA Ann. Rev.*, 1925, 109).

Years passed during which ulcers received less mention, if not less attention; but they never left the mission-village scene. During World War I, the War Office forbade the export of bandages, forcing the missionaries to improvise with rags and natural materials. Dr. Wigan dressed ulcers with raw local cotton and beeswax or palm oil. The scale of the problem is suggested by statistics from Likoma Hospital in 1920–21, where ulcers and other injuries accounted for 60 percent of all disease reported. Intestinal worms (10 percent), yaws and gangosa[3] (7 percent), and bilharzia (5.5 percent) came next. Assessing the status in 1924, Dr. Wigan noted that "a very large proportion of our cases has always been ulcers," although in this year fewer cases had been noticed, especially the "foul fungating tropical ulcer" (*UMCA Ann. Rev.*, 1924, 101, 103).

A sense of the sheer magnitude and endemicity of ulcers throughout Malawi can be gained from reports by other mission hospitals, including those of the Dutch Reformed Church. In 1924, the Dutch Reformed Church

Mission claimed to have treated 75,000 patients at its hospitals, a third of whom presented with ulcers (King and King 1991, 130).

Meanwhile, a government report confirmed the enormity of the problem and set out the "three classes" of ulcers seen in the protectorate. In addition to the "tropical" variety, there were ulcers caused by local injury, and those associated with diseases such as yaws, syphilis, and leprosy. Lower risk groups included males who had become essential workers in the evolving colonial system. Accordingly, this group was comprised of "houseboys," dispensers, native police, and other "natives working in contact with Europeans" who were "obliged to be more cleanly" because they allegedly had less contact with the fecal contamination that plagued rural villages. Since they received wages, some observers thought such workers might be better fed than villagers.[4]

Tropical ulcers apparently had declined by the UMCA's final decade in Malawi.[5] Whereas ulcers and injuries reportedly accounted for 60 percent of disease in 431 Likoma patients (island and mainland) in 1920–21, they reportedly dropped to 8.5 percent in 1950. Hookworm cases exceeded ulcer cases by six times in 1950 (*CA* 69 [1951]: 197). In 1954, the mission treated more than 1,000 patients in its sphere for ulcers, but this represented only 14 percent of the five major diseases. Ulcers placed ahead of bilharzia (9 percent), and behind malaria (32 percent), hookworm (31 percent), and "venereal" disease (14.5 percent) among the 7,037 major cases presented for treatment at UMCA facilities. At first glance this altered pattern suggests that the identification and treatment of ulcers had become more routinized and effective during the missionary decades. Hookworm, on the other hand, was a telling sign of poor progress with sanitation and hygiene in Malawian villages, and possibly even around the station compounds. Yet ulcers did not retreat for long, if at all, as improved statistics soon indicated.

Reliable statistical indicators of Malawi's public health have always been scarce due to the difficulties of making definitive diagnoses and maintaining accurate, consistent, and complete records.[6] In 1963, Dr. Robert Brown compiled the most comprehensive annual statistics on disease and health services utilization ever assembled during the UMCA's history in Malawi. Brown, an American recruit, analyzed conditions recorded at the mission's then six hospitals/dispensaries and three stand-alone dispensaries as part of his Annual Report.[7] The result is a valuable biomedical snapshot of certain health conditions prevalent in the UMCA's domain on the threshold of its effective departure from Malawi.[8] This information is a key source for evaluating change.

UMCA health workers handled 29,189 individual cases in 1963, divided among seventeen diseases. Although what proportion of these "cases" may have been "re-attendances" is not clear, attendance by outpatients had apparently been the greatest ever recorded.[9] Ironically, in 1963 tropical ulcers once again became the most frequently reported disease.[10] By rank, malaria, conjunctivitis (the "weeping eyes" of 1894?), hookworm, and bilharzia followed ulcers. This surprising result suggests that disease ecology, specifically the interplay of poverty and environmental conditions, mission treatment, and control of ulcers, had come full circle in the preceding sixty-five years. Was the end only the beginning?

Comparison of ulcer cases (N = 8,238) with regard to Malawi's exploding population offers necessary perspective on the prevalence of this disease. Paradoxically, the prevalence rate may actually reflect some measure of success. That ulcers ranked first in recorded disease rate in 1963—even ahead of malaria—may mean that more sufferers were coming in for treatment than ever before. Also, the apparent decline in ulcers reported in 1954 may reflect careless underreporting of the real situation. Alternatively, the findings may simply point to the failure of the UMCA (and protectorate government) to make significant inroads into altering the broader, root causes of this ancient, debilitating malady.

The Scottish Livingtonia Mission reported circumstantial evidence of links between seasonal hunger, undernutrition, and ulcers on the west side of Lake Malawi. The Scots enjoyed more abundant medical resources, including doctors and trained African staff, and enjoyed a professional edge over the UMCA in terms of progressiveness and number of trained medical practitioners. Nevertheless, the Scots' statistics from their dispensaries in one district show that in 1949 ulcers (N = 777) continued to rank high on the list of diseases treated, in third place behind cough (1,548) and hookworm (1,083). While the MO's report noted "no signs of actual starvation," with the onset of the rains there had been "an increase of tropical ulcers suggestive of vitamin deficiency."[11]

Ulcers act as a highly sensitive barometer of fluctuations in rainfall, food shortages (during the rainy season), and human nutrition. Vitamin and protein deficiencies, with consequent lowering of resistance to infection, together with bacterial agents, are widely accepted elements of a narrowly defined etiology of tropical ulcers. However, solving the affliction demands systemic attention to the political ecology of food production and diet quality. Given its central purpose and available resources as a colonial mission, these broader, complex issues received little attention from the UMCA.

People everywhere had a profound dread of smallpox epidemics. Stirred by the unprecedented scale of population mobility and social contact, variola invaded both population centers and remote places in many areas of colonial

Malawi. Outbreaks took one of two forms, mild variola minor and severe variola major, the latter with around 20 percent mortality.

Circumstantial evidence suggests that the UMCA's steamers, along with government and commercial vessels, contributed to smallpox dispersal while transporting people for hundreds of miles between the dozens of small ports and anchorages that dotted the lake's coastline. Most of the infected survived, yet several times, even as late as the 1950s, deaths in a single epidemic of variola major often reached many hundreds. In addition to causing pockmarked faces and limbs, if the infection spread to the eyes corneal ulceration often produced blindness. When Dr. Howard assumed his duties as the UMCA's Medical Officer at Likoma in 1899, he literally walked into an epidemic that was spreading through the country via routeways from German East Africa, Zanzibar, and the Zambezi and lower Shiré valleys. Concurrent severe epidemics of whooping cough (both sides of Lake Malawi) and mumps added to people's misery.[12]

With smallpox on the rise, Howard made several "vaccinating tours" to the mainland. The Association for the Supply of Pure Vaccine Lymph, Pall Mall East, provided the mission with "a regular 6 weekly supply of [glycerinated calf] lymph." However, it was difficult to keep both glycerated and unmodified human lymph active in the warm local environment, and the earliest vaccination attempts failed miserably due to deteriorated lymph. Supplies of lymph from the Scottish Mission in Blantyre did not arrive until the end of 1900. While all 141 African adherents on Likoma had been vaccinated (smallpox had died out on the island), this small number could not check a serious epidemic from developing on the adjacent mainland coast and into the Yao country.[13]

Some Africans living in areas beyond the reach of the first vaccinators played "Russian roulette" by inoculating smallpox into the back of the hand on the web between the forefinger and thumb. Dr. Howard recorded that in one lakeside village ten males died from the smallpox, but in another place "a large amount of vaccination was successfully done by the natives from two persons vaccinated at Chia during [his] first *ulendo* (medical safari)."[14]

Collaboration, including experimentation, notably among the Scottish and UMCA missions, finally produced some successful vaccination campaigns in which up to "95% efficiency" of coverage was reported. Using African workers, the UMCA vaccinated 4,350 people in 1899–1900. Vaccinations by the mission continued into 1903, when 348 more people received lymph. Poor lymph quality continued to frustrate efforts to vaccinate enough of the population to stop smallpox from breaking out. Vials sent out from the Jenner Institute "failed completely," and it was difficult to find good vaccinators.[15]

During the next five decades intermittent smallpox epidemics suddenly burst out in places and then burned out. In the Dedza district on the Rift escarpment, a survey of about 6,000 people by Dr. Davey in 1913 revealed that 95 and 9 percent of adults and children, respectively, "had signs of past smallpox." Locally children received traditional variola inoculation. At least seven outbreaks, apparently independent of each other, occurred between 1908 and 1960.

Smallpox was "rampant" in the coastlands around Malindi station in 1908, and the mission tried to vaccinate everyone in sight. Since all mission children had been vaccinated and school boarders had dropped to fifty, Dr. Howard concluded "it will not break out here." Near the station, but well beyond the compound, the mission set up a smallpox camp that took in over three hundred cases. This time Likoma was largely spared, except for a married woman. She was kept "isolated in a hut on the rocks . . . and her husband looked after her."

In the first months of 1909 UMCA workers vaccinated 3,178 people on Likoma and Chizumulu Islands, and in four settlements on the mainland (*CA* 27 [1909]: 22, 93). In 1911 smallpox moved into Mtonya district in P.E.A., north of Malindi. Only one death occurred at the station, but many in the surrounding countryside died. Smallpox struck again in 1921, this time south of the lake near Likwenu. It lasted several months and one village was quarantined. Many died, especially children, and UMCA staff were forbidden to sleep in the village or hold services (*UMCA Ann. Rev.*, 1921, 19).

By 1926, the protectorate Medical Department had deployed a small cadre of traveling vaccinators, armed with imported lymph, in all of Malawi's administrative districts. While "theoretically under the direction of a Medical Officer, Sub-Assistant Surgeon, or the Resident," these men had little if any supervision. The Medical Director assumed that the vaccination returns he received were "correspondingly unreliable." Overall, 43,475 people reportedly received successful vaccinations, and another 28,754 experienced a "modified" result. Vaccination failed in nearly 32,000 instances, while another 6,131 were not seen. In Kota Kota and Ft. Johnston, two districts with UMCA medical facilities, approximately 36 and 28 percent of the vaccinations were considered successful.[16] Mission efforts at this particular time remain opaque.

Since it was always greatly understaffed, the protectorate government rarely if ever properly discharged its public health responsibilities. Such a statement is much less a condemnation of the Medical Department's staff than it is a reflection of the intentional no investment, pay-as-you go, minimizing system perpetrated by Whitehall and the Colonial Office. By the immediate post–World War I period the template for managing serious public health problems amounted to autocratic, strong-arm policing to gain African compliance with smallpox control, including mass vaccinations and destruction of people's property.

The next smallpox epidemic of record in Malawi began in 1928 and continued at least through 1930. Vaccine for 120,000 vaccinations was distributed by the government and administered in the first year by 46 African vaccinators. In 1931 the protectorate's African population was around 1.6 million, thus yielding a vaccinator ratio of 1 : 35,000 (Kuczynski 1949, 2:556). While the virus eventually retreated, the movement of people during the tobacco-buying season hampered its control.[17] Likoma and Chizimulu Islands had another small outbreak in 1933, including some severe cases. Overall, the threat was moderated by the mission's aggressive decision to vaccinate over two thousand inhabitants of the islands (*CA* 52 [1934]: 104).

Further smallpox outbreaks followed during the 1940s, including a prolonged epidemic in Msumba Archdeaconry in the UMCA's heartland in 1947. According to the bishop, in this instance the spread was checked and deaths kept lower because the government promptly supplied the mission with lymph, enabling its hospital staff to undertake a vigorous vaccination campaign (*CA* 66 [1948]: 131). Such good fortune bypassed many other places. Drs. Michael and Elspeth King (1991, 57) found evidence in government files that smallpox epidemics continued on "relentlessly" into 1949 and beyond.

Malawi's changing political economy, including the government's emphasis on estate labor and cash-crops and inattention to food crop production, was directly linked to why and how communities became exposed to epidemic smallpox. In southern Malawi in 1949, the disease was fueled by one of the protectorate's frequent famines, by the reactive migrations of people into central parts of the country, and by the long-institutionalized flows of migrant labor to Rhodesia and beyond. These processes led to overcrowding and decreased resistance. Mortality reached 25 percent in Lilongwe. The protectorate's Medical Department carried out over 740,000 vaccinations, including large numbers of people on the Zomba Plateau. According to a mission nurse at Malosa, the 1949 smallpox epidemic was a terror that "raged with virulence." Isolation camps were badly understaffed. When the infection had run its course there, "they brought in the maimed who were generally children with abscesses with deep pustules, some were blind and all needed a long convalescence with good food" (ibid.).

Human responses to the horrors of smallpox often rendered its control extremely difficult. Villagers knew from word of mouth or direct experience that the Medical Department, upon discovering a confirmed case, would

close off their villages, burn the houses, and destroy the crops. Conceal-
ment of symptomatic individuals thus became a common tactic for preserving what little they possessed. Following a pre-dawn raid of one village,
a government health inspector observed that 75 per cent of the huts were
infected, with families "hiding cases in the bush from sunrise to sundown"
(58). Individual government officers might voice humanitarian concerns
about African welfare. Nevertheless, apart from military-style vaccination
campaigns aimed at smallpox prevention, government assistance with the
reconstruction of shattered families and livelihoods carried little weight in
colonial circles. As in many other aspects of community health, smallpox
was essentially a nasty disease that the administration attempted to manage
when it was left without a choice.

Smallpox gradually receded during the 1960s, punctuated by scattered
small outbreaks. Between 1960 and 1962 an isolation hospital near Lilongwe
supervised 1,488 cases, where the death rate was still high at 11 percent.
Smaller outbreaks occurred elsewhere until 1971, when that year's nine cases
became Malawi's last (ibid., 5). On the UMCA front, three cases at Malindi
and one more across the lake at Kota Kota in 1963 were the last smallpox
cases the mission handled.[18] As in other areas of its medical purview, the
UMCA's African and European staff did everything they felt was possible
in good faith. They stretched scant resources, isolated cases, provided vaccinations and palliative treatment, and comforted the sick according to their
understanding of Christian principles. The mission's mandate and philosophy did not encompass responsibility for the eradication of smallpox. On the
other hand, its health workers' actions generally reflected a strongly imbued
principle of compassion for individual patients. Compassionate treatment,
one of the mission's more abundant resources, was a basic premise guided
by personal religious belief and ideas of Christian character.

Influenza, also called Spanish Flu, entered Malawi in 1918 just after
World War I as part of the raging global pandemic. It lasted into 1919 and
returned in 1923. Lack of experience with the disease placed Malawi at
an equal immunologic disadvantage with many other parts of the world.
Influenza had features in common with smallpox since it could bring havoc
to African social and economic life, and it rapidly became "common to
every station."

Dr. Wigan reported that Likoma was hit harder by influenza than most
places in the country, while Mponda's and Likwenu also "suffered terribly" (*UMCA Ann. Rev.*, 1919, 12). Grim conditions prevailed around Mtonya
station in P.E.A., with daily wailing—"*malilo, malilo, malilo*"—for the dead.
Nearly eighty deaths occurred on Likoma, and many more had been stricken

and recovered. There was practically nothing the mission could do to assist people. It had been unable to establish regular medical work in this Portuguese-administered part of the diocese, and during World War I the site itself had become overgrown and derelict. For UMCA visitors from lakeside, it was "heart-rending to see the helplessness of the people . . . during this pestilence; there are no doctors, nurses, no hospitals, no medicine, no nourishing or suitable food, no blankets, no comfort" (*CA* 37 [1919]: 88).

At Likwenu and its outstations, the UMCA temporarily closed all schools and churches in an effort "to stay the spread" of influenza. Despite many sick people, the death rates remained low around this locality. Meanwhile, nearby Zomba, the protectorate administrative headquarters, had become "a city of the dead." The entire village was laid low at once. Extensive crop losses occurred in some places because there was no one to do the weeding. The government supplied necessary drugs to the missions as well as to its own bomas (stations), where people could come in and get what they needed. "All our time," said a UMCA staff member, "is spent taking drugs to the villages and ministering to the more severe cases" (ibid., 92).

To the missionaries, Africans appeared "grateful" for the collaboration that occurred between government and the missions against their common influenza adversary. It was also clear to a writer in the UMCA's *Diocesan Chronicle* that in Likwenu district, at least, the mission was making substantial progress in reducing African fear of European medicine and lessening the hostility of Muslim villages to Christianity. Refusals of flu medicine were restricted to just a few villages, which reportedly then suffered the highest death rates. Yet underneath the outward signs of greater openness to Western medicine brought on by the pandemic, a UMCA source reminded readers of *Central Africa* that traditional responses to disease still threatened progress. Around the mission stations one still heard rumors "of magic and evil spirits" causing influenza, by more than "cared to express themselves openly; . . . but even so . . . the epidemic has taught people quite definitely that they can trust us in time of sickness" (92–93).

Once influenza abated, missionaries who read the "Station Notes" began to realize the implications of the "long roll of deaths" among the African Christians. "War, influenza and then famine, are not allies to the work," said Bishop Fisher (109). Moreover, there had been a long foreign war in which Africans had no stake. And all over the protectorate, large quantities of locally produced food, instead of being available to help Malawians cope with their nutritional needs during the influenza epidemic, had been diverted away from African families to support the European war. Thousands of tons of staple foods (especially maize) were demanded for shipment to the front in Tanganyika and elsewhere. Profiteering and hunger followed in large regions of Malawi such as the Nyasa Vicarate, worked by the White Fathers and White Sisters.[19] Then came the final and worst year of the war and its destructive aftermath: "Weakened by lack of food, Africans in the Protectorate were overtaken by two devastating epidemics, smallpox and Spanish influenza. With most of the remaining maize being turned into beer a combination of famine and disease accounted for the deaths of hundreds of Malawians" (Linden 1974, 110).

During World War I the mission's staff and programs had been drastically slashed. The *Chauncy Maples*, commandeered by the Royal Navy at the beginning of the war, was not yet returned to the UMCA. Influenza had eaten away in society's fabric like a cancer. A drought soon followed, ensuring still another famine in Malawi. Those whose conscience or faith conditioned them to care about African welfare saw their hands tied. According to Malindi's new priest-in-charge, it was "terrible to hear on all sides the complaint of hunger, and be unable to do anything" (*CA* 37 [1919]: 109). Added to the other pressures on the mission at the end of 1919 was the worst financial crisis in its history (177).

It is clear that epidemic disease and hunger in Malawi went far beyond merely neutral, unprovoked "environmental events." The protectorate government had no alternative to supporting the war effort. It simply took many decisions in which people were manipulated without regard to the consequences for production, or drought, or extraordinary population movements. The British colonial system was never effectively challenged about its ruthless exploitation of the African population. Its collective shamelessness in appropriating local food stocks and forcibly sending tens of thousand of men (*tenga tenga*) to carry supplies to the front, exposing them to disease and death, was never really questioned. The government's decisions were justified by the reining presumption of the time, that African interests and progress coincided with European interests.

For their part, some of the UMCA missionaries abhorred the racist behavior of officers in charge of the British and South African troops stationed in Malawi. Certainly they also objected to the poor and confusing moral example many of the troops exhibited, and they might recoil at the brutalization so many Malawians experienced during the war. But apart from seeking new converts these Anglican missionaries did not view themselves as change agents. A few apolitical commentaries about the *tenga-tenga* crisis did appear in *Central Africa*. In general, the actions of UMCA Europeans almost invariably reflected their rationalization that the survival of their own vocation and way of life depended on keeping as much as possible out of the affairs of state. Public political stands and efforts to influence policy-making that affected African life were best left to others.

In contrast, the Roman Catholic White Fathers and White Sisters did try to become activists on behalf of some African interests. For example, much friction developed between their priests and Nyasaland Protectorate officers over the mistreatment of Africans. The priests had attempted to help "countless tenga-tenga . . . on an individual basis," some of whom had been treated as animals by the military. Reduced to "skin and bone," many of the men who returned from the front were severely ill with dysentery and enteritis, and too weak to travel on to their homes. Even government nurses reportedly refused health care for needy Africans. In contrast, the White Sisters cared for the sick throughout the war (Linden 1974, 111). As tensions continued to grow, however, the Catholic clergy received a direct order from their superior, Father Guilleme, "never to interfere in Government affairs. Limit yourself to pointing out to the relevant authorities those abuses of which you are absolutely certain. By acting in this way you will stay in the role of the missionary which cannot be that of a policeman" (quoted ibid.).

Influenza revisited all UMCA stations in 1923. Likoma's archdeacon made daily rounds to oversee the distribution of "literally gallons of medicine." It evidently did not taste well. Exclaimed a chief who arrived on the island from "down south": "Do not my people prefer to die of the sickness rather than of the European medicine?"[20]

Following the 1923 outbreak, and another in 1935, major influenza epidemics apparently receded (*CA* 54 [1936]: 175). The UMCA's experience with this disease from 1919–23 is an important illustration of the conceptual and structural weaknesses in its medical organization and goals, in Malawi and in London. The mission was simply not set up to effectively cope with most of the diseases and complicated health issues encountered in its vast sphere. Measures taken to stop, manage, and heal disease also depended on African acceptance—and to some extent understanding—of European medicines. Such regard developed at different paces among various population groups and localities.

In truth, of course, influenza was a global problem. Few if any places, with or without a good health infrastructure, escaped its effects. To their credit, the historical materials also reveal that many UMCA medical workers sought to live in the spirit of "pressing on" with the day and problem at hand. Ideally, this attitude to work and mission grew from commitment to a private faith perspective that was publicly nonnegotiable. A practiced, spiritual focus helped to preserve a missionary's integrity and sanity. It aided in strivings to be exemplary and compassionately centered, and it reinforced the personal meaning of the daily work performed by the nurse, dispenser, and doctor.

Yaws produces gruesome skin lesions and scarring on many parts of the body, including the soles of the feet. Many sufferers spent long periods with uncovered sores and dirty bandages, exposing them to other infections. Left untreated, yaws can invade deeper body structures, producing crippling bone damage. It spreads easily through direct contact with an infected person, through an abrasion or cut in the skin, or by flies. Yaws, which was biologically identified in 1905, has caused enormous human suffering over the centuries. It is virtually the only scourge of record that was endemic over large areas in the Diocese of Nyasaland at the beginning of the missionary period, and virtually eradicated by its end. The absence of yaws from UMCA hospital and disease reports by 1963 is striking.

Government campaigns played a major role in the spectacular successes against yaws. Mission health staffs, whose drug supplies usually came from the protectorate government, also made crucial and unheralded contributions of their own. Yaws had been rife in many lakeside villages, as well as in the surrounding mountains.[21] Practically speaking, the UMCA was the only source of Western-type medical care available for hundreds of miles, from Milo in mountainous southwest Tanganyika, to Ft. Johnston just beyond where Lake Malawi drains into the Shiré.

Improvements in yaws therapy spanned a period of about thirty-five years. Prior to World War I, UMCA medics had success with potassium iodide, in tandem with the antiseptic Lysol and copper sulfate. As word of this therapy's effectiveness spread, people who had previously feared missionary medicine began to seek it out at mission hospitals and dispensaries. The fact that it might require months of waiting for the potassium iodide to really clear away the symptoms of yaws did not deter chronic sufferers. Meanwhile, severe wartime shortages of staff and drugs, and related turmoil, greatly hindered efforts to control any chronic diseases. For example, in the neighboring UMCA Diocese of Masasi in Tanganyika, most Africans who had been "cured" with potassium iodide before World War I reportedly experienced relapses (Ranger 1981, 266). It was apparently much the same in Malawi.

Soon after World War I new "wonder drugs" for the treatment of trypanosomes became available in Malawi. Research into organic arsenic compounds by Dr. Paul Ehrlich in Germany had yielded Salvarsan 606 in 1909 (injected intravenously) and its derivative Neosalvarsan 914 (cheaper than Salvarsan and injected intramuscularly). These chemotherapeutic agents replaced mercury and iodides. At first, it seemed that their ability to cure yaws and syphilis was immediate, dramatic, and potentially life-changing. People flocked to hospitals and dispensaries for the injections. The "magic" of the hypodermic needle quickly revolutionized expectations among Malawians as well as other colonial African societies. Demand for injections (*dawa ya sindano* in Swahili) dramatically grew. Unless accompanied by "the needle," pills and most other forms of treatment for illness and injury came to be seen as inferior or inadequate. Meanwhile, the White Fathers had decided the new arsenicals were too expensive for the huge number of yaws sufferers in their sphere. They chose instead Castellani's Mixture, an injection combining a compound of antimony and iodine. The protectorate's Chief Secretary arranged for this drug to be sent out to the White Fathers periodically, along with wages to pay mission dressers who visited the villages on bicycles. At one point in 1922, Father Sarrazin informed the Medical Department that there was an increase of 1,000 yaws cases around Ntakataka Mission alone.[22]

An appeal by the UMCA in Britain for help in purchasing the drugs met with a "generous" response in 1920. UMCA medical staff set to work to provide the injections bolstered by the extraordinary possibility, if not yet confirmed reality, that "nearly every case [is] now curable with a single intravenous injection" (MO's Report, *UMCA Ann. Rev.*, 1920–21, 78). Indeed, following one of the painful arsenical or antimony tartrate (for bilharzia) injections, patients generally experienced rapid, marked improvement.[23] Regarding this revolutionary therapy, Dr. Wigan remarked that "it is difficult to think that there is in existence at all any more direct and visible benefit in a physical sense that can be conferred on a sick person than the injection for Framboesia" (*CA* 42 [1924]: 122). However, many people were fooled into believing that they would experience a dramatic reduction of symptoms with one injection. It turned out that a one-shot cure for yaws was generally inadequate. Believing they had been cured, people often quit the injections and thereby opened themselves to a relapse. They also remained potentially infectious to others on a continuous basis.

UMCA medical staff gave 5,001 injections of arsenicals for yaws to 3,814 patients between 1924 and 1926 (*UMCA Ann. Rev.*, 1925, 111). Patients, many assisted by relatives and friends, were expected to pay about five shillings (a month's wage) for these injections, which roughly covered the cost of the drug to the mission (King and King 1991, 126). By 1923 potassium iodide had become an obsolete drug against yaws. Salvarsan or Neosalvarsan were now the drugs of choice. Neosalvarsan cured, but the treatment was reported to take longer and cause painful swelling (Simpkin 1926, 43). Those injecting Salvarsan had to receive special training for the intravenous method, and demonstrate skill and good judgment.

In varying degrees, endemic disease was deeply embedded in the local cultural ecology and social fabric of most places in the Diocese of Nyasaland.

Patterns reflected both the ancient endemic causes of high morbidity and new health threats stirred up by the actions of the colonial regime. According to a government source, yaws was most common in populations located between the shoreline of Lake Malawi and 1,800 feet above sea level.[24] Yet in the late 1920s, Dr. Wigan expressed dismay because yaws, syphilis, and hookworm were so "rife" at Milo, situated some 5,500 feet above the lake. At this time, the UMCA's three stations in Tanganyika seemed to have the lion's share of endemic disease. By Wigan's estimate, "about 60% of our treatment has been in Tanganyika Territory" (CA 45 [1927]: 90). Within a few years yaws would begin to recede noticeably. Even by 1930 cases at Milo Hospital, opened under British auspices in 1925, had been "greatly reduced." Also, fewer ulcers—a proportion of which were caused by old yaws cases—were seen (CA 49 [1931]: 125).

By 1936 the protectorate's Medical Department, in response to an inquiry from Jamaica's Board of Health, advised that mass treatment had led to "a great reduction" of yaws in the Malawi.[25] Yet the disease persisted for another two decades, and the 3,237 cases reported in the protectorate in 1949 was certainly an underestimate (King and King 1991, 126).

Penicillin's introduction in the 1950s offered a "final" solution to yaws. Its unprecedented action against bacterial infections came in the form of a one-injection, long-acting "silver bullet." Yaws was soon rapidly eradicated in Malawi, and for their commitment to the process the UMCA deserves great credit.[26] A similar effect was documented in the neighboring Diocese of Masasi in Tanganyika, where the drug also produced miraculous healing. But as the missionaries there discovered to their dismay, this victory over disease was, in Ranger's phrase, an "ambiguous triumph" (Ranger 1981, 267). Patients with yaws came into the mission hospital for the injection (often from long distances), but most did not feel a reciprocal obligation to convert to Christianity.

Schistosomiasis (bilharzia) and hookworm had long been endemic in many areas of precolonial Malawi. Risk of exposure to schistosomiasis was and is often greatest in villages sited near reed-infested areas of Lake Malawi's shoreline. Many people also had sustained contact with snail-infested waters through their domestic and recreational activities (wading, working, swimming, canoe-handling) in inshore waters, slow-moving streams, river margins, and water pools. These environments exposed unsuspecting children and adults to the snail-shed cercariae, which rapidly penetrate the legs or another exposed body site.

Unhygienic disposal of human feces also exposed people to the risk of hookworm infection. Hookworm (and roundworm, or Ascaris) were perpetual co-residents wherever more than a few people clustered together in sedentary settlements. When places near compounds were used for defecation, feet became contaminated with feces. Given the requisite soil, temperature, and moisture conditions, infective hookworm larvae were then spread across the ground into adjacent domestic spaces. In this manner larvae penetrated the feet of unsuspecting villagers, beginning the infection cycle.[27]

Schistosomiasis and hookworm, both communicable diseases, were undoubtedly both present, even if not consistently identified, in many of the first Africans treated by UMCA medical staff. Dr. Howard observed in 1910 that urinary schistosomiasis (*S. haematobium*) was the preeminent parasitic disease. He estimated that nearly half the male population was infected, and it was also common in females. In Howard's opinion, that "persons of all ages and both sexes are extremely fond of bathing" was a major risk factor (Howard 1910, 68).

At the same time, mild hookworm infections with clinical symptoms also commonly occurred in the smaller villages. Unsanitary conditions generally worsened as settlements grew in size, and in large villages such as Kota Kota, with thousands of residents, hookworm caused widespread severe anemia. Poor hygiene and sanitation ensured that schistosomiasis and hookworm significantly added to the precolonial burden of ill-health. Colonial rule produced a growing population (after World War I), larger settlements, and unprecedented mobility. These factors further opened the door for the intensification and spread of helminthic infections, so long as public health efforts to eliminate them remained of low intensity or nonexistent.

After World War I, both the UMCA and the protectorate's Medical Department initiated campaigns that employed newer drugs to treat selected populations burdened with endemic hookworm and bilharzia. Measures intended to change the maladaptive practices that maintained endemicity were also introduced. Reported case loads at hospitals and dispensaries varied from considerable to massive, and between mission and government accounts. Intestinal worms, a catch-all term, accounted for 10 percent of reported disease at Likoma in 1920–21 (*UMCA Ann. Rev.*, 1920–21, 76). Meanwhile, in 1922 the protectorate's Medical Department estimated that hookworm infected about 80 percent of Africans, but did not compare the rate of infection with actual levels of hookworm disease.[28] Said the DMS at this time: "We have to confess that we have little knowledge as to the extent or prevalence of any of these [major endemic] diseases."[29]

Two years later the protectorate's Chief Sanitary Officer reported that "at least 90% of the native population was infected with Ankylostomiasis . . . and that a substantial proportion of these infections [were] sufficiently heavy to cause material disability." He noted that "for all practical purposes, anaemia in a native means Hookworm."[30] UMCA staff also noticed a "great increase in the number of cases under treatment" at hospitals. Following the belated introduction of microscopes, helminthiases diagnoses grew nearly threefold.[31] By the 1930s, hookworm, together with syphilis, had become the most common causes of miscarriage and birthing difficulties in UMCA hospitals.

Carbon tetrachloride became the drug of choice for mass treatment of hookworm in the early 1920s.[32] Up to this time no effective therapy existed. Two decades later Oil of Chenopodium was also used at Likoma and other stations.[33] Both drugs proved extremely unpleasant to take. The government adopted carbon tetrachloride on the basis of "very favorable reports," and the administration heavily promoted its attractive features, claiming "1 dose, cheap, side effects rare, and simple to administer."[34] Stockpiles were distributed free to government hospitals and rural dispensaries, missions, and employers of labor. In 1930, the government treated 18,305 people with carbon tetrachloride in its own facilities.

Maintaining the work capacity among adult African males in the labor force was a great government concern. Hookworm symptoms such as "lassitude and a discomfort suggestive of dyspepsia" affected Africans, although reports downplayed their severity. Nevertheless, said the protectorate's DMS, even "these slight symptoms are sufficient . . . to interfere with his output of work."[35] In a letter to the manager of a European estate employing African laborers, the DMS assured him that in its "pure drug" form carbon tetrachloride was "harmless." Beer-drinkers were the one exception: the "evil effects of carbon tetrachloride in heavy beer drinkers are proved clinically and must be remembered in further campaigns." Clinical symptoms in such beer drinkers included severe epigastric pains, vomiting, liver tenderness, and jaundice.[36]

After a dozen years of mass administration of "harmless" carbon tetrachloride, the government apparently reversed its view and adopted a far more cautious, skeptical position. Writing to the UMCA's Dr. Wigan in 1936, the DMS advised: "As you know carbon tetrachloride is a dangerous drug and should only be given after accurate diagnosis and under supervision. Its use en masse is not likely to be of much benefit unless accompanied and followed by a campaign for the improvement of sanitary conditions."[37]

Four decades into the century, no informed observer could argue against the need to treat the root causes of hookworm. That sanitation practices in African settlements were poor to nonexistent was hardly a revelation. More holistic approaches to public health demonstrated that curative medicine by itself was an impractical solution to the eliminating the infection. Yet the cure was cheap and expedient, and there could be no guarantee that digging a pit latrine for every household would resolve age-old behaviors and hookworm eradication. Carelessly used latrines, certainly a common feature of public places, readily supported ongoing hookworm infection in a community.[38] In 1939 at the UMCA leper settlement at Likwenu, for example, over fifty patients lived in dispersed huts and cultivated their own food on three-acre plots. The mission provided "one latrine among two or three patients," which would certainly have far exceeded anything then typical in African villages. Nonetheless, hookworm disease was present and patients required examination and treatment. The visiting Secretary of BELRA advised that latrines be placed closer to the huts and made deeper.[39] It is not known whether this suggestion was implemented.

By the mid-1930s the government reported that new latrines were "visible in almost all the villages" of Malawi. But the latrines lacked supervision, and the free movement of Africans to estates and the cotton markets spread an epidemic of acute bacillary dysentery that caused a high mortality.[40] Latrine construction was not an unmixed blessing, for it could create other problems, not least the contamination of their immediate surroundings. Disgusted by insanitary conditions, some people simply avoided latrines. A survey of the large village of Jalasi near Malindi in 1938 reported that latrines about eight feet deep were "reasonably well-supplied," but their bottoms lay on bedrock. Consequently, "they stink abominably and breed large quantities of flies. Pollution of [Jalasi's] three wells is inevitable."[41]

Hookworm continued to rank high among all reported morbidity in the UMCA's sphere right up to Malawi's independence. Likwenu Hospital, south of the lake, reported an "appalling" prevalence rate in 1944. Treatment alone was useless: "Nearly every patient has hookworm or bilharzia or both; they get treated and become re-infected solely because the drinking water is infested and they do not understand sanitation" (*CA* 65 [1947]: 56).

Hookworm accounted for 50 percent (5,043 cases) of all major diseases reported in 1950. It "easily takes first place," said the UMCA's Dr. Maclean. Syphilis was a distant second with 14 percent of cases (*CA* 69 [1951]: 197). Proportionately fewer cases of hookworm were seen in mission centers during 1954, but it is by no means clear whether these returns are reliable. The 2,156 reported hookworm cases represented 31 percent of all disease, second only to malaria at 32 percent (*CA* 73 [1955]: 246). Hookworm ranked fourth overall in 1963, but new cases eclipsed those of the previous decade by more than 50 percent.[42]

Over the years the UMCA showed a growing commitment to treat patients with hookworm. As population grew the numbers of people coming in for therapy also increased. Yet mission efforts (and those taken by the protectorate government) seem to have been little more than a holding action, a "finger-in-the-dike" response. Once treated, people returned to their villages only to reexpose themselves to the parasite. Thus, despite the investment in latrines that gradually occurred around the protectorate, the UMCA did not curb hookworm in its sphere. It lacked the resources needed to couple its treatment of patients with sustainable public health measures in the villages. Regardless of the availability of more powerful drugs, beginning with Nilodin in the 1950s (*UMCA Ann. Rev.*, 1951, 29), in 1990 hookworm remained a prominent element of the disease profile in densely populated lakeside settlements such as Malindi. The same was true of schistosomiasis, which along with cholera remained endemic because people used the lake-shore as a toilet.[43]

Schistosomiasis (or bilharzia, a blood fluke infection) remained seriously endemic in and beyond the lake zone. At Likoma Hospital in 1921, 151 people were diagnosed and given 1,500 painful intravenous injections of antimony tartrate. Apparently 100 of these heavily-dosed patients were cured (*UMCA Ann. Rev.*, 1921–22, 97). Dr. Wigan noted that "treatment...is taken as a matter of course now and three times a week there is a small queue waiting for intravenous injections" (*CA* 41 [1923]: 248; Wigan added that "queues always sit down in Africa"). Schistosomiasis was rife around Kota Kota on the west coast, where the UMCA and government both had medical facilities. Over half of the children surveyed had the infection (King and King 1991, 101), which pointed to their frequent water contact. In one batch of 172 urine specimens examined in 1930 revealed 84 percent positive for *S. haematobium*. The rectal form of infection spread by *S. mansoni* was also present, but stool samples revealed prevalences below 10 percent.[44]

Bulinus and *Biomphalaria*, the primary snail hosts for the schistosomes, found favorable habitats in pools and sluggish streams away from the lake as well. Jalasi, noted earlier for its poor latrine system, was up in the hills ten miles inland from Malindi. In 1938, a medical survey of this village found eight hundred huts highly infested with hookworm. By comparison with bilharzia, however, hookworm had become "a minor factor in the deterioration of health [in Jalasi village]." Instead, bilharzia had become the "principal cause of general ill health."[45] Jalasi illustrated what was by now a general process: endemic disease was increasing "hand in hand" with the growing population. Mean haemoglobin levels in Jalasi had fallen below 65 percent of normal.[46]

Reports and scattered control measures continued. In 1949, bilharzia ranked first among major communicable diseases on Likoma. By then

Dr. Maclean, the mission's MO, had seen enough. He announced that "a war has been declared on the island against preventable diseases" (*CA* 68 [1950]: 204). While affirming that "a very large proportion of the population was infected" with bilharzia, hookworm, malaria, tick fever, TB, and leprosy, Maclean also lamented that in public health measures "cooperation of people tends to be passive only . . . with the exception of the Boy Scouts."[47] Community participation, the most critical element of a viable public health campaign, proved difficult to muster let alone sustain. As Maclean had discovered, considering all of the other demands on their lives, Likomans found it easier to live with the "devils" than find the considerable time, energy, and understanding needed to root them out. And controlling snail populations was an extremely difficult challenge under any conditions.

Development of irrigation schemes in the Lower Shiré Valley after World War II greatly facilitated the further spread of bilharzia, the disease linked to slowed-down waters. Newer, more effective drugs, including Nilodin (triostam) and Ambilhar became available by 1950, but their side effects could be worse than the disease. In 1951 and 1952 Burroughs Wellcome Co. gave the UMCA enough free supplies of Nilodin to treat one hundred people. Whether this gift was "generous," as reported, or not, the number of infected people was in the tens of thousands. Only a small fraction of cases were identified at the mission's hospitals (*UMCA Ann. Rev.*, 1951, 29, and 1952, 25). UMCA statistics show that on the eve of independence in 1963, schistosomiasis cases ranked just behind malaria, hookworm, conjunctivitis, and ulcers.

The mission did identify schistosomiasis as a major threat to African health. Staff believed they could at least make a dent in its prevalence among small population groups, and devoted considerable effort to that end. As with malaria, however, the disease yields slowly under poverty conditions. By independence, reports indicated that nearly three times more people received treatment for the infection than in 1954. A note of caution here is required. Inconsistencies and artifacts in the UMCA's reports preclude great confidence in any interpretation of them. Attendance fluctuated for many reasons, greatly undermining the ability to assess disease prevalence. When the mission ran out of drugs, it simply sent away people who sought treatment. By 1980, schistosomiasis infected an estimated two million of Malawi's 6.5 million people. Depending on the locality, prevalence ranged from 15 to 50 percent of the population (King and King 1991, 102).

Malaria was of extraordinary concern to the mission in the early days when European survival was at stake. In 1897 the standard list of medicines "necessary for the treatment of malarial fever in its various forms" included

twenty-six tablets and solutions, ranging from four types of quinine to lau-
danum and strychnine. This list came with a caveat that "No one should go
to Africa without these" (Cross 1897, 200–201). Malawians and millions of
other Africans had lived with and died from this menace for millennia. Constantly enlarged spleens persisted up to five years of age, with accompanying
high morbidity, mortality, and impoverishment (Howard 1910, 66).

Permanent eradication of malaria presupposed unattainable affluence
and political mobilization. It is an intensely seasonal infection virtually everywhere in Malawi. Arrival of the rains brings an explosion of natural and
man-made habitats favoring anophelines. The mission's position on these
breeding places had always been that "it is not practicable to control them,
without incurring enormous expense, except in a few areas such as the
ridges of Milo and parts of Likoma and Malindi (*CA* 67 [1949]: 91). In 1922,
the government viewed its own stations at Liwonde, Karonga, Kota Kota,
and Ft. Johnston as places that "are and must remain veritable hot beds of
malaria, and the only solution is their [the population's] removal to other
sites."[48] Such resettlement never occurred.

Statistics suggest that utilization of government dispensaries for malaria
treatment increased over time. Nonetheless, there is no escaping the fact that
people dealt with the malaria burden mainly at home, away from medical
facilities. For its part, the government treated a mere 3,022 cases in 1926, or
only 2 percent of all cases seen. Malaria cases treated in government centers
rose to 8,200 in 1930, when the disease accounted for 3.8 percent of recorded
deaths. Reports also surfaced that Africans of different socio-economic backgrounds were beginning to make greater use of quinine. Policy now held that
quinine packets should be made available free of charge to "any native at any
Government hospitals or dispensaries."[49] For financial reasons, the UMCA
and other missions restricted quinine treatment to Africans who showed
acute symptoms. Mass prophylactic use was not advocated because it could
cause a loss of immunity among those who survived attacks as children and
thus increase the risk of a serious epidemic.[50]

Malaria cases reported at UMCA facilities are fragmentary and markedly
stagnant over a period of several decades. Moreover, the mission's figures
inaccurately suggest that malaria cases slightly decreased from the 1920s to
the 1950s.[51] Then, as now, the reality was that most malaria cases never got
reported. The disease cannot be confirmed other than microscopically. Its
true extent was masked by a general diagnosis of fever, or *homa*. Reported
cases jumped over 70 percent to 2,250 in 1954, when malaria ranked first
among endemic diseases treated by the mission. During the next decade
malaria cases treated nearly tripled, with 6,221 cases reported in 1963.[52] This

apparent surge of cases parallels the near-doubling of Malawi's population between the end of World War II and independence.[53]

It is fair to say that colonialism and missionary medicine had virtually no damping effect on malaria as a public health problem. Most children with cerebral malaria who desperately needed treatment with drugs and a blood transfusion typically remained too far from a hospital to receive help. Some individuals certainly did benefit. At the UMCA's Liuli Hospital in 1955 about three-quarters of the mothers who delivered in the hospital had cots with mosquito nets for their infants in their homes, which seemed to reduce the frequency of malaria infection. The missionaries attributed these outcomes to the fact that the men who lived around Liuli had been to South Africa for work. Exposure to European practices there, they reckoned, provided the example that led these Malawians to use part of their incomes to purchase cots and nets for their children.

Palliative treatment of malaria with quinine and, beginning in the 1950s, new synthetic antimalarials such as chloroquine could ease suffering and even save lives.[54] Unfortunately, within a few years of chloroquine's availability in the tropics the *Plasmodia* started to develop resistance to it, prompting renewed reliance on quinine. Meanwhile, anophelenes began to adapt to the insecticides aimed at them. Since then, grand proposals to eradicate malaria in Africa, and globally, have been continuously thwarted by weak political will and poorly targeted health care funds.

Finally, tuberculosis (TB) requires mention, because it mirrors the changing social conditions under colonial rule. Although allegedly absent before Europeans arrived, some cases of TB were known when the protectorate was founded. Dr. Howard termed it "a rare disease" around Lake Malawi in 1900, present "only in those villages situated along the slave and trade routes, whither infection was carried from the coast" (Howard 1910, 67). Yet within the next decade the disease greatly increased. This was primarily attributed to the ever-growing pool of men leaving home to work in the European-owned mines in South Africa or Rhodesia (see chap. 5). Sooner or later, large numbers of them returned to Malawi exposed, infected, or sick with TB. If seen at a mission or government hospital in the protectorate, a symptomatic person would typically be sent home, where he could readily infect others. Effective drugs did not exist, and it was believed that many cases would "benefit by the open air treatment" still common in Europe (*CA* 51 [1933]: 150).

The UMCA's Alice Simpkin blamed the spread of TB squarely on the actions of Europeans, and observed that "the African goes under very quickly when it takes hold of him" (Simpkin 1926, 27). Thirty years later, the UMCA referred to TB as the "menace of Rhodesia" and the greatest killer of all in that colony. Rhodesia had some 6,000 to 7,000 cases by 1951, and was in need of an "impossible" 5,000 hospital beds to treat it. TB mainly affected Africans (including Malawian migrants), it was believed, because they lacked inherited immunity, had few workable ideas about hygiene, suffered over-crowding in mine camps, and were slow to seek medical care (*CA* 74 [1956]: 62). Back in Malawi, the UMCA reported ninety-four cases treated at mission hospitals in 1949, most of them at remote Milo and Liuli in Tanganyika, and Msumba.

In 1955, the protectorate government estimated the annual incidence of TB at 32 per 100,000 people, a rate which more than doubled to 80 per 100,000 by 1982. Over 8,000 new cases were reported in 1988. During the 1990s, TB ranked eighth among the most common causes of death in Malawi's hospitals, but many also died at home (King and King 1991, 79–80). Despite new drugs, the synergism between TB and HIV has enormously contributed to their tragic proliferation today, and to the corresponding burden on families, the health-care system, and society at large.

When the remaining UMCA missionaries started packing their bags in the early 1960s, most patients coming to mission hospitals and dispensaries typically showed "multiple symptom complexes" such as malaria, malnutrition, anemia, and hookworm. Medical staffs had been both committed and appreciated by Africans, and by World War I they had discerned much about disease ecology. Despite these advances, the mission had little choice but to concentrate its efforts on the small proportion of the population that had both access to care and the social and cultural readiness to use it. Regarding this last point, informal evidence suggests that matrilineal descent among the Nyanja and Yao peoples, and adherence to Islamic practice among most Yao, contributed to lower rates of medical care utilization in the UMCA's sphere than could be expected among the patrilineal and non-Muslim societies of south-central Africa. This applied especially to females in those societies, for whom matrilineal descent and Muslim custom imposed the requirement that women and girls had to obtain the consent of their uncles (mother's brother) or an adult male surrogate from the matrilineage before they could attend a medical facility.[55]

Not through lack of effort, the mission's overall efforts at revolutionizing medical care and public health amounted to the proverbial drop in the bucket.[56] In this light the missionaries had much company among the several religious and secular agencies whose aims included good works.

ARTS AND SCIENCES:
DRUGS, MEDICAL TECHNOLOGY, AND SURGERY

Mission Links to Medical Science

Before 1890, malaria, treated with quinine, was really the only disease with a specific drug remedy. Treatment of conditions such as pneumonia, meningitis, and syphilis depended primarily on the quality of nursing care and patient characteristics.

The most useful drugs among the pioneer doctors included quinine, morphia, chloroform, local anaesthetics, digitalis, local antiseptics, and vaccine lymph (King and King 1991). D. Kerr Cross, a Scottish missionary doctor and later MO for British Central Africa, described what a well-equipped, tropical medicine kit in the late 1890s should contain. He listed sixty-eight medicines, including six "hypodermic" drugs such as morphia and ether, plus another twenty-three items for surgical purposes. As much as possible, said Cross, supplies should be in tablet form so they could be accurately administered without scales, and easily swallowed and absorbed. Cross was also well aware of certain strategic aspects of drug marketing. He strongly recommended that doctors purchase drugs from Burroughs, Wellcome and Co., an efficient company that paid "special attention to foreign export." Their hypodermic medicines were also "all that could be desired" (Cross 1897, 200–203). In reality, before World War I most Africans had little if any access to systematic treatment with such remedies.

Developments in antisera therapy began at the Koch Institute in the late 1880s and 1890s. Modern chemotherapy was based on derivatives of aniline dyes. Even before World War I, European doctors going to the tropics could obtain "magic bullets" such as Salvarsan. Many new drugs eventually became available in Malawi, if only irregularly, but the long distances could render the drugs extremely costly.

By 1903 Dr. Howard had been in Malawi for nearly four years as the UMCA's MO. He spoke with delight about the new dispensary established at Malindi, and claimed that the *dawa* had "in it everything that is needed, from a grain weight to a huge jar of sulphur, so we can do our dispensing, and fumigate our houses if necessary" (*CA* 22 [1904]: 37). Restocking was not cheap, however, given transfer costs. Drug prices in the protectorate had inflated "almost beyond comprehension." For example, a 5-pound package of potassium iodide used for treating various conditions including yaws, tumors, and asthma[57] cost £21s 6d, and a bottle of 500 tablets £11s (*CA* 22

[1904]: 142). Also, with so many people suffering multiple ulcers, shortages of dressings, especially old linen and rags, strained the mission's resources to the break point. For the benefit of British readers Dr. Howard wrote that "the nurses have been beseeching us to turn over our wardrobes and hand over everything we can, while they watch with eagle eye the clothes as they go to the wash in the hope that they can suggest that some old and valued friend in the shape of a coat or cassock has really qualified for use in the dispensary!" (*CA* 22 [1904]: 142).

Apart from Salvarsan, the new breakthroughs in drug therapy did not become available in Central Africa until after World War I. Meanwhile, hygiene and skilled nursing clearly saved African lives and reduced suffering among the relatively small numbers who had access to and actually utilized mission services. As noted, by the 1920s Neosalvarsan began to have a dramatic effect on yaws, and potassium iodide was phased out. Intravenous injections of antimony tartrate, though painful, offered hope to schistosomiasis sufferers for the first time. Despite the introduction of the new anti-schistosome drugs, Miricil and Nilodin, by the late 1940s and early 1950s, effective treatment of humans for this recurrent water-based infection was still decades away. No drug by itself could control schistosomiasis in the absence of improved drainage, snail destruction, widespread education, and changes in human habits.

Bayer 205, available in Malawi by the early 1920s, was praised by the UMCA's Dr. Wigan as a "most successful" cure for sleeping sickness. In his view, this development was "as important as the discovery of '606' [Salvarsan], and "especially important to the British Empire" (*CA* 42 [1924]: 43). The vector *Glossina morsitans*, the "savanna" tsetse, spread *T. rhodesiense*, the primary trypanosome in Malawi.[58] Early attempts to save sufferers relied on a toxic arsenical drug, Atoxyl, which was ineffective and could cause blindness. The seriousness of this disease in Malawi was recognized in 1906 when a high-profile research team from Europe, including Robert Koch, arrived to conduct a Sleeping Sickness Survey and make recommendations for controlling its spread (King and King 1991, 115–16). In 1907 a few screening posts were set up to try to monitor trypanosomes in the blood of travelers who entered Malawi from other tsetse-infested territories.

Intensified human environmental interference through population and game movement, bush clearance, and road development in the first decades of the twentieth century had already begun to change the sensitive dynamics of tsetse ecology. Several serious epidemics of human trypanosomiasis occurred in the protectorate before and during World War I, yet mention of sleeping sickness in UMCA reports is unusual.[59] Today, vigilance against tsetse spread remains an essential element of public health in Malawi.

Colonial deeds also helped to stir up tick-borne relapsing fever, which was spread through human contact with the domesticated, spirochete-harboring *Ornithodorous moubata*. Opportunities for control dramatically increased in the 1950s due to the development of BHC (Gammexane). Methods and targets of application included spraying people, clothing, and blankets, as well as the inside of huts and rest houses, where the ticks hid in cracks in walls and attached themselves to domestic fowl. The UMCA responded slowly because it lacked funds to buy the insecticide.

Leprosy was largely "entrusted" or delegated by the colonial authorities to missionaries and their African dispensers and dressers. In the 1920s and 1930s, hopes grew among both missionaries and lepers that injections of natural oils, including moogrol and hydnocreal (used into the 1960s), and Alepol, would lessen symptoms and promote healing. But these "bulky and irksome" injections caused great pain and generally provided little benefit (*UMCA Ann. Rev.*, 1952, 25). Considering its poor performance, Iliffe (1987) asserts that "hydnocarpus [therapy] was, literally, a confidence trick" that lasted for decades (225).

Effective anti-leprosy drugs did not materialize until the transition from colonial overrule was already well under way. Sulphone drugs, notably dapsone, finally enabled leprosy treatment to become "primarily a medical rather than a charitable enterprise" after World War II (ibid.). Here, too, setbacks followed. Leprosy bacilli had developed resistance to dapsone by the 1970s. Sooner or later, each new leprosy drug encountered resistance. Paradoxically, as more powerful drugs became available in Malawi, the size of the population with leprosy also grew. In 1908, the government's estimate that 769 people had leprosy was far from the reality. Estimates increased to 30,000 in 1955, and to 80,000 by independence, placing Malawi among countries with the highest leprosy prevalence (227–29).

Most of the powerful antibiotic compounds including Prontosil, penicillin, streptomycin, and tetracycline, did not enter Western medical therapies until the end of the colonial missionary era. The Salk polio vaccine was available in Malawi in 1957, but parents frequently refused to have their children vaccinated until after new cases began to show a marked upswing. The more easily administered Sabin oral vaccines arrived in 1962, just before independence. A survey in 1979 found about 17,500 of Malawi's 2.5 million children (6.5 per 1,000 survivors through age nine), with "residual paralysis from Polio, usually of the legs" (King and King 1991, 161). UMCA records on polio are scarce before 1960.[60]

Bush Microscopy

By 1900 a few of Nyasaland's mission and administration doctors had access to optical microscopes, but the UMCA did not introduce them until end of World War I. In 1924, Dr. Wigan began training twenty-five African senior school students at Likoma, some as young as fifteen, to become dispensary assistants, capable among other tasks of identifying hookworm eggs and bilharzia flukes. Under Wigan's supervision, many of the trainees became quite skilled at identifying specimens. In the early stages most of the microscopic work was done primarily by two men, Edward and Lester, who during eleven months in 1923 examined and reported on most of 848 specimens collected at Likoma.[61] By 1924 a microscope was available at each UMCA hospital, and in 1925 Likoma acquired the mission's only relatively high-powered microscope for use with an oil-immersion type lens.[62]

While they represented "a decided advance" because they permitted more definitive diagnoses, most of the microscopes the mission received could not be used with an oil immersion lens. Consequently, examinations of blood films for infections such as malaria, tick fever, or sleeping sickness, and analysis of specimens for tuberculosis and leprosy bacilli, still had to be sent the long distance to the government laboratory in Ft. Johnston. This routine was tedious and impractical, particularly in cases of acute illnesses.

Low-power microscopes nevertheless became an important tool in the mission's efforts to upgrade its medical care. For African hospital assistants, the medical officer, and nurses, they helped remove some of the guesswork of diagnosis, particularly in the identification and specific treatment of debilitating helminthiases. During a visit to Likoma in 1930, the UMCA's Bishop of Masasi in Tanganyika observed that "the microscopic work done by their [Malawian] dispensary boys by itself suffices as an instance of the wonderful efficiency that has been attained" (*CA* 48 [1930]: 136). However, after a decade of training and familiarization in the 1920s, references in mission reports to this mode of diagnosis rapidly taper off. In the absence of sustainable public health interventions, medical staffs had to cope with the population's repetitive exposure to and reinfection with hookworm, bilharzia, and other infectious agents.

Surgery

Unlike injections, Africans in the UMCA's sphere accepted Western surgery much more slowly and with much greater apprehension. The first European doctors in Malawi carried a set of pocket surgical instruments and chloroform. They served as "jacks of all trades" and adepts at improvisation (King and King 1991). In 1876, at Bandawe, Dr. Roberts Laws of the Livingstonia Mission was the first to operate on an African under general anesthesia, using a chloroform-soaked cloth spread over the patient's nose and mouth. With the patient asleep, Laws amazed onlookers by removing a tumor. He wrote that news of this demonstration quickly spread "far and wide," attracting many other surgical cases whose needs ranged from teeth extraction to major operations (ibid). Chloroform, said Laws, was "one of the greatest surprises to the natives, as it was the greatest help to us" (Laws 1934, 121).[63]

Laws, a progressive in his time, believed that European medicine should be "at the service of the natives" (120). At the same time he recognized that in African minds the new medicine was readily "mingled with superstition," and that medical missionaries had to exercise patience to "safeguard the future." He believed from the start that Africans ought to be trained to do surgery, sooner rather than later. In the early days, Laws's strategy was to undertake "only comparatively simple operations, the results of which were likely to be successful. In this way the faith was established in the minds of the people regarding the skill of the European doctor" (121). Laws also oversaw the establishment of a comparatively extensive system of Presbyterian hospitals and dispensaries in northwest Malawi, with the headquarters at Livingstonia.

In contrast with the UMCA, the Livingstonia medical mission benefited from greater financial support, several staff doctors at any given time, a more extensive capability for training African staff, and often more sophisticated equipment. For example, the Scots mission installed the protectorate's first x-ray machine in 1927, made possible through donations from Scottish Sunday Schools (King and King 1991, 45). Within a few years the other major Scottish missions, at Blantyre and Zomba, also acquired x-ray equipment. In contrast, the UMCA never got such technology.[64]

In his reminiscences, Laws recalled that Livingstonia's David Gordon Memorial Hospital, which opened in 1910 with a "splendid operating theatre, male and female pavilion wards, and a nurses' house with provision for European patients," "has been an untold boon for the carrying on of medical work. Patients come from the other side of the Lake seeking treatment" (Laws 1934, 125). In time, despite initial resistance, successful cataract operations using a localized cocaine anesthetic proved to be among the most dramatic medical interventions at Livingstonia (King and King 1991, 43).[65]

Surgery was by no means a daily occurrence at the main mission hospitals for many years after they had opened. In 1894, the UMCA's Dr. Robinson observed that "the native has an inherent antipathy to the knife" (*CA* 12 [1894]: 139). And there was more to surgery acceptance than overcoming Africans' understandable fear and prejudices toward it. Such procedures could not be undertaken without reference to the guiding social principle that negotiations had to involve numerous matrilineal kin, who acted as a kind of therapy managing group:

> So many relatives have to be consulted; but the person of most importance is not the mother or the father, whose influence is quite secondary, but the mother's eldest brother, called the *Mchibweni*. In the case of Rebecca (Hepatic abscess), as she was grown up, it was *her brother*. However, he was unwilling until Rebecca turned to her husband and said, "you are my husband and must decide." (Ibid.)

Shortly after assuming his post as the UMCA's MO in 1899, Dr. Howard successfully operated for four hours on a nineteen-year-old boy whose mastoiditis was endangering his brain. Such major operations, including obstetrical surgery, remained exceptional and the subject of widespread popular mistrust (King and King 1991, 45). During World War I, surgery was further curtailed by the mission's lack of surgical instruments, which caused Dr. Wigan "a great trial." Frequently, operable cases had to be turned away, and there was no prospect of procuring any equipment until after the war. The Germans reportedly took away a large supply of the useful surgical instruments they had stocked in their Tanganyika mission stations, thus denying them to their British successors (*CA* 35 [1917]: 218).

Even after World War I, operations under anesthesia in UMCA hospitals amounted to a modest 77 in 1924, 105 in 1925, and 95 in 1927.[66] However, the great bulk of this surgery fell into the lap of the UMCA's only doctor—who by 1930 had responsibility for nine hospitals spread across a north-south distance of over four hundred miles. In 1922, when Dr. Wigan dared to take a furlough, all operations had to be delayed until he returned from England (*CA* 41 [1923]: 95). Prayer had to suffice for emergency cases during the interval. When Wigan was again furloughed for most of 1939, surgery lapsed once more, although some cases got referred to government hospitals such as Ft. Johnston. Wigan's share of the medical work was partly absorbed by three new nurses, whose arrival in the diocese was a stroke of luck since

World War II had already commenced (*UMCA Ann. Rev.*, 1936, Medical Officer's Report; and 1939, 32).

In contrast to Malawians' distaste for surgery in general, requests for cataract operations increased dramatically before World War I. In 1912 a nurse at Likoma observed that people with cataracts were arriving

> one after another, all prepared and wishful for operation. These cases usually make many demands upon the temper of both doctor and nurse, for it is difficult to impress upon them the necessity of keeping absolutely still at the time of operation and after, and here again comes the great need of trained native nurses to look after such cases. Our last cataract case even went so far as to remove the bandage, so anxious was he to know if he could see, and in spite of this, he can. (*CA* 31 [1913]: 96)

As African confidence in mission medicine grew after World War I,[67] so did the demand for surgery. Interest in operations was shown even at the remotest stations such as Milo. In 1936 the surgical case load at Milo was likened to Likoma's, and Dr. Wigan went and remained there for three months to operate on patients.[68] By then the overall medical task in the diocese was far beyond any one person's ability to manage. Fortunately, a few of the senior African dispensers showed remarkable skill after being taught certain kinds of surgery (*UMCA Ann. Rev.*, 1927). Some became so proficient that they were lauded as "a credit to any plastic surgeon" (*CA* 60 [1942]: 20). At the same time, their ongoing instruction and practice was also the doctor's responsibility, and on his time. Despite the undisputed value these dispensers gave to their individual African patients, they too had large workloads, and sometimes they were overwhelmed by a persistent and growing demand. In 1939, Wigan expressed relief that he did not have to assume all responsibility for the expanding surgical needs in the UMCA's sphere. He noted that "for some time, Government medical officers at Fort Johnston have been keen surgeons, they are there all the year and rightly attract most of the patients" (*UMCA Ann. Rev.*, 1939, 32).

Records at the close of the colonial era suggest that major surgery requiring general anesthesia was not a preoccupation of the UMCA doctor, despite the fact that he performed major operations while attending to his many other responsibilities. In 1963, the doctor performed 64 surgeries under general anesthesia, 625 under local anesthesia, 506 tooth extractions, and 219 "other" operations.[69] Surgery requiring local anesthesia thus accounted for nearly ten times as many operations as that requiring general anesthesia, yet in reality this amounted to about 2.5 operations per day, excluding weekends, when distributed across all UMCA hospitals and dispensaries. African assistants assumed responsibility for a large number of these procedures. These statistics should be not be interpreted as in any way discounting the humanitarian and life-preserving work that the UMCA was able to accomplish. Rather, the numbers underscore the mission's extended but relatively small-scale and low-intensity hospital and surgical capabilities.

In comparison, by 1951 only three government hospitals (Blantrye, Zomba, Lilongwe) existed to serve the whole of Malawi. Generally larger than UMCA facilities, the three hospitals accounted for 535 major operations (333 at Zomba) and 2,039 minor surgical procedures.

In the 1930s, European staff at the government hospital at Fort Johnston (adjacent to the UMCA's hospitals at Mponda's and Malindi) reported that African surgical patients and other inpatients tended spontaneously to get out of bed and move outside to get exercise and fresh air. This behavior was believed to reap benefits such as reduced instances of fever, postoperative infections, vomiting, and chest problems. It also contrasted markedly with patients in British hospitals, where the prevailing health culture kept people confined to their beds (King and King 1991, 46).

Attempts to evaluate the contributions of surgery to the UMCA's medical mission suffer from a scarcity of narratives, while the population base for the incomplete statistics remains largely guesswork. Whenever appropriate the mission relied on the *Charles Janson* and *Chauncy Maples,* until 1928 and 1953 respectively, to transport surgical cases from their homes to the nearest hospital. While the UMCA was the only mission that intentionally integrated steamers into its system of medical care, it is interesting to speculate on whether a different allocation of medical resources would have produced more positive and profound changes in the mission's medical and health productivity. Some other missions in colonial Malawi, including Livingstonia and the CSM-Blantyre, were not only considerably better off in terms of equipment and staffing. Their territorial sphere was also smaller, comparatively less cumbersome, and more efficient to administer than the UMCA's huge fishhook-shaped region.

Whereas government hospitals eventually exceeded what the UMCA accomplished in terms of hospital beds and numbers of people treated, this did not extend to the superior quality of caring for patients that was generally credited to missionary hospitals and dispensaries. In theory and practice, the missionaries emphasized that emotional and spiritual support remained indivisible from healing bodies. These values remain a lasting legacy to Malawi's church-related hospitals today.

What the UMCA was unable to accomplish must not obscure a more complex truth. That is, a fair and accurate account of the medical mission's contributions acknowledges the personal heroism displayed by its doctors, nurses, and dispensary assistants through the years. Remembering Dr. Wigan, who did not retire until nearly 71 years of age, the Bishop of Nyasaland spoke about "his unerring and patient skill as a doctor and a surgeon; the high standard, personal and professional, that he has set himself and demanded of his staff, and his scrupulous financial economy" (ibid., 65). Much later, King and King concluded that the influence of both Doctors Howard and Wigan spread "far beyond their own patients. Slowly thousands of people around the lake came to understand the value of Christian humanitarian attitudes and of modern scientific medicine" (ibid.).

As the tenure of the remaining European members of the mission came to an end in the 1950s and early 1960s, they could legitimately claim to have successfully implanted their legacy of Christian values respecting the care, treatment, and recovery of the sick. Unfortunately, this tradition of care and sympathy for the whole person did not slow or mitigate the UMCA's continued slide into medical obsolescence. Primitive hospitals, equipment, and diagnostic capabilities proved progressively inadequate to the task. Despite their medical skills, commitment, and ingenuity, the professional and intellectual isolation of Dr. Wigan, in particular, and the British nurses from mainstream medicine and public health also exacted a toll on the mission's medical preparedness.

Long before Malawi's independence, the UMCA's infrastructure of health care had begun to experience "sad deterioration." No new staff accommodations had been built for many years. Medical personnel lived in mud-brick housing with thatch roofs and dirt floors, which had "outlived their usefulness as adequate dwellings."[70] Such sacrificial living conditions reflected a de facto policy of placing the desire for evangelism and church growth ahead of even basic missionary material supports. The mission's overextension of its medical outreach capabilities reflected this attitude of always squeezing big feet into small shoes.

One patient's experience of obstetric surgery at Likoma in 1962 illustrates the often necessary resort to seat-of-the-pants procedures. A woman maternity patient arrived at the hospital after a canoe trip from the Portuguese mainland, where a male nurse had given her two ampules of oxytocin. She had reportedly begun labor three days earlier, and needed a Caesarean section. Both mother and infant, an attendant said, survived "by a narrow margin. The baby was revived partly by the African method of burning rags being held under its nose (not really to be recommended in an operating theatre where ether is being used, since an ether/air mixture is highly explosive) and partly by mouth to mouth respiration from the Sister" (*CA* 80 [1962]: 121). Thus while some medical care might often be preferred over none, a favorable outcome from Western-style medicine was not assured.

According to Dr. Robert Brown, who became the mission's new (American) DMO in 1963, conditions of surgery in UMCA facilities contributed greatly to the public's display of antipathy toward such procedures. There was, he said, "an extreme reluctance on the part of the local population to submit to surgery."[71] Furthermore,

> when one considers the limitations we are faced with, open ether and chloroform anesthesia which was abandoned in the western world fifty years ago, no blood available for transfusion purposes, limited supply of instruments, and the necessity to operate by paraffin lamp at night, one hesitates to advise surgery except in circumstances where non-intervention is sure to result in the death of the patient.[72]

Similar concerns about obsolescence had been raised fifteen years earlier by Mabel Drew, a newly arrived nurse at the mission's Likwenu Hospital. The medical books she found there were

> very, very aged. Surgery in 1890 was different from what is done today [1947]; books on drugs go out of date very rapidly; our book on Tropical Diseases is dated 1925. I know we have to use methods ten years behind England, but it would be a help to have something modern to look up. (*CA* 65 [1947]: 58)

Drew's perspective is invaluable. New to the diocese and ready to plunge into the work, she was irritated by the antiquated resources she found at Likwenu. Her comments, together with others above, suggest that UMCA medical staff had grown complacent with the status quo ante. Even though the mission's doctors and most nurses had received first-rate training in Britain prior to arrival in the mission field, over time they apparently were worn down by the effort required to stay professionally current in Malawi. Why these circumstances took over is probably deeply seated in the psychological profile of mission culture and race relations. Sustained by their religious faith and socialization, one could say that the mission accepted two geographies and two standards of preparation and readiness. UMCA missionaries placed a high value on maintaining a collective optimism about their current resources and future capabilities. On the medical side, however, they could not sustain the vision or the exemplary standards of professionalism and organizational skills Dr. Howard had supplied the diocese from 1899 to 1909.

Because it is significant to several aspects of the UMCA's legacy, not least medical services, I end this chapter with an overview of the mission's political stance during the years that brought the birth and early death of the Central African Federation. This effort to impose regional hegemony by white colonizers was led by Southern Rhodesia, with the participation of Northern Rhodesia and Nyasaland. I suggest that during this tumultuous period theUMCA botched a crucial opportunity to build closer political, social, and spiritual ties with its African supporters in what would soon be called Malawi.

THE CENTRAL AFRICAN FEDERATION

In 1953, the race-driven politics and uncertainty surrounding the imminent vote on the Central African Federation (CAF) had bred alarm, distrust, and protest among Africans. Many Africans came to believe that the UMCA had become synonymous with the colonial powers, and they showed their displeasure by refusing to attend church. The European missionaries preferred to think that this behavior resulted from "the African confusion of Christianity with colonial rule" (UMCA n.d., 1). From an African perspective, the UMCA, instead of yielding to God, was giving in to the White-dominated concept of the CAF, which was first raised in the 1920s by Europeans in the Rhodesias and Malawi. Many Africans now began to feel that the CAF had little to offer them except continued subordination, low-wage labor on farms and mines, endangerment of their lands, and the possibility of a South African-style apartheid regime.

The UMCA's "soft" stance toward the CAF and its unwillingness to assume any real risk on behalf of African welfare contributed to the latter's sense of the mission's collusion and betrayal.[73] Bishop Thorne of Nyasaland epitomized this "onlooker" mentality. While he reflected honestly on the times, the bishop spoke as if he was a powerless nonparticipant. He observed that educated Africans, who had mixed socially in English homes and Scottish colleges during long-term stays abroad, were rarely ever asked to dinner in a private European house in Malawi. The bishop said that he knew of "no hotel in Nyasaland where one could take an African guest," and admitted that "it is colour, not culture, that we [British] make the principle of discrimination" (*UMCA Ann. Rev.*, 1953, 12). Yet he did nothing more than make this admission.[74] The UMCA's passive acceptance of the political status quo[75] dramatically contrasted with the proactive, pro-African fight against the CAF by leaders in both branches of the Scottish missions in Malawi and in Britain (Sindima 1992).

Unsettled conditions during and immediately after the CAF period contributed to reductions in hospital and outpatient work, compared with 1950. The CAF's collapse in 1963 caused an exodus of expatriate government staff, and produced an "acute shortage of medical staff" in Malawi. According to the UMCA, many of these doctors and nurses lacked a basic Christian outlook, and they "did not look upon their service to the African community as a vocation" (*UMCA Ann. Rev.*, 1963, 35). There was thus an urgent need to recruit Christian health workers for Malawi.

Missionary medical staff did not remain oblivious to factors that had begun to impinge on their approach to African health needs, even before World War II. However, it was an exceedingly difficult task for them even to imagine how their customary medico-religious model might be adapted to a world where the secular ideology of "modernization" was rapidly becoming the new prescription for achieving social and economic development. Planners for a UMCA diocesan conference at Masasi Diocese in 1947 frankly raised some of the outstanding questions concerning the UMCA's medical mandate:

> Medical work was started to meet immediate needs, partly to look after the health of English missionaries, and partly because the Mission could not be blind to the presence of so much suffering all round it. Gradually there grew up the idea of medical work as an evangelizing force, but this seems to be getting swamped by the increasing 'professionalism' of our hospitals. Is the job of the doctors and nurses to run as efficient a hospital as they can (contrast the idea popular in some quarters that any old thing is good enough for Africa), or are they to limit their professional work in order to give themselves time to be 'missionaries' in the ordinary sense of that word? What is the best method of recruiting Christian medical staff, and can we plan for the day when there will be African doctors working with us? How can we get more co-operation between the medical staff and other members of the Mission? (*CA* 65 [1947]: 78)

These observations reveal a clinging to the traditional rationale for mission medicine, with its insistence on healing as complementary to evangelism. While it was not quite the old days, when the mission often encouraged patient stays of weeks and months and lost few opportunities to proselytize in hospital, the drag of medical custom and social privilege is evident. There is a persistent, paternalistic certainty about who should continue to provide physician care, and it is not Africans. The statements clearly do little to lift the level of dialogue, and the anguish associated with a slow but an inevitable transition in health care philosophy and control is palpable.

NOTES

1. Following independence in 1964 the African-run government did little to improve Malawi's conditions of extreme poverty ($170 per capita GNP in 1998), very high infant mortality (140/1,000), and serf-like wages. For instance, wages on tea plantations remained US$10 per month until 1989, when as a result of external pressure they were increased to $14. For GNP per capita and IMR, see Population Reference Bureau 1998.

2. Geoffrey Irvine, M.D. (ret.). Church of Scotland Mission, Chogoria, Kenya. Interview May 20–22, 1991. Naivasha, Kenya.

3. A late sequel of yaws and endemic syphilis characterized by "massive, grossly mutilating ulcerative destruction of the nose, soft and hard palates, and pharanx" (Miller and Keane 1987, 498).

4. Another environmental hypothesis about the rural pattern of ulcers was based on time of day and risk zones. People in the villages defecated, usually twice daily, in patches of high grass near their houses at times when there was little light. Their feet or shoes got contaminated, serving as a vehicle that spread disease organisms through the village. In general, villagers' feet and other areas of skin contained deeply engrained dirt. A relationship between Klebs-Löffler bacillus or diphtheroid organisms and tropical ulcer was suspected but not proven by laboratory methods. H. G. Wiltshire, "Notes upon the Association of Klebs-Löffler Bacillus or Diphtheroid Organisms with Ulcers seen in Nyasaland," Nyasaland Protectorate, Med. Dept. Ann. Rep., 1928. Appendix II. M3-1-4. MNA.

5. Ulcers often proved intractable. Even if the human and environmental conditions that produced them remained largely unaltered, professional experience and advances in cleaning, disinfecting, and bandaging ulcers certainly reduced healing times. In the 1890s, the standard mode of treatment included applications of permanganate of potash and Vaseline. Use of Lysol, for cleansing ulcers and killing the spirochetes associated with them, and applications of potassium iodide, had become standard treatment procedure by 1910. By 1933, the government medical service was apparently similar to mission treatment: the ulcer was cleaned with normal saline solution and zinc ointment was applied to the raw surface wound. The lower leg was then encircled with a zinc oxide plaster. After a week, or when the odor became "too objectionable," the process was repeated. See Diocese of Nyasaland, Med. Dept. Ann. Rep., 1910, 25-MAM-6-1-1, MNA; and Nyasaland Protectorate Medical Lab, Zomba, to Director of Medical and Sanitary Services (hereafter, DMS), August 8, 1933. MNA.

6. We may assume that traditional societies in Malawi passed on accounts of epidemics, famine, etc. to successive generations through their oral histories. However, there is practically no evidence or reason to suspect that any society in precolonial Malawi kept written health-related records.

7. Diocese of Malawi (Nyasaland), Med. Dept. Ann. Rep., 1963.

8. Hospitals and dispensaries: Likoma, Kota Kota, Malindi, Mponda, Likwenu, Matope. Dispensaries only: Chizumulu, Cididi, Mkope Hill. Liuli, Manda, and Milo Hospitals in Tanganyika, which were once included in statistics for the Diocese of Nyasaland, were removed from jurisdiction before this time. Longitudinal comparisons of total annual returns are thus problematic.

9. N = 394,843 outpatients and 3,526 inpatients, respectively. Some 35,833 patient-days were recorded. Diocese of Malawi (Nyasaland), Med. Dept. Ann. Rep., 1963, 15. Published records for the preceding ten to twelve years are of course sketchy at best.

10. Likoma claimed well over half of all reported ulcer cases in the diocese.

11. G. Currie, MO, to Provincial Medical Officer, Central and Northern Provinces. Annual Report on the Work of the David Gordon Memorial Hospital, 1949. M3-1-80. MNA.

12. Diocese of Malawi, Medical and Surgical Reports, 1899–1900. 145-DOM-10-4-7. MNA.

13. Ibid.

14. Ibid.

15. Ibid.

16. Nyasaland Protectorate, Med. Dept. Ann. Rep., 1926. M3-1-3. MNA.

17. Nyasaland Protectorate, Med. Dept. Ann. Rep., 1930. M3-1-5. MNA.

18. Diocese of Malawi (Nyasaland) Med. Dept. Ann. Rep., 1963, Hospital Statistics. MNA.

19. Major stations closest to the lake included Dedza, Bembeke, Mua, and Ntakataka.

20. Diocese of Nyasaland, Medical Officer's Report, 1923. UMCA A3 143, p. 4. MNA.

21. His cut-off date off date of 1920 notwithstanding, Gelfand (1964) is strangely silent on this major public health issue.

22. PMO to MO, Dedza, Aug. 9, 1922; and Fr. Sarazzin to Med. Dept., March 19, 1922. M2-5-22. MNA.

23. There was some debate about the number of injections required. Dr. Wigan, thinking of costs, said that "fortunately" only one injection of Novarsan was needed. *UMCA Ann. Rev.*, 1921–22, 97–98. RHL.

24. DMS, Zomba to Supt. MO, Jamaica Central Bd. of Health, Kingston, April 28, 1936. MNA.

25. Ibid.

26. Some areas of tropical Africa were experiencing a resurgence of yaws by the 1970s. This reflected fundamental weaknesses of poor coverage and resource scarcity, and "poor management systems in the face of a population still woefully lacking in basic health knowledge" (Ofosu-Amah 1980, 316).

27. Moving through the bloodstream, hookworm larvae migrate into the lungs en route to the pharynx. Here they are swallowed, finally taking up residence in the small intestine as mature worms daily producing thousand of eggs.

28. Nyasaland Protectorate, Med. Dept. Ann. Rep., 1922, 192. M3-1-1. MNA.

29. Ibid.

30. Sanitary Officer, Aug. 2, 1924. M2-50-10. MNA.

31. From 1924 (425) to 1926 (1,191). These numbers could only have been a tiny fraction of the actual population burdened by the infection.

32. At least one UMCA station in coastal Tanganyika had adopted oil of Chenopodium, given by mouth, as the routine remedy. It was said to kill the worms and "the patient gradually recovers his health" (CA [1923]: 248).

33. Diocese of Nyalsaland, Med. Dept. Ann. Rep., 1949. MNA.

34. Hookworm Campaigns, Aug. 2, 1924. M2-5-10. MNA.

35. Nyasaland Protectorate, Med. Dept. Ann. Rep., 1928. M3-1-4. MNA.

36. Hookworm Campaigns, Aug. 2, 1924. M2-5-10. MNA.

37. DMS to Dr. Wigan (UMCA), Aug. 12, 1936. M2-5-10. MNA.

38. Unless latrines are kept clean, their introduction may actually increase hookworm disease. On the other hand, if someone goes in the bush the feces tend to dry up on the ground fairly quickly. Personal communication, Dr. Geoffrey Irvine, Naivasha, Kenya, May 1991.

39. Report Submitted by Dr. E. Muir, BELRA, 1939, 5-6. M2-5-13. MNA.

40. Medical Dept., Chiradzulu, to DMS, Zomba, Nov. 7, 1936. MNA.

41. Medical Survey of Jalasi Village, June 1938. M2-14-2. MNA.

42. Diocese of Malawi, Med. Dept. Ann. Rep., 1963. MNA.

43. Based on conversations at Malindi with Mr. H. Kangundo, Clinical Officer, June 1990.

44. Nyasaland Protectorate, Med. Dept. Ann. Rep., 1930. M3-1-5. MNA.

45. Medical Survey of Jalasi Village, June 1938. M2-14-2. MNA.

46. Three groups of the village population showed a 48 to 65 percent prevalence of *S. haematobium*. Many Jalasi children who were treated had blood in the urine, whereas adults showed more spleen enlargement and neuritic and lumbar pains. Medical Survey of Jalasi Village, June 1938. M2-14-2. MNA.

47. Diocese of Nyasaland, Med. Dept. Ann. Rep., 1949. M3-1-80. MNA.

48. Nyasaland Protectorate, Med. Dept. Ann. Rep., 1926. M3-1-3. MNA.

49. Memo on Malaria and Use of Quinine in Nyasaland. April 16, 1931. M2-5-14. MNA.

50. DMS to Chief Secretary, Zomba, June 23, 1938. Consumption of Cinchona Alkaloids in the Empire. M2-5-14. MNA.

51. For example, despite the population's growing population, for 1922, 1949, and 1950, the mission reported only 1,611, 1,377, and 1,311 cases of malaria, respectively, in all its facilities. Sources include *CA* (1922, 1950, 1951, 1954); Diocese of Nyasaland, Med. Dept. Ann. Rep., 1949. M3-1-80. MNA.

52. Diocese of Malawi, Med. Dept. Ann. Rep., 1963, 15. UMCA. MNA.

53. Republic of Malawi, Department of Census and Statistics, Malawi Population Census, 1966: Final Report, Zomba, n.d.

54. The chloroquine compound unwittingly remained in German labs during the war.

55. In Chewa/Nyanja the term for the oldest male guardian in authority is *mwini mbumba*.

56. In 1963, for example, mission facilities recorded 480,000 outpatient attendances (all categories including dispensary, antenatal, and leprosy), up from 430,000 in 1962. Total outpatients (other than antenatal and leprosy patients) reportedly increased by 17,420, or 50 percent, over 1962. This large jump suggests significant "improvement" in

patient confidence and access to care. However, the report does not explain what factors produced the alleged growth of patients. Using the published data and for the moment assuming patients were distributed equally across the diocese's nine dispensaries, each facility averaged 5,811 outpatients annually. Each dispensary then received around 484 patients monthly, and about 22 people per day (five-day week) with a new episode of illness or injury. Adapted from Diocese of Malawi, Med. Dept. Ann. Rep., 1963, 14–15. MNA.

57. See Diocese of Nyasaland, Malindi Native Hospitals, 1910: Patients in Hospital on January 1st. 25-MAM-6-1-1. MNA.

58. Most flybelts occurred on the western and southern sides of Lake Malawi, and in the Shiré Basin south of Blantyre.

59. An outbreak of trypanosomiasis occurred around 1929 in Kota Kota, killing ten of the mission's cattle and others owned by local herders. Drs. Wigan and Vost provided a course of antimony injections to try to cure the epidemic, but the outcome is unknown.

60. Polio is not mentioned in the Medical Report for 1949, but forty-two cases were listed for 1963. Diocese of Malawi, Med. Dept. Ann. Rep., 1963. MNA.

61. *UMCA Ann. Rev.,* 1922–23, 98. RHL; Diocese of Nyasaland, UMCA Medical Officer's Report, 1923. UMCA A 143. RHL.

62. *UMCA Annual Rev.,* 1924, Medical Officer's Report.

63. Chloroform was widely useful in trauma cases. Locally, large numbers of people received wounds from fights with spears and maulings by wild animals; others suffered with tumors and needed amputations.

64. Not all European doctors working in Africa felt handicapped without x-rays. For example, Dr. Geoffrey Irvine of the Church of Scotland Mission, Chogoria, Kenya, said that x-rays were "far from essential because they often do little more than confirm a correct clinical decision. They're jolly nice to have, but not essential, even for TB." Interview May 20, 1991, Naivasha, Kenya.

65. At Livingstonia Hospital 93 cataract operations were performed in 1911, and 117 in 1924.

66. *UMCA Annual Rev.,* Medical Dept. for 1925, 111; and 1927. MNA.

67. This change was observed at Likoma just after World War I. *UMCA Annual Rev.,* 1919–20, Med. Officer's Rept., Oct. 1919–Sept. 30, 1920.

68. *UMCA Annual Rev.,* 1936, 31.

69. UMCA Med. Dept. Ann. Rep., 1963. MNA.

70. Diocese of Malawi (Nyasaland). Med. Dept. Ann. Rep., 1963, 6.

71. This observation contrasts with the positive reports about operations made by the missionaries in the 1930s.

72. Diocese of Malawi (Nyasaland), Med. Dept. Ann. Rep., 1963, 5. There is little evidence that there was any concern about the use of chloroform by the UMCA medical staff. In contrast, Dr. Geoffrey Irvine, formerly of the CMS Chogoria Mission on Mt. Kenya, spoke of the dangers involved: "We had nightmare experiences with chloroform induction and ether—rag and bottle—dropping it onto a mask. People would stop breathing, and there was little you could do about it except jump on their chest. . . . [Dr. Dorothy Irvine] and I went to Ireland on one occasion for a OB/GYN refresher course, during which we learned to incubate (pass a tube into the trachea) and that to me was one of the biggest advances I'd ever made because you could

control respiration. The moment you could put a tube down and inflate the cuff the you could . . . artificially respire them for a long as you wanted. That wasn't a new discovery in the field of medicine; it was an enormous advance in our own practice. I am astonished that we were ever released into the registered medical work without that skill." Interview May 20–22, 1991, Naivasha, Kenya.

73. In contrast, the militant Scots missionaries in northern Malawi had long struggled to create a nonracial society of Christian artisans and leaders throughout the country. They associated the CAF with the "spirit of white supremacy" that prevailed in South Africa, and by extension Southern Rhodesia. See Mufuka 1977, 147–59.

74. For an apparently different conclusion, see ibid., 204.

75. For support for this conclusion, see UMCA, S.F. Series, 29, XIII, "Confidential" files, General Secretary, UMCA, London, to Bishop F. Osborne, Sept. 1, 1952: "There is a good deal of differences on view on many points. Some think that Federation ought to be postponed, or dropped, and others that it should be carried through, but *there does seem to be agreement that the Church ought not officially commit itself to either view.* This is what I think myself" (emphasis added).

CHAPTER TEN

The Rise and Fall of Missionary Medicine

RACE MATTERED

Studies of colonizers and colonized cannot avoid a confrontation with issues of race or ethnic difference. From the mid-nineteenth century onwards there is abundant evidence that European attitudes, assumptions, and behavior reflected a deep-seated racism toward Africans (Hammond and Jablow 1992). This prejudice operated on conscious and subconscious levels, infecting individuals and groups. Relations on the cultural frontier, and particularly the technological tools and symbols arriving from Europe, reinforced the "correctness" of the inferiority stigma Europeans bestowed on so many things African. It is debatable whether such prejudices were less raw or overt among missionaries than within secular European communities.

Certainly among many Europeans there was a pretense of "scientific certitude" about the received and virtually predestined position of Africans on the evolutionary "ladder." No less an intellect than Sir Harry H. Johnston, Commissioner and Consul-General in British Central Africa in the 1890s, summed up the physical and mental characteristics of the Negro of South Central Africa. A century later, the harsh tone of his language is shocking and repugnant, and the conclusions seem absurd to reasonable minds. The Negro, Johnston said, "is a fine animal, but in his wild state exhibits a stunted

mind and a dull content with his surroundings which induces mental stag-
nation, cessation of all upward progress, and even of retrogression toward
the brute" (Johnston 1897, 472). He believed it quite possible, had the Arabs
and Europeans not broken Africa's isolation from the outside world, that
"the purely Negroid races, left to themselves, so far from advancing towards
a higher type of humanity, might just have actually reverted by degrees to
a type no longer human, just as those great apes lingering in the dense
forests of Western Africa" (472). Yet the condition was not hopeless because,
Johnston believed, "the black man, in all his varieties but two or three of the
most retrograde" was still "not too far gone for recovery and for an upward
turn upon the evolutionary path—a turn which, if resolutely followed, may
with steady strides bring him upon a level at some future day with the white
and yellow species of man" (ibid.).

Whereas this investigation has not used a systematic psychological framework to understand the processes and outcomes of religious and secular
imperialism, the psychology of race relations is never "off the subject."
In writing this book, I have often acutely sensed that many important
clues to understanding the behavior and interrelationships of missionaries
and Africans lay deeply embedded in complex individual and institutional
psyches. These states of mind took shape from, and reflected, myriad spoken
and unspoken racialist attitudes and actions. Three examples from earlier
chapters support these observations.

In Malawi, the advent of white missionaries in self-received possession of
a mandate to blunt the slave trade and Christianize Africans helped push
questions about race and human capabilities into the foreground of social
consciousness in the region. For purposes of residence and worship, the
missionaries actually grew more segregated from Africans as the Diocese of
Nyasaland developed. By 1900, new knowledge about malaria transmission
provided an epidemiological rationale for maintaining a buffer zone of about
a half-mile between European houses, in the central mission compound, and
African settlements on the periphery.[1] By 1917, separate worship sites for
Europeans and "natives" had become official UMCA policy in Malawi. In
a letter to one of his priests, Bishop Fisher presented a detailed, forceful
argument to the effect that the oppressiveness of African hygiene and their
festive worship styles made joint worship unacceptable to Europeans. However, he said, to preserve a semblance of "unity despite race," Europeans
and Africans races might meet together on special occasions in suitable buildings. Fully aware of the inherent contradictions and racism in this policy,
and its potential embarrassment for the mission, the bishop wrote on his
letterhead the admonition: *N.B. No part of this letter to be printed in* [UMCA]
Magazines.[2]

Ironically, the missionaries pointed to the *Chauncy Maples*, which they alternatively called "The White Ship," to symbolize their sense of European superiority. This racial appellation was meant to distinguish the *C.M.* from "all the other transport ships" operating on Lake Malawi during World War I. Lacking any trace of sublety about the status of Africans in European minds, use of "The White Ship" was intended among other purposes to impress readers of *Central Africa* in Britain. The name was also said to originate in part from the "character" of the steamer's African crewmen, whom the missionaries and other whites continued to call "boys," in the derogatory fashion of the times. Said one writer in *Central Africa*, "The White Ship" reflected the words of its skipper, who reportedly said "I have taught those boys; I have prayed with those boys; I have beaten those boys; and I will keep them white" (*CA* 42 [1924]: 161).

The third example of racial climate concerns the UMCA's cowardice during the Central African Federation crisis in the 1950s, about seventy-five years after contact. The mission chose to ignore and thus not to hear the requests of its Malawian followers to have their fears and arguments voiced. After so many decades in relationship with their own parishoners, in particular, the mission's decision to stand aside and not contest Malawi's imposed federation with the white settler- and corporate-dominated Rhodesias produced shock, anger, and dismay among African church and community leaders. African public opinion, already stirred by the rise of nationalism following World War II, generally and vigorously opposed federation. They saw it as an arrangement intended to further subjugate the protectorate to apartheid-style white minority rule. It would drain away cheap labor and other resources from Malawi and only strengthen European economic and political domination from Salisbury (see chap. 5).

GOVERNMENT-MISSION RELATIONS

Within a decade of its establishment, the Diocese of Nyasaland came under the formal umbrella of British colonial rule. Overall this relationship, while not of equals, produced positive benefits on both sides.[3] For instance, the UMCA, along with the FCSM, CSM, DRCM and few other missions, provided basic medical services for Malawians who could access them for at least two decades before the protectorate government began to act on its own responsibilities in this area. Starting in the 1920s, the government also periodically assisted the UMCA and other medical missions with key drugs needed to treat diseases such as yaws, hookworm, leprosy, and bilharzia, either through grants-in-aid or by selling them. It occasionally served as a go-between when relations grew tense between the UMCA and officials in Portuguese East Africa. Individuals in both government and the mission also reciprocated various courtesies of the kind exchanged by fellow countrymen who were far from home.

Since the UMCA had relatively harmonious relations with other missions, it made few demands on the government to resolve disputes that might arise. The UMCA's peculiar lakeside situation, and the spatial relations that followed, meant that its evangelism initiatives provoked minimal territorial conflict with other missions. Generally speaking, British DOs whose responsibilities included UMCA territory spent little time adjudicating disputes between it and the other missions. In contrast, DOs assigned to other districts sometimes became embroiled in mission politics while they tried to resolve conflicts over the location of mission schools, churches, and clinics. As mediators, the DOs could encounter a climate where doctrinal differences spawned harsh competitiveness and unyielding pettiness. For instance, such arguments marred relations between the Dutch Reformed Church and Catholic White Fathers Missions southwest of Lake Malawi. As with the Scots Livingstonia Mission, the UMCA's early arrival and relative location permitted it to more effectively observe a policy of "live and let live."

PERSPECTIVES ON TECHNOLOGY, AFRICAN HEALTH, AND SOCIAL CHANGE

The foregoing chapters raise key questions about the historical, geographical, and social significance of the UMCA's medical mission in colonial Malawi, Mozambique, and southwest Tanzania. In conclusion, I revisit four questions that reflect on the study's central themes and goal.

Western Technology: The Steamers

On balance, as an imported technology, what did the steamers contribute to the UMCA's medical mission? To African welfare?

Technology was writ large when the UMCA introduced the steamers *Charles Janson* and *Chauncy Maples* to Lake Malawi. Little evangelism or medical work could have been carried out along the coast or in the adjoining mountainous districts without the steamers during the mission's first thirty to forty years of existence. Many settlements would have otherwise remained inaccessible for a very long time. The steamers thus predisposed, enabled, and, for several decades, reinforced the UMCA's quest to "stake out" territory wherein Christianity might be spread. However, whereas the steamers played a major role by bringing near and far-flung settlements under UMCA influence, they also contributed to the mission's declining ability to achieve and sustain itself as a positive force in African health and social change.

Initially, given the availability of fuelwood, the steamers' basically unlimited range enticed the mission into the trap of geographical overextension. Within a decade of their introduction the steamers had profoundly helped knit together a long, looping network of places identified as "UMCA" villages, with their varied clusters of schools, churches, hospitals, and dispensaries. A lack of human and material resources to support evangelistic efforts in each new place was viewed, in missionary culture, as a challenge to the work ethic. Such scarcity was an impermanent condition that would be rectified with Christian patience, faith, and finally divine providence.

Second, the steamers' ultimate promise was only partially realized because of the lengthy down-time for repairs, inadequate contingency plans in the absence of another steamer for back-up, and the Royal Navy's long sequester of the *C.M.* during World War I. Roads, a presumed responsibility of the three colonial governments under which the UMCA operated, remained practically nonexistent and of little practical consequence for mission communications on the eastern side of Lake Malawi.

Meanwhile, the *C.M.*, the mission's remarkable "flagship" and veteran of thousands of sailings with freight, stores, and passengers, including those in sickbay, was sold away shortly after its fiftieth anniversary. For many African church leaders, this unilateral act by the real powers in the mission symbolized a breaking of faith with them and their congregations. As noted, these years also witnessed the rise and fall of the doomed Central African Federation. The trust and goodwill that had taken decades to build between the mission and African Christians was severely undermined. With African self-determination visible on the horizon, the UMCA's European staff began to fade away.[4]

Medico-religious Pluralism: Continuity and Expansion

Colonial Malawi served as a test case where UMCA missionaries attempted to demonstrate their ability and commitment to exploit the power of what they believed was a vastly superior system of medical treatment and healing arts. On balance, then, what was the outcome of their sometimes heroic efforts, continued for over sixty-five years, to transmit the benefits of Christianized, Western medicine in the midst of Central African medico-religious values, resources, and methods?

With the possible exception of a widespread aversion to surgery, Africans in the UMCA sphere did not need long to discern that missionary medicine could offer distinct technical advantages over indigenous healing systems. They generally and cautiously began to welcome the material and technological accouterments of biomedicine, including injections with the hypodermic needle, new drugs, and the cottage-style hospitals that provided freedom and security for recuperation from illness. Significantly, Africans began to weave these features of Western-style medicine into an expanding medical pluralism. For most people, the new medicine provided a selection of valuable "add-ons" to existing indigenous healing beliefs and practices, rather than full replacements for them.[5]

Some African healers developed reputations as specialists who treated one or two kinds of affliction effectively. For their services *asing'anga* received payment in money or goats. Many colonial Malawians continued to consult with and pay substantial sums to *asing'anga,* often as their first resort, interspersed with visits to clinics or hospital outpatient departments (*CA* 62 [1944]: 80).

While skills and reputation vary greatly, today, small villages and the largest cities in Malawi have many resident and itinerant practitioners of traditional healing. Many Malawians, notwithstanding their considerable exposure to Western education and values, confirm that important elements of their indigenous medico-religious heritage persist. This is particularly true with respect to human agency as a factor in explanations of illness, including beliefs about the possible exercise of harmful witchcraft and sorcery. Western-educated Malawians may also believe that some traditional healers employ "discovery" techniques to explain sudden or unusual illness. Some powerful diviners or other specialists also provide "protection" for specific individuals and organizations (e.g., politicians and football teams), and can bring loss and disappointment to others (Ciekawy and Geschiere 1998).

Over the years Malawian and other African colleagues have offered useful reflections on the phenomenon of their navigating two cultures inside one mind. I do not know if African traditions remain more indelibly imprinted, or less malleable, than those of other great culture spheres. What does seem irrefutable is that most Africans cannot willfully or readily discount their cosmological and medico-religious inheritance. Twenty-five years ago the Kenyan legal scholar Mutungi (1977) asserted that the belief in witchcraft, whether unconscious or intentional, knows no educational, social, or occupational limits. In 1980 a theological student in a Malawi college observed that from a very young age "the existence and fear of witchcraft is hammered into our minds" (Hopkins 1980, 56). A survey of twenty-five students of Christian theology at the same institution offered evidence of the existence of a pervasive witchcraft syndrome that powerfully influenced their attitudes and behavior (ibid.).

Despite missionary disapproval, pervasive use of charms and amulets continued in use as a means to ward off trouble or to attract something or someone desirable. Every baby and toddler wore some kind of "protection" around the neck or waist. Muslim charms typically consisted of pieces of paper on which Arabic phrases from the Koran had been written. A list of charms used by UMCA schoolboys in 1935 included various objects that would make people invisible, attract a lover, improve a hunter's luck, protect against wizards in your bed, help exorcise spirits, aid flying, protect against poisoning, and help secure a job (*CA* 54 [1936]: 15–16).[6]

Missionaries took a more benign view of Africans' use of medicinal plant preparations (*miti shamba*), perhaps because they considered them less threatening to their efforts to inculcate Christian spirituality. However, in the African milieu herbs were much more than natural substances with pharmacological activity targeted on specific ailments. Preparation and administration of herbal medicines was and often remains a lengthy and intensely religious process, empowered by an immanent God through the human practitioner. Herbs typically lack the power to heal on their own; they acquired potency when transformed through proper preparation and rituals. In one sense this process parallels the conversion of bread and wine in Christian Communion (Good 1987).

During the missionary period African rites were usually quietly practiced in villages or special sites away from mission stations. Various government Witchcraft Ordinances (1911, 1929) criminalized witchcraft and might have been expected to give aid and comfort to missionaries. While the UMCA praised the government for "making the whole thing criminal, and criminal under heavy penalties" (*CA* 30 [1912]: 3), there is little evidence that the mission gained any advantage from these laws. Because no one had ever seen a witch or developed a working definition of witchcraft, efforts to suppress such elusive practices using methods even remotely reminiscent of English law proved confusing, fruitless, and even counterproductive. In 1938, the District Commissioner (DC) for Mlanje District, a liberal man with sensitivity to African realities, reported to his government superiors:

> Further cases occurred in which the services of a witchdoctor brought no harm to anyone but only relief from mental and bodily suffering to one woman and two young girls (self-confessed witches) and an elderly man who had long been an invalid; yet in these cases the course of official action

demanded by the law would have deprived these unfortunates of the relief from their suffering. There is something wrong; it cannot be right that a District Commissioner should have to choose whether to disregard the law or apply it knowing that its application would be a piece of senseless cruelty.[7]

This same DC included in this report a statement made by the head of the Church of Scotland Mission, who emphasized:

> The time is ripe for a reconsideration both by Government and Missions of their traditional attitude toward Native ideas of witchcraft. They can only be counteracted by long continued and patient teaching of truer ideas, Christian and scientific.

Writing to the protectorate's Chief Secretary in the following year, the Mlanje DC complained that the advice of Lord Hailey and other informed observers had been ignored in the final recommendations of Nyasaland's "Witchcraft Committee." He observed that "the law concerning witchcraft has been made, and amendments recommended, without reference to the only community it affects." The DC pleaded for the government to admit its mistake, repeal and not replace the Witchcraft Ordinance, embody ordeal trials in the Penal Code, and leave all other matters to the Native Authorities and Courts as coming under native law and custom.[8] Thus, on the secular side, the Mlanje DC was one of a small number of unusually insightful and empathetic European civil servants who had the first-hand knowledge, cultural awareness, and requisite skills to think outside the confines of his own civilization.

From the missionaries' viewpoint, the Christian injunctions they tried to impose reflected ancient precedent in the law of Moses:

> When thou art come into the land which the Lord thy God giveth thee, thou shalt not learn to do after the abominations of those nations. There shall not be found among you *any one* that maketh his son or daughter to pass through the fire, *or* that useth divination, *or* an observer of times, or an enchanter, or a witch, or a charmer, or a consulter with familiar spirits, or a wizard, or a necromancer. For all that do these things are an abomination unto the Lord; and because of these abominations the Lord thy God doth drive them out from before thee. Thou shalt be perfect with the Lord thy God. (Deuteronomy 18:9–13, KJV)

UMCA hostility to "pagan" healing practices ensured that they remained fenced off, out of bounds, and unacceptable for mission Christians. Some missionaries showed interest in learning about traditional practices, hoping to better counter them. But only the rare individual acquired the necessary perspective to make space for the co-existence of medico-religious practices of the people they sought to convert. As late as 1955 the UMCA published books in London with such titles as *War with the Witchdoctor* (advertised in *CA* 73 [1955]: 300).

Any parishioner who defied UMCA standards of behavior could expect sanctions. Missionaries aimed their disgust and wrath primarily on traditional practices used to maintain social control. It was unacceptable for anyone connected with the mission to participate in accusations of witchcraft or to seek witchcraft protection. It was also improper for church adherents to engage in oathing and ordeals, worship ancestral spirits, attend *vinyao* spirit dances, or visit sacred groves or other places where "heathen" rites were observed.

Missionary strategy to gain and retain converts by attempting to cast out African beliefs and practices may be seen as self-limiting precisely because it trampled on what Gray (1990, 5) defines as

> one of the deepest and most enduring desires of all African societies: the anxiety to eliminate evil.... Evil was experienced as that which destroyed life, health, strength, fertility and prosperity. African cosmologies had little if any room for the secularized concept of pure chance or misfortune ... the dualism so deeply rooted in Judaeo-Christian thought was seldom present. Evil of sorcery, witchcraft, and misuse of spiritual power posed the greatest threat to many African peoples.

Powerful, culture-bound supernatural forces remained the unquestioned cause of much illness and misfortune in Malawi and elsewhere in Africa. Kenyan theologian John Mbiti writes of the Akamba "saturation" with beliefs, fears and superstitions:

> Every Mukamba, whether Christian or otherwise, has a dormant or active share of these beliefs. The people have not been sufficiently armed to fight against witchcraft and sorcery, in spite of many years of contact with Christian teaching and Western education. (Mbiti 1971, 9)

A British social anthropologist called the persistent witchcraft beliefs of the Nyakyusa people of southwestern Tanzania "the standardized nightmares of a group" (Monica Wilson, in Hautvast and Hautvast-Mertens 1972, 407). Efforts to annul them by the UMCA or other colonial missions proved fruitless.

Gray asserts that Christianity "was often seen as a fresh source of supernatural power. It could enhance and support existing concepts and structures; it could challenge and endanger the status quo; it could bring liberation in various forms" (Gray 1990, 6). In Malawi's paternalistic and color-divided colonial setting, access to Christianity as a universal promise of hope and freedom from fear provided, as did Western medicine, an alternative system of reference.

Yet within the Diocese of Nyasaland, Christianity provided insufficient tools for Malawians' to "win" the struggle with evil and realize their "enduring desires" to rid their societies of it. This assertion is borne out by the UMCA's tenure in Malawi, the unfulfilled expectations of its missionaries in Tanganyika's Masasi Diocese, and other mission spheres. Neither Christianity nor missionary medicine could annihilate Malawians' practical problems of evil nor supplant the ancient claims of the old culture. Even if Western medicine had been abundantly provided under colonialism, there would still be little basis for imagining that a mere several decades of simple "medical provision" (Ranger 1982, 338) could neutralize or supplant deeply held medico-religious beliefs. For Africans to absorb and fashion biomedical ideas about disease, healing, and public health into a practical, more or less exclusive paradigm, much longer and more sustained contact was required. For this hypothetical result to become reality, African societies would have to stop valuing the benefits of choices available to them through the practice of medical pluralism.

Some missionaries did recognize, but not without ambivalence, that it was necessary to move closer to African thinking if the mission was to provide more effective medical care. As late as 1963, the UMCA's General Secretary observed that Europeans

> find it so hard to grasp that for an African, body and soul are really one entity, always interacting—as they are in the Bible. An African expects spiritual treatment to accompany the physical treatment and tends to regard a European doctor as inferior to a witchdoctor if the former only gives him half treatment. Perhaps he is right. . . . And yet the baleful influence of the witchdoctor is still very strong and a great hindrance to both medicine and evangelism. (*CA* 81 [1963]: 147)

In retrospect, beginning in the 1880s two medical and technological systems converged on each other in the Lake Malawi region. Both were culture-bound systems, although Western-style medicine offered a blend of secular and missionary forms. Any assumptions that the newly imported medical system would neutralize or replace African healing through the sheer force of its presumed technological, cultural, and moral superiority proved incorrect. To the contrary, Parrinder is correct in his assertion that the introduction of European ideas and customs further and profoundly unsettled African societies. The widening gap between rich and poor, and other new sources of insecurity, only added to the power of belief in witchcraft, which was blamed for "unknown and incalculable dangers" (Parrinder 1963, 129).

What Kind of Mission Medical Care?

Was the UMCA's attempt to develop medical and health services largely a misguided gesture? Did the mission's actions, de facto, mainly serve colonial objectives and ignore Africans' aspirations for development and improved standards of living?

In principle, the UMCA, with its social, economic, and ecclesiastical roots in the Church of England, had access to a large population of Britain's best trained doctors and nurses, and to Western medical knowledge and practice of world standard.

Except for its early pioneering years up to World War I, I have suggested that the UMCA mission to Malawi, and the headquarters in London, grew to accept an antiquated, third-rate system of medical care. Many questions arise from this assertion. Was it unavoidable that the UMCA settled for a medical system that was substandard even in relation to other "mainline" missions in Central Africa, such as the Presbyterian institutions at Blantyre (CMS) and Livingstonia (FCSM)? The answer, of course, is no. Did the mission's London headquarters knowingly follow a policy, or subconsciously operate on the premise, that any initiative it undertook in Central Africa was, at least, more than had been there before? Furthermore, did the mission's failure to commit greater resources for African health reflect an assumption on its part that colonial and mission Africans had little inclination to expect, or possess the requisite power to negotiate, more for their own communities? Did they at some point conclude that UMCA's African Christians would not "make a fuss" about something that seemed beyond their control?

Intuitively, based on circumstantial evidence, I believe that such attitudes were plausible and did influence the amount of effort expended, both in London and Malawi, on the development of medical resources. At the same time, it would be ridiculous to think that when mission leaders started medical work in 1899 they intended to be satisfied in the end with a generally marginal accomplishment. Rather, attitudes that produced acceptance of the status quo developed incrementally, as shortages of professional and financial resources, and years of severe scrimping, became part of the UMCA's conservative subculture both in the mission field and in Britain. However, even when medical outreach and practical education increasingly fell behind, evangelism, the real purpose of mission, was always a trump card that no one dare fault.

The approach of political independence brought stocktaking and re-assessment of the inherited health systems in virtually every African country. In Malawi, government medical services had never reached more than a small fraction of the population. A large share of the health infrastructure consisted of mission hospitals, dispensaries, and mission-trained African and some European staff. Availability, outreach, and quality of care varied considerably among the mission societies. Immediately following independence, efforts got underway in Malawi and many other African countries to promote collaboration and enhance the quality of Christian and government medical work. The main goal was to rationalize the inherited colonial foundations and improve the population's access to higher quality medical and health services. In Malawi, it was decided in 1966 to promote such development with the creation of the church-related Private Hospital Association of Malawi (PHAM).

Readers will have noticed that my assessment of the UMCA's medical record at Lake Malawi includes a strong critique of its numerous internal contradictions and self-defeating policies. Pollock's assertion about the interpretation of history also applies to historical geography: "to be properly understood [it] must not overlook values held when events took place, erroneous though they may be by later standards" (Pollock 1971, 5). Put somewhat differently, it is important us to recognize "the right of the past not to be colonized by the present, not to be politicized by what is our very parochial tendency to see all things in terms of power distribution" (Bowman 2000, 18).

Criticism of missionary medicine with respect to their motives, foot-dragging in the training of Africans, and curative emphasis is valid and sustainable. Nevertheless, there were also missionaries who aimed to promote a quite different scenario for mission health work. For example, documentation shows that by the 1920s there was alive in the leadership of the wider missionary community a realization that African health standards could not be raised and sustained through curative medicine alone.

"Towards a Healthy Africa" was a major theme at the widely publicized International Missionary Conference held at Le Zoute, Belgium, in 1926. Discussions at Le Zoute also featured substantial nonmissionary participation. First and foremost in its report, the Conference recognized that under European influence African society was "in a process of disintegration over large areas" and "paying a heavy price" for the exploitation of the continent's resources. Many viewed the "enormous, shameless," and deleterious "Drink Trade" as "second only to the slave-trade in its evil effects" on African society (Smith 1926, 21, 17–18). Opening up Africa and imposing taxation had created unprecedented and harmful demands for labor. Taxation had forced Africans to leave their communities to find work. Consequently, Europeans had to accept responsibility for the expanding place-to-place spread of diseases such as tuberculosis. Civilization's "influx" had undeniably worsened African health conditions (17, 21, 76).

Second, providing "bricks and mortar" represented only one part of the kind of health campaign Africa needed. Dr. J. Gilks, Kenya's Director of Medical and Sanitary Services, emphasized:

> We are not going to improve the general state of public health in Africa by building more hospitals. Even if we were called upon to build all the hospitals needed we could not get the funds.... The proper way to go on, the most economic way, is to prevent people from getting sick... We must get down to a public health program. (77)

These and other observations at Le Zoute, including the high priority of improving African diets and housing, suggest that by the early mid-stage of colonial rule numerous missionaries and government medical authorities alike knew what approach was needed to engage Africa's poverty and declining health standards head on. Concerning "what missionaries can do," the Conference heard from the Phelps-Stokes Commission representative that the "mission school" was the most potent weapon available to them "for the destruction of disease in Africa" (79). Improvements in public health depended on expanding educational opportunities.

No single factor can adequately explain why in missionary accomplishments in health care and health promotion fell short of what was needed and possible. General explanations cannot ignore the overwhelming magnitude of the task at almost any scale. Several decades proved an inadequate length of time to promote massive structural and cultural change even under the best of financial and other circumstances. Mission boards and colonial governments often failed to commit appropriate financial and human resources. In the UMCA's case, despite their pleas for more, medical personnel in the field typically failed to receive enough resources to sustain their hospitals and dispensaries even at the minimal level of support needed. Well-meaning rhetoric of the mission's leadership in London and in Malawi rarely generated the financial support and supply of medical professionals expected of the Home Church.

For example, from the 1940s to the 1960s there was a continuous turnover of mostly short-term medical staff, with impairment of continuity. In 1946, the "urgent need for doctors, men and women, to run native hospitals, train African assistants, and supervise district dispensaries" was extensively advertised in British medical publications. Confidentially, the UMCA's general secretary wrote to Nyasaland's bishop saying that they were even "prepared to consider married doctors and also that there was the possibility of a small salary" for them, plus maintenance." Out of twenty-eight enquiries from British and other doctors about this position handled at London headquarters, only one, "a charming young Hungarian with exactly the right spirit" actually volunteered his services. However, he was turned down because he was not a Christian.[9] A decade later, the mission's continuing "grave shortage" of medical staff, teachers, and priests prompted the bishop to fly to England to personally appeal to the "Church at home" for assistance with the recruitment of "3 priests, 4 teachers, and a doctor." Two months later, despite an exceptional on a BBC broadcast, no one had answered the bishop's pleas.[10]

The good-faith efforts and aspirations of UMCA doctors and nurses were often undercut and rarely rewarded. A climate of fateful acceptance frequently prevailed among the medical staff. This situation was infrequently punctuated by outbursts of complaint in public settings about the lack of support for the work in Central Africa. Other frequently cited obstacles to the fuller development of medical missions include the financial cutbacks, acutely experienced in England also, imposed by two World Wars and the global Depression.

By the 1930s, when the UMCA and other medical missions began to react to the social changes induced by colonialism, new demographic forces and patterns ensured that the scope and complexity of their task had become staggering. By World War II there was keen awareness that "the field open to medical endeavor is so vast that anything the Mission can do will no more than touch the fringe. The larger resources open to the government will not carry them much farther" (*UMCA Ann. Rev.*, 1942, 23).

Many self-imposed and external constraints led the UMCA to accept a diminished medical potential and to persist in obsolescence. The mission generally failed to translate new ideas about public health into real benefits for their poor African parishes. Nevertheless, as the following excerpts dating from 1942, 1943, 1945, 1948, and 1949 reveal, for the mission staff the 1940s were a time of rapidly growing sensitivity, at least, about the importance of preventive work and various strategies for introducing it:

> There is always a good deal of illness in the villages, especially among the children...lessons on hygiene and cleanliness need to be given.... Prevention is better than cure and there is certainly a very great deal that can be done in Africa to remove the causes of disease. Foremost among these we may place malnutrition, bad housing conditions, and low wages. (*UMCA Ann. Rev.*, 1942, 25)

> Preventive medicine is only in its very early stages [and] much of the curative work done in our hospitals is almost immediately undone by the patients' return after cure to the same infected conditions at home which originally caused the disease. (*UMCA Ann. Rev.* 1943, 34)

> School meals have been introduced at all the central stations in Nyasaland: a meal is given at midday to all children in the higher classes or standards who will also be reading again in the afternoon. The entire cost at the rate of 1d. per child per day is borne by Government. The meal is already making a perceptible difference in the health and alertness of the children. (*UMCA Ann. Rev.*, 1945, 31)

> Not only must there be a re-orientation of the [African] mind towards causation and prevention of disease, but the price that Nature demands must be paid in self-discipline, self-help, and the development of a sense of responsibility toward the community as a whole; and there must be more solid integration of profession and practice.... Health clubs can be encouraged. (*UMCA Ann. Rev.*, 1948, 13)

> Medical conferences were held and recommendations on medical policy were made to the Bishop who approved them in principle. The recommendations were based on the principle that the preservation of health and the relief of suffering were essential functions of Christian Missions, and emphasis was laid on the importance of developing family welfare services at all stations where co-operative groups of people were found. Preventive work...is being carried out....A contributory scheme for family welfare has been begun at Liuli. (*UMCA Ann. Rev.* 1949, 21)

Clearly, the fundamental issues had not materially changed since Le Zoute.

In the UMCA's case, the record confirms that most of the critiques of medical mission have degrees of truth about them. Still, fairness demands perspective, and greater discrimination than a sweeping rejection of the complex motives, efforts, and results of the UMCA medical mission spread over seventy years. It is necessary to interpret actions and outcomes in their fullest possible contexts.

It is crucial to remember that the UMCA was not established as a professional medical service or as a development agency in the present sense. No one ever attempted to pretend that evangelism was not the greatest priority, not even when material and health needs could legitimately lay claim to a greater immediacy. Proselytization defined the UMCA's purpose, even in those few periods when there was broader scope to focus extra attention on building hospitals, conduct small-scale campaigns to eradicate bilharzia, train African laboratory workers or nurses, and respond to outpatient demand.

As late as 1963, the official UMCA position continued to express great dissatisfaction with the level of resources available for medical work. The fact that many other missions enjoyed considerably greater success in recruiting doctors than the UMCA (whose institutional ineptitude and futility on this particular score was legendary), remains perplexing. We repeatedly hear the mission doctor and nurses describe the medical work as "exciting," but also "exasperating" since "it is always done on a shoestring and because it is still desperately difficult to get staff" (*CA* 81 [1963]: 147). Certainly on this account there was enough angst and hand-wringing among mission personnel to go around. Following a field visit to the dioceses in 1963, the UMCA's London-based Medical Secretary highlighted in his trip report that they all greatly lacked Africans trained as priests, doctors, nurses, and teachers, "Christian or non-Christian, and there is still a great need for them to come from outside" (183). In contrast:

> Other Christian denominations are able to pay their workers good salaries and put a lot of money into their work. This cannot be said of the Anglican Church, but though I did not meet anyone who complained of the meagreness of the pocket money, all were driven frantic by the lack of funds for their work, particularly in hospitals and schools. Some life saving drugs prescribed in our hospitals are possible only because drug samples have been sent out. . . . I could see the mounting frustration of highly trained people who are being prevented from the practical exercise of their skills by inadequate facilities and by the shortage of workers. (143)

In his conclusion, the secretary questioned the Home Church: "Is it not humiliating that after so many generations, Bishops still have to exhort us in Britain as St. Paul exhorted the Corinthians when he asked for help for the

Macedonians?—do we still have to be ashamed into supporting our sister Churches?" (ibid.). In fact, the UMCA's insolvency in Malawi grew so severe that only large subventions ($30,000 promised annually) from the Episcopal Church of the U.S.A. kept it going from 1964 to 1966 (*CA* 81 [1963]: 42–43, 169).

To suggest that the UMCA did not install community-based health care ignores the crucial facts. Before the 1940s, no agencies anywhere in the world had systematically and effectively integrated the tools of prevention and health promotion into their development programs. Perhaps one way of placing the UMCA's successes and failures in objective perspective would be to compare them, dollar for dollar, year for year, against the World Health Organization's (WHO) accomplishments in the post-colonial era. In terms of a single intervention, nothing in the history of disease control can match the WHO-engineered success with smallpox eradication. Important gains in the areas of maternal and child health have also been made. Nevertheless, the WHO's overall record of converting billions of dollars into direct and indirect health benefits in both developing and developed countries reveals few clear-cut or sustainable gains for Africa. Illustrating the magnitude of the challenges are the WHO's varying rates of success in its "Health for All in the 21st Century" program (successor to "Health for All by 2000"), and in its efforts in Africa and elsewhere to control STIs/HIV/AIDS, malaria, diarrheal diseases, and TB.[11] This is not a cynical view of the record. Nor does it minimize the importance of ongoing international health work that is compassionately pursued today by many thousands of health profession-als, academicians, and others. Instead, the point once again highlights the enormous sociocultural, political, and environmental constraints that hinder sustainable interventions for even the most basic health needs.

Health and Social Change

On balance, what conclusions can be drawn from the evidence about the UMCA's record in fostering African health and social change in Malawi?

From their founding, UMCA stations, hospitals, and dispensaries served as key places of public exposure to new ideas and foreign material culture for Africans and missionaries. Intentional and spontaneous social exchanges began at these places in which Western education and literacy, health care, evangelism, and mixing of African and non-African cultures occurred simultaneously at varying rates. Meanwhile, except for their all too frequent down times, the steamers *Charles Janson* (from 1885) and the *Chauncy Maples* (from 1901) linked the far-flung stations together fairly efficiently. Particularly in the early years, these smoke-belching vessels with their loud steam engines and horns inspired awe and curiosity. Undoubtedly, the arrival of steamers at coastal villages drew many onlookers who eventually associated in one or more ways with the mission.

The steamers served the mission's political and psychological strategies aimed at converting a contested African-missionary frontier into a UMCA domain. Steamers never made canoes obsolete, but canoes obviously posed no match for the steamers in terms distances covered, speed, load factors, and safety. In this way steam technology can be said to have been a powerful catalyst that aided the dispersal of novel information, attitudes, and behavior into villages up and down the lake. At the individual level, UMCA missionaries naturally showed delight when acculturating Africans demonstrated their ability to replicate certain revered English manners and mores, not least the tea ceremony![12]

Despite extremely limited access to mission and government-run schools for the overwhelming majority of Malawians before independence, formal education stimulated profound changes in the nature of African social and spatial relations. Few would disagree with Isichei (1995, 229), who observes that "it was an enduring paradox of Christian life that mission education created new inequalities."

Gender bias was among the most pronounced forms of exclusion, existing from the start in both African societies and among missionaries. In contrast with females, male Africans able to attend mission or government schools in colonial Malawi generally realized a degree of upward job and class mobility. Both African and European attitudes of the time produced a gender bias that fell harshly on the educational opportunities for girls and women. Overall, the most significant factor minimizing the post-primary advancement of Africans was the fact that Nyasaland had no secondary schools until 1940 (King and King 1991, 132). This was no accident, for secondary education would have undermined the protectorate's status as a labor pool for private estates and government needs. A small number of adventurous men improved their lot by leaving the protectorate, usually first as migrant laborers. Later, through wits and sheer determination, handfuls found secondary or technical schools to attend in Rhodesia or South Africa. Today, it requires little imagination to think what could have been accomplished in the areas of public health and medicine alone had African education interests been a priority of government and missions.

At all scales, health-related developments generally intertwined with broad social changes reflected in patterns of housing, clothing, labor migration, diet, transportation, education, perinatal practices, and child-rearing.

Several illustrations of social change from 1936 to 1963 depict the diversity of scenarios and social forces at work. They reveal that virtually any aspect of social change also had consequences for individual and African community health. A report from the highland Milo station (Tanganyika) in 1936 during an influenza epidemic illustrates the numerous mundane, incremental changes that characterized the missionary period. *Central Africa* had published a special appeal to UMCA supporters in Britain for wooly vests or frocks for babies and small children in the Livingstone Mountains. Since European contact, mothers who lived nearer the station or a small township had increasingly discarded the wearing of skins in favor of cotton cloth. Customarily, they had also carried their babies in skins on their backs (most still did), which protected them from the cold morning mists and winds. By changing their mode of dress, the missionaries worried that mothers also exposed their babies to new and undesirable health risks (*CA* 54 [1936]: 175).

By the 1940s, Kota Kota Hospital had the largest and most developed midwifery work, with over fifteen babies born in some weeks. Mothers' postnatal hospital stays typically ran from seven to twelve days, in marked contrast with the near-zero confinement practices in the village. European nurses also tried, with only marginal success at this point, to get mothers to drink cows' milk from the mission's herd and to give it to their babies as well. While well intended, such demands for change in lactation and nutrition amounted to an assault on sound African cultural practices, apart from unusual cases where breastfeeding was not feasible.

One of the biggest problems identified at Kota Kota just after World War II was the deleterious effect of labor migration on young married couples. As the missionaries understood it, the sanctity and stability of marriage was severely compromised by the colonial economy and the behavior it encouraged. As soon as the wife became pregnant, the husband wanted to leave for the mines in Rhodesia or South Africa, maintaining that he would send for her when he was making enough money. A husband, it was reported, rarely stayed around home until the baby's birth. Once separated from his wife, the temptations to stray became great for both parties (*CA* 64 [1946]: 45). This situation (directly related to colonial tax policy) greatly stressed the couple's commitment to the monogamous ideal of Christian marriage and the two-parent role in child rearing. From the mission's perspective, the new generation of children would not be well served by the secular values (broadly European-inspired) then spreading across colonial Malawi.

After World War II lakeside Kota Kota remained one of the protectorate's largest African settlements, as it had been during the nineteenth-century slave trade. It held the district administrative offices, schools, the UMCA mission, and a port for steamers. Justus Kushindo, an African teacher in the local UMCA school, observed that Kota Kota was home to "thousands of boys and girls of the Chewa tribe." Religiously divided into Christians, Muslims, and pagans,

> these boys and girls wander about like sheep without a shepherd. It is a pity that though there are thousands of these, few . . . come to school to learn. Most who came to school are Xtians. The Islams are the ones who hate or dislike education the most. Girls . . . are not keen in their work. They often leave school before they are over-age . . . many leave school just because they want to get married. Among the Islams sometimes a girl of twelve may be married to a man of forty. The boys are not as clever as they should have been, because they smoke the leaves of a certain plant called 'Chamba.' After smoking this poisonous tobacco, they look very stupid and sometimes mad. (*CA* 65 [1947]: 13)

Allowing for the teacher's own biases, what remains is a powerful portrait of indirect, European-induced social-structural disintegration symbolized by the youths' use of cannabis, their underemployment and lack of direction, and the implicit fraying of the society's traditional moral fabric. Public health implications apparent in this scenario included drug addiction, STIs, teen pregnancies, and family conflict.

On Likoma Island, decades of close contact between Africans, missionaries, and the steamer traffic had contributed to many changes in education, housing, hygiene, domestic customs, and other social patterns. Improvements in housing generally signaled the presence of other enhancements in the quality of life. In 1928 practically all housing on Likoma consisted of windowless round huts made of wattle and mud daub. A fire burned in the middle of the floor with no outlet for the smoke except through a low doorway. A UMCA nurse arriving to attend a sick patient recalled she "would first of all be half-blinded by the smoke, and then would have to wait a few moments before her eyes got accustomed to the gloom and she could make out the form of her patient lying on a mat on the mud floor" (*CA* 64 [1946]: 100). A few houses were built of sun-dried bricks in 1928, but by 1946 local housing had been transformed by new materials and forms: "practically all the houses are built of these . . . bricks: they have wide verandahs and good-sized windows [some glassed] which really let in the light and air." Houses generally had "a sitting room in the middle with a bedroom on each side, and [wooden] bedsteads are largely used now . . . strung with

plaited palm-leaf rope. . . . Quite a number of people too use mosquito nets"
(ibid.).

Yet in the UMCA's sphere Likoma was exceptional. On the mainland,
ordinary villagers had little access to improved materials or money to buy
them. A scattering of men had learned to produce sun-dried bricks and do
simple bricklaying, but poverty was deep and demand limited. A report in
Central Africa in 1947 noted that housing quality remained

> appallingly low. Huts are badly thatched, and inhabited long after they
> should have been condemned. Nearly always they are devoid of ventilation
> and are therefore dark and smoky. . . . They are generally overcrowded,
> and often infected with ticks [vectors of relapsing fever] and bugs. This
> poor housing standard must surely be the second greatest factor in the
> poor health of the people, counting on malnutrition as the first. (*CA* 65
> [1947]: 82)

Mkope Hill Station was remotely situated in the dry savanna on the
southwestern coast of Lake Malawi. A recounting of advances that occurred
there between 1920 and 1950 helps to underscore the point that fundamental
change is much more than the sum of new forces. Apart from the rising lake
level, which had driven many African villagers to the higher ground of the
mission, the district's greatest infrastructural change had been the building
of a north-south motor road connecting Mkope Hill with Cape Maclear,
Monkey Bay port, and Ft. Johnston. By 1953 this road had begun to attract
a few Europeans who had started buying quarter-acre lots for holiday and
weekend houses and businesses (*CA* 72 [1954]: 99).[13] By 1950, Cape Maclear
received a weekly flying boat from England, providing four-day service each
way for £250. Villages and families had to cope with far fewer men, with
large numbers of them away for long periods in the Rhodesias or South
Africa. Remittances from the thousands of absent husbands and relatives,
and the earnings of the growing number of men by then in government
or other European employment, placed more money in circulation. Yet
for local Africans there was little affordable surplus food for sale in this
agriculturally risky zone. Station notes for 1919 recorded

> hunger in the country: there still is. The new contact with the outside
> world has not changed that. All along the Lake the soil is sandy and not
> of much use for growing crops. The people now, as then, spend half of
> the year from four to ten miles inland, producing their years' food . . . on
> scattered fields . . . they dare not leave . . . untended because they are liable

to be destroyed in the twinkling of an eye by baboons...and wild pigs. Some of the villages are almost deserted during these months. (*CA* 68 [1950]: 174–75)

Padre Hicks, the UMCA's priest at Mkope Hill in 1950, concluded that in more than thirty years

no improvements have been made in agricultural methods, and there is no surplus of food to provide for teachers and school meals for children, many of whom walk up to ten miles a day to and from school on an empty stomach.... One year is put down to drought and another year to too much rain. (178)

Mkope Hill was and remains a marginal environment for agriculture. There is little doubt that colonial labor policies, which extracted male labor and forced the bulk of agricultural labor and production onto women and children, directly contributed to the area's further marginalization that was manifest in the downward spiral of food deficits, malnutrition, and underdevelopment. The UMCA was hard pressed to do more than try to blunt some of the forces that hammered away at the population's persistent poverty, and attempt to "humanize" local hardship.

At Mponda's station, on the lakeshore south of Mkope Hill, the UMCA's social concerns and self-limiting modus operandi persisted unchecked in 1953. "Very disquieting revelations" about two sexually explicit initiation dances had come to light. According to the missionaries, all Christian girls had no alternative but to attend what was "an essentially a Muslim affair," but which also had "according to all the Yaos present...a great deal of evil in its teaching." It was "urgently necessary" to gain the co-operation of Christian elders in the congregation, especially older women, to find a Christian substitute rite (*CA* 72 [1954]: 99–100).

At the same time, the UMCA had removed its nurse at Mponda's for economy reasons. Consequently, the amount of work being done for women had considerably diminished. This was seen as a loss that greatly limited efforts to persuade adolescent girls to refuse their customary sexuality training, which the missionaries saw as harmful to their character development. Station notes for 1953 record that the departing nurse had made "real contacts with the women and the Mission's influence penetrated deeply into the family by her acts of disinterested charity. Now that most valuable missionary activity has been removed, and [despite the adjacent government Hospital at Ft. Johnston] nothing has taken its place."[14] Once again, the constraints revealed in this example demonstrate the near-impossibility for the missionaries to develop sustained and meaningful public health activities, even if they had been inclined to do so. Whether one agrees with the missionaries' strivings at social engineering is beside the point.

There is yet another factor concerning mission social objectives. It is reasonable to think that by the 1950s the mission would have attempted to train and deploy Christian African women to carry on the work of reeducating adolescent girls about "appropriate" expressions of sexuality. That this was apparently not even a consideration points to the continuing power of women in the matrilineages who had traditional responsibility for inculcating adult mores and expectations in adolescent girls before marriage.

When the mission era ended, it was clear that the secular and religious forces of colonialism had instigated many changes in African social patterns and material culture, including the visible landscape. Helen Taylor, a UMCA missionary in the diocese from 1932 to 1945, returned to Malawi after an absence of eighteen years. Her recounting of a visit to the Kota Kota district in 1963 captures landscape elements of Malawi's emerging "limited opportunity," or "veneer," capitalism (*CA* 81 [1963]: 165). Kota Kota was now posted, including signs for various villages, the jetty, rice mill, government offices, and tourist attractions ("Arab Slave Market"). While most roads remained untarred and dusty, they had been improved and road traffic had greatly increased. Lorries and private cars driven by Africans frequently overtook each other. In the old days people would jump with fear and disappear into the bush at the sight of an approaching car; now they moved at their own speed to the side of the road. Many more shops had opened with a much greater variety of goods, yet as before most sold the same items—"from a toothbrush to a suit of clothes." Africans appeared to own about half of these shops, unlike the old days when Indians owned practically all of them. Another major change that "hit me in the eye," said Taylor, was the multitude of sign-posted advertising "in the shop windows, on boards outside, nailed up on the trunks of trees—everywhere you are invited to drink Coca Cola or Fanta, to smoke Tom Tom cigarettes, to take Aspro for your aches and pains, to buy a Raleigh bicycle, a Singer sewing machine, or Caltex petrol. The modern world has indeed come to Kota Kota" (165–66).

In 1963, housing at Kota Kota reflected "the greatest mixture of the old and new" in Africa. Better-paid residents lived in three- to four-room houses built of brick with plastered interior walls, glazed windows with good frames, and "pretty gay curtains." Tables, chairs, a bookcase, and a gramophone or transistor radio furnished the inside. However, since the cost of aluminum and iron was nearly prohibitive, most of these "modern" houses still had thatched roofs. Higher quality houses were interspersed with the ubiquitous, unhygienic old style houses lived in by the poor majority. They featured pole and reed walls plastered with mud, no windows, and usually a dilapidated grass roof. Interior furnishings amounted to little more than a few mats, native bedsteads, possibly a stool or two, cooking pots, and a hoe and axe.

Taylor also noticed that "a much greater gulf" had opened between rich and poor people since 1945 (167). Rich people might earn £20–30 or more a month, while the poor, self-employed peasant farmers who produced maize and rice had no fixed wage. Instead, they obtained what earnings they could from the sale of crops at the local market. Meanwhile, rice prices continued to fall.

People at Kota Kota dressed better in 1963. Women and girls had taken to cotton frocks and bright head scarves. Many more people wore shoes. Taylor thought that teachers dressed smartly, although the preference of the men in Malawi and elsewhere in British Africa for "dark suits, collars and ties," though smart, "seemed less suitable for the climate."

She noticed two other "changes for the better" that had "lightened the daily toil of women: the introduction of piped water through the town and the opening of a maize mill. Both innovations conserved women's energy and time. Water-stands had eliminated long and sometimes dangerous walks to the lake or a stream, which was often polluted. Access to cleaner water would reduce diarrheal and other water-borne diseases. Milling the staple food greatly reduced the tiring hours women spent in food preparation. Said Taylor, one "no longer hears the constant thud of the old wooden pestles and mortars" (ibid.).

Up to this point Taylor emphasized that her account only described "superficial changes." In her view Africans, as people, seemed fundamentally unchanged since 1945, but in fact deeper changes had occurred that proved more difficult to measure. Among the more educated, for example, she perceived "a feeling of unrest and anxiety about the future." Yet as she traveled to other parts of the country she found it heartening that "so much progress has been made towards a higher standard of living" (183).

In January 1965, the UMCA was formally merged into the United Society for the Propagation of the Gospel (USPG).[15] Financially, at least, the UMCA had little alternative.[16] The UMCA's General Secretary rationalized that the merger meant greater efficiency and coherence of support in the future. UMCA dioceses, he said, would not be overshadowed by the USPG's wider interests, and there was no reason to fear that the merger would weaken personal links with friends, stations, or dioceses in Africa (*CA* 82 [1964]: 180).

To its credit, the old mission had made useful, positive accomplishments in education and medical services in its Nyasaland Diocese. Scores of well-educated and dedicated UMCA missionaries, both men and women, had given themselves to further the church's purposes. In this process, they directly and indirectly facilitated the exposure of many Africans to influences of the rapidly changing world outside Malawi. Whereas they had made contributions to African welfare, they had also exposed Malawians to new vulnerabilities.

A small proportion of the missionaries had spent their entire lives, or at least working lives, on African soil. Some lay in gravesites near the lakeshore, alongside African clergy and parishioners. The old European missionary system had come and gone. It had left an indelible mark on past and present generations of African Christians, and on others who became involved in mission functions. Now it was the Malawians turn to build on the missionary foundation: to administer, finance, maintain, and build-up the work in the diocese and its parishes. To the extent possible, the legacy of UMCA interests in Malawi would from then on be represented in the form of various grants for project and expatriate personnel support administered by the USPG.

It is important to reemphasize the fact that collectively, the UMCA and other Christian missions in Central Africa arrived on the ground much earlier, and were more effective, than the protectorate government in providing medical services and concern for African health. That is true regardless of the extent to which health services and evangelistic goals were intertwined. In missionary eyes, it would have been a perversion of Christian doctrine to intentionally separate the two realms. Even the most introspective and skeptical UMCA missionaries could be expected to view the mission's record in Malawi with a sense of considerable accomplishment.

On the other hand, the mission's record speaks for itself regarding the achievements within its medical mandate. Overall, the progress as measured at the end of the UMCA's tenure was not favorable, even in the mission's own terms. Dr. Robert Brown, the American physician based at Malindi who had been recruited on a fill-in basis in 1963–64, put together the most comprehensive annual hospital statistics ever compiled for the diocese. (It was at this time that the American Episcopal Church stepped into the breach with a relatively large contribution over three years to stave off bankruptcy.) The new data revealed that hospital admissions had grown by more than 30 percent since 1953. Some 3,526 inpatients (or 441 per hospital) generated 35,833 inpatient days. Hospitals that drew the most inpatients at the end of the colonial era included: Likwenu (917), Kota Kota (878), Likoma (685), Malindi (582), Mponda (373), and Matope (95) (fig. 4.9).[17] By now, however, the work of the old European-directed medical mission was finished forever. Future policy and development would be guided not by the UMCA, whose absorption into the USPG was imminent, but by the African-run Anglican diocese of independent Malawi and the new Private Hospital Association of Malawi (PHAM).

The dramatic improvements in medically related statistics indicated above reflect a belated effort to shift away from old medical mission habits to create a more comprehensive system of health. The impetus came much less from within the UMCA and more from new staff with proactive dispositions, including Dr. Mumford (a retired English physician who returned to help the mission in 1962) and especially Dr. Brown (table 7.6). The mission recruited them to oversee its medical services during the period of transition to an independent Malawi. In addition to hospital statistics, they gathered comparatively comprehensive data on African health, including place of birth, baby clinics, abortions, diseases, anesthetics, tooth extractions, and home visits. Their approach reflected the biomedical and public health worlds outside colonial Africa, with emphasis on greater professionalism and accountability. The new doctors' training and interests were grounded in an ethos of public health principles. They introduced more comprehensive and targeted statistical analysis of health information to facilitate the rational planning of health services.[18]

What the newer doctors such as Dr. Mumford and Dr. Brown uncovered in the diocese was a "sorry state of decay, and neglect" at Likoma."[19] In 1964, four doctors were needed for services to function effectively, but since its inception the diocese had never been able to recruit more than one full-time medical officer, and an occasional additional part-time doctor. Over large parts of the diocese medical facilities were spread extremely thin, and thousands of people in its sphere lacked physical access to care. Moreover, existing hospitals were "greatly handicapped" because they did not feed patients. As elsewhere in British Africa, this practice required that anyone admitted be accompanied by two or three relatives to prepare the patient's food and collect the necessary firewood and water. Such inefficiencies resulted in many premature voluntary departures; this included TB patients whom in leaving endangered themselves and exposed others to the risk of resistant infection.

In the UMCA's Portuguese mainland sphere there was only one dispensary within sixty miles of Likoma Island. In addition, many of the mission's medical facilities had been poorly located. A rising lake level forced several to move to a different site. For anyone ill or lame, reaching Likwenu Hospital was a tough challenge because it was necessary to climb a steep hill.

Dr. Brown called it "a difficult climb for a person in good health." Most of the local population had moved away from Matope, the poorly sited station on the banks of the Shiré. Likoma, already suspected of harboring chloroquine-resistant malaria by the early 1960s, was extremely difficult to reach since the government steamer stopped only once every seventeen days. During the frequent periods of rough water travel by canoe and other small craft practically halted. On the coast opposite the Likoma, the local north-south track was passable by Land Rover but only in the dry season.[20]

At the south end of Lake Malawi, no medical facilities existed north of Malindi for fifty miles. From a doctor's perspective, Malindi's St. Martin's Hospital, with forty-five beds, was itself a source of great "professional frustration" since only 60 percent of one's knowledge could be put into practice. It was nearly impossible "to adequately diagnose and treat illness because of the severe limitations imposed by the lack of facilities."[21] According to Dr. Brown, for every seriously ill patient who entered St. Martin's, "at least five remain to die in the village."[22] Kota Kota Hospital, established in 1904, now supplied thirty-three maternity beds and provided the mission's only training school for midwives. Yet in 1963 it had no doctor in residence, and none was closer than Lilongwe, the capital, located a tedious four hours away by car.[23]

By the early 1960s the wards at Kota Kota had become "grossly over-crowded." "Severely overtaxed" nursing sisters and facilities were further compromised by the "great wastage among the students who leave because of pregnancy and marriage."[24] Kota Kota took in all obstetrical cases and reportedly served "effectively as an adjunct" to the nearby government hospital. This place, one of the three earliest UMCA hospitals, had no doctor. In his short-term role as Diocesan MO, Dr. Robert Brown brought the critical eye of an outside professional. There is no suggestion that he was expected to come out to the lake, offer up a "well-done, hip-hip-hooray!," and spare the medical mission from a report on the realities of its existence after sixty-five years. Instead, he offers transparency, putting the UMCA on notice by exposing the long-term consequences its idiosyncratic philosophical positions and self-imposed isolation from modern professional and intellectual currents in medicine and health care. Brown rebuked the mission for its acquiescence to continuing mediocrity, at best, and the obsolescence of its medical programs in 1963. Thus,

> while there is a certain amount of romantic fascination for the 'bush hospital,' and the surgeon who operates by a hurricane lamp, to continue to tolerate these conditions, and in fact glamorise them, impresses me

as being nothing more than a sophisticated evasion of responsibility. It is our duty not to say so much we have done, but to expand every effort to achieve decent and adequate standards of medical practice.[25]

This severe indictment arrived as the colonial period ended. It was too late to awaken the UMCA's old guard to future action. However, Brown's report directly complemented a wider analysis of the status of all medical missions in Malawi that was undertaken in 1965 for the Malawi Christian Council by the World Council of Churches (WCC).

Overall, the WCC report indicated that at independence Malawi had neither records of vital statistics nor of maternal and infant mortality. At this time there was "little evidence of any organized plan aimed at preventive measures," with the exception of three externally initiated and supported measures: leprosy eradication, TB (University of North Carolina), and blindness (Israeli government). Virtually all doctors (est. 1 : 60,000 people) and supervising nurses were expatriates. A small training program for nurses (above the Assistant Nurse level) had just opened at Blantyre; but the country lacked programs to train Public Health Nurses, and diagnostic facilities were "very inadequate."[26] The WCC report also commends the work of Roman Catholic missions for providing over half of all mission hospital beds. Among the best equipped and run hospitals were Malamulo (Seventh Day Adventist) and Lunzu, "the best planned facility in Malawi" (Montfort-Marist Sisters). Mkhoma (Dutch Reformed Church Mission) was among "the best staffed and operated," with three expatriate doctors and five nurses. Mzuzu (Medical Missionaries of Mary); and Likuni (White Sisters), which had begun "a dynamic program under the imaginative leadership of Dr. Sorenson," a U.S. doctor and lay-volunteer, also received plaudits and ranked high in mission hospital standings.[27] Apart from the reference to maternity work at Kota Kota, and the "quite unsatisfactory" hospital at Likwenu, it is telling that no UMCA medical station or program received favorable treatment in the Christian Council's report. Certainly one finds reasons to believe that overall the UMCA's medical program was not in vain; yet in truth its imprint seemed to grow fainter with the progression of time. Having used its steamers and relative location to great advantage in creating a mission sphere of influence, the UMCA actually went too far in its evangelistic ambitions. With considerable initial success, the missionaries engaged and contested African cultures on both the spatial and, less successfully, mental frontiers. They were largely successful in defining what was UMCA territory, and strategically imprinted its vast landscape of Rift, lake, and mountains with central stations, churches, schools, hospitals, dispensaries, and outstations.

However, in doing these things the mission also permitted itself the unfortunate indulgence of continuously overreaching its limits—limits set by its human and financial resources and self-limiting philosophies. Examples of the latter include isolation from ideas and professional standards, exclusion of married persons and children from the mission field, dependence on volunteers for all professions, and generally inconsistent and ineffective fund-raising in Britain for medical work it proposed to do in Central Africa.

Once again, contexts of place and real lives remain central in this analysis. The European doctors, nurses, and other staff who volunteered for service in Central Africa, together with the African dispensers and nurse-midwives they trained, generally carried out their medical responsibilities with great energy, responsibility, and dignity. Despite the scarcity of human and material resources, many applied great skill and compassion, and tirelessly labored even to the point of exhaustion. Dr. Robert Howard entered upon the scene in the critical early years when disease exacted an exceptionally high toll on missionary life, threatening the mission's very survival. He served brilliantly. His practical interventions and leadership in malaria and environmental health may have prevented the UMCA's failure for a second time. Howard regularly traveled by steamer to treat patients in the hospitals at Malindi, Kota Kota, and Likoma, whose establishment he oversaw. En route he often visited a number of lakeside villages to identify the most needful cases. He and Mrs. Howard, obliged to leave their work in the Diocese of Nyasaland after they married, were permitted to continue their respective medical and nursing professions under Bishop Weston in Tanganyika and Zanzibar. Howard received acclaim for building up the UMCA's hospital and surgical capabilities in Zanzibar. They retired to England after World War I, and Howard became a UMCA treasurer until his death in 1947 ("In memoriam: Robert Howard," *CA* 66 [1948]: 12).

Dr. Wigan also became a legendary, if somewhat less innovative, figure. He worked as Medical Officer for forty-seven years, virtually entirely without support from a second doctor. When he was not at a hospital—seeing patients, in surgery, or consulting with nurses—he was traveling by steamer, donkey, or on foot to get to one. With a single doctor responsible for the entire diocese, the overwhelming bulk of work with ill or pregnant patients fell to the European nurses and, in time, African dispensers and midwives.

Rather than focusing on doing several things well in a few places, apparently by default mission administrators in both Malawi and London allowed staff in the field to spread themselves too thinly. Such actions diluted the potential of the few resources the UMCA secured for its medical work in Central Africa. The consequences of this kind of expansion came as no surprise to the staff on the front lines with responsibility for accommodating the growing numbers of Africans seeking treatment. By the early 1920s, at least, staff at mission hospitals such as Mponda's, which had only one nurse and periodic itinerant visits from the mission's lone doctor, were reportedly "all but overwhelmed" by patient demand (*CA* 42 [1924]: 104).

In terms of the mission's desired objectives and capabilities, its watered-down, "minimalist" strategy produced disappointing results. In fact, it opened places for medical services and then allowed them to languish. To help avoid a growing overall financial crisis in the diocese, in 1954 Bishop of Nyasaland Frank Thorne sold the *Chauncy Maples*. This action, as interpreted by Thorne's successor in an address to the UMCA's General Council in London in 1963, "at one stroke severed the head from the body of the diocese" (*CA* 81 [1963]: 35). Despite a special grant of £20,000 from its London headquarters to help relieve the shortfall in Malawi, the mission had remained mired in debt. Within five months of the new bishop's arrival in Malawi in 1962, auditors informed him that the diocese had an accumulated deficit of £21,000. For each of the seven previous years spending had exceeded income by about £6,000, and an overdraft at the bank continued to increase by £500 a month. Audits had been abandoned to save money. While no intentional misuse of budget authority was claimed, "things had gone wrong" in Malawi ever since the loss of the *C.M.* and the resulting isolation of both Likoma and Mponda's from the rest of the diocese. Without the steamer, the bishop and administrative offices had become "hopelessly isolated." These circumstances had "burst wide open the whole method of running the diocese" (36).[28]

Paradoxically, over the course of some fifty years the *C.M.* contributed mightily to the mission's rise and its fall. In the end, the mission's exaggerated claims to world prominence for its number of converts from Islam to Christianity could not counteract the effects of its lack of human and financial resources (ibid.) These formidable circumstances directly contributed to the UMCA's rapid self-isolation within the Lake Malawi basin. As colonial rule drew to an end in 1964, a growing psychic distance also separated UMCA Africans, white missionaries, and supporters of the mission in Britain. For over eighty years the mission had contributed to the creation of new human geographies within the Lake Malawi region, and between it and the outside world. With Malawi's independence imminent, the mission's human and financial resources diminished more rapidly than they could be locally replaced.

To paraphrase a more general study of colonialism, the UMCA's attitude toward the declining fortunes of its Central African diocese was not one of cynical disregard. Yet its stance on issues of race, culture, and development reflected the peculiar ethnocentrism that so often permeated British relations with Africa (Hammond and Jablow 1992, 15). Despite genuine heroes, important accomplishments, and good intentions, there apparently was a quality of institutional indifference about the UMCA that eased its walk away from the hopes and expectations it had instilled among the African faithful, five thousand miles from London.

NOTES

1. This created a domestic, nocturnal *cordon sanitaire*. Some malaria experts recommended an alternative approach that did not rely on segregation of the races. See chapter 7.

2. See Fisher to Winspear, Nov. 24, 1917. UMCA 1/1/2, MNA, and chapter 5 for other details. Emphasis in original.

3. While the UMCA's aims and methods in Malawi certainly differed from those of the protectorate government and British policy-makers, as I write in chap. 1, they did produce their own "geography of imperialism" in the sense that they promoted and sacntioned unequal relationships between themselves and the African population. They also marked and guarded "their" territoral sphere; helped to alter indigenous patterns of settlement, movement, and communications; and changed the cultural landscape by imposing/adapting important symbols and paraphernalia of the English state church and European civilization.

4. In the UMCA's Masasi Diocese in Tanganyika, the replenishment of European staff was markedly down around the time of Uhuru in the early 1960s. "Unfortunately, at this time of opportunity, when the new [African] leaders are giving our hospitals every encouragement to expand, the flow of missionary nurses and doctors has contracted to a trickle. The African Church should be able to provide its own doctors and sister-tutors in perhaps 20 years time, and its own staff of nurses in perhaps 10 years time. But *now*, God is calling us" (quoted in Ranger 1981, 34).

5. In comparison, Ekechi asserts that among the Igbos in eastern Nigeria, "receptivity to European medicine was predicated on its practical results." The Igbo allowed an important space for Roman Catholic medical work during the colonial period, and their pragmatism enabled the new medicine to have a "measurable" influence on their society. The missionaries cut into the medicine men's (*nde dibia*) established income source, which in turn won the missionaries the "relentless" hostility of the traditional practitioners. Reportedly, Igbo still consult traditional medicine men but "rarely resign themselves to fate" (Ekechi 1972, 224–25).

6. Even as colonialism was ending, UMCA missionaries reacted incredulously to the fact that "many Christians are prone to place faith in charms, and to wear them secretly under their clothing" (Winspear 1960, 71).

7. Annual Report on the Mlanje District for the Year 1938. Extract. S10101-38. MNA.

8. DC, Mlanje, to Act. Chief Secretary, Zomba, Dec. 11, 1939. S1-101-38. MNA.

9. "He said that he respected Christians doing good work," but that he could not be a church member. Meanwhile, one of the recruitment lessons was not the absence of Christian doctors, but that "so many of them seem to be married with young families." Paragraph source is UMCA, S.F. Series, X–XIII. UMCA General Secretary to Bishop Frank, Nyasaland, July 10, 1946. RHL.

10. UMCA, S.F. Series, XV–XIV, typed note by [Bishop] Frank, Nyasaland, April 9, 1956; and XVI, Position of UMCA Nyasaland in 1956 re: Bishop's special appeal (undated).

11. World Health Organization. Fifty-first World Health Assembly. Agenda Item 19, Health for All Policy for the Twenty-first Century. WHA 51.7. 16 May 1998.

12. Just after World War II an English nurse and guest were invited to the home of a Hospital Assistant and his Standard III bride (third year of primary school) for tea. Upon reaching the house, situated on a hill in one of Likoma's many small hamlets overlooking Lake Nyasa, they were entertained in a room reminiscent of an English country cottage. They were charmed by the un-African ambience, unerring display of courtesy and English tea-time manners, and the ritual of drinking tea out of beautiful "willow-patterned tea-cups." A "pretty print cloth" on the table, a gramophone on a side table, books and a clock on another, and pictures on the wall, rounded out the scene. *CA* 64 (1946): 101.

13. A decade later, President Banda's policies began to attract increasing numbers of whites on holiday from apartheid South Africa to this same part of the lakeside, prompting the development of a few small resorts and a curio trade along the road.

14. *CA* 72 (1954): 100, citing Mponda's Notes, *Nyasaland Diocesan Chronicle*, August, 1953. Reference to the government hospital emphasizes that the work there is "at the best . . . little more than attending to the body."

15. The USPG, headquartered in London, is an umbrella organization of the Anglican and the United Churches. It is currently active in fifty countries worldwide, including Malawi, supporting many mission programs that provide for support of professional and lay personnel and training, and funding for projects in health care and development.

16. By 1961 there could be no question about the self-compromised status of the diocese's educational as well as medical programs. It had been in financial delinquency for decades. Only three of its African priests had passed their Standard VI (elementary level) exams, and apart from two places it had no matriculated teachers in any of its schools. No Anglican Africans from the diocese were known to be among the "100 or so" Malawian students "doing degrees and higher professional courses overseas and in Rhodesia." Unflattering comparisons were drawn with other missions in Malawi, such as the Roman Catholics. UMCA, S.F. Series, XVI, Bishop of Nyasaland, London, to Canon Broomfield, Dec. 2, 1961.

17. Also in 1963, there were some 395,000 outpatient attendances, over 53,500 visits to antenatal and baby clinics, and 1,730 babies delivered in the mission's facilities. People with leprosy made 35,277 outpatient visits, and accounted for 38,653 hospital days. UMCA, S.F. Series, Hospital Statistics, 1963. A separate reported claimed, correctly, that church attendances remained large, and that "every single day over 1,000 outpatients are treated in the hospitals of the diocese" (*CA* 81 [1963]: 37).

18. Diocese of Malawi (Nyasaland), Med. Dept. Ann. Rep., 1963. Mimeograph. 16 pp. Data from p. 15.

19. Ibid., 7. Bishop Thorne wrote: "Poor Dr. Mumford was quite horrified by the primitive state of Likoma Hospital: nobody else [there] could see why there should be such a fuss about moving the maternity patients around when it rained, as until last year they had always done it *all* the patients! I think almost all the staff houses are in the same condition everywhere" (emphasis in original). UMCA, S.F. Series, XVI, Bishop Donald, Malawi, to Canon Kingsnorth, UMCA, London, March 8, 1962. RHL.

20. Diocese of Malawi, Med. Dept. Ann. Rep., 1963, 7.

21. Ibid., 11. The author visited Malindi on several occasions in 1989 and 1990. Administered today by the Diocese of Southern Malawi with the assistance of the United Society for the Propagation of the Gospel (USPG), St. Martin's hospital serves a densely populated, desperately poor region, over 80 percent Muslim, along the lake coast and up into the adjacent mountains. It has ninety beds plus thirty to forty "floor beds" and twenty maternity beds. Staff, paid by the Malawi Government with indirect support from the USPG in Britain, includes one chief clinical officer (3+ years medical training) a matron (sr. nurse-midwife), three medical assistants, and seven enrolled nurse-midwives. Since 1964 physical improvements had included a few new externally funded brick blocks (for inpatients, a small lab, isolation, maternal and child welfare, office space). The hospital's needs (1990) were a throwback to the impoverished conditions accepted by the UMCA. Thus, no motorized transport was available to or from the hospital, only a "Bush ambulance" (a home-made stretcher mounted on two bicycle wheels). There had been no telephone for a long time, but the old wiring remained sticking out of the wall. The operating theater was a colonial structure from the 1930s, lighted inside by a thirty-watt bulb. The hospital had no x-ray capability and no laundry. The water supply system off the mountain was precarious, while the inshore lake water was often polluted and an important source of bilharzia and cholera. The lab, interfaced with a USAID-funded malaria project, needed upgrading and expansion. In- and outpatient loads had expanded greatly, but the quantity of drugs supplied from the diocesan medical headquarters (Malosa)—especially antibiotics and chloroquine—had remained at the old levels. Finally, and symbolically, St. Martin's lacked a morgue. Of necessity, the dead are sometimes simply laid out on a table in the Clinical Officer's office until the family can collect the body. (Field notes.)

Postscript: In 1998–99, St. Martin's physical facilities were considerably improved with leadership of a USPG Special Skills Programme. The improvements include a water system, nurses' housing, sanitation, medical equipment, drugs, and a morgue. The latter addition was especially critical. In 1990 there were normally just a few deaths per month at the hospital. By 1999, because of the "desparate HIV/AIDS associated death rate rate . . . it is not unusual for there to be three deaths in one day." USPG, Project News, "Health Care in Southern Malawi," Project 282, Bull. 30 (August 1999), 1–2.

22. Diocese of Malawi, Med. Dept. Ann. Rep., 1963, 9.

23. USPG, Project News, "Health Care in Southern Malawi," Project 282, Bull. 30 (August 1999), 1–2.

24. Ibid.

25. Ibid., 12.

26. World Council of Churches for Malawi Christian Council, "Survey of Christian Medical Work in Malawi, Central Africa, July 31st–August 15th, 1965," 1–3 (mimeograph).

27. Ibid., 4 and 7.

28. In 1962, in the hope of staving off the closure of its medical and educational work, and to give its new bishop "a year to move in and lays his plans for the long pull," the UMCA, London, agreed to increase the Nyasaland overdraft from £5,000 to £10,000, and also give another £5,000 from 1962 legacies. UMCA, S.F. Series, 30. I, Nyasaland Finance, General Secretary, UMCA to Bishop Stephen F. Bayne, Jr., Oct. 31, 1962.

Bibliography

Archival sources include those in the Malawi National Archives (MNA in the notes) and in the Rhodes House Library, Oxford (RHL in the notes). The latter has the UMCA's monthly, *Central Africa*, vols. 1–82 (1883–1963), the *UMCA Annual Review*, and the *UMCA Annual Reports* for the same years.

Akerele, O., I. Tabibzadeh, and J. McGilvray. 1976. "A New Role for Medical Missionaries." *WHO Chronicle* 30:175–80.

Allen, R. 1927. *The Place of Medical Missions*. London: World Dominion Press.

Anderson, H. G. 1956. *The New Phase in Medical Strategy*. London: Church Missionary Society.

Anderson-Morshead, A. E. M. 1955. *History of the Universities Mission to Central Africa*, vol. 1: *1859–1909*. 6th ed. rev. London: UMCA.

———. 1991. *Lady of the Lake: The Story of Lake Malawi's M.V. Chauncy Maples*. Blantyre, Malawi: Central Africana. Facsimilie reprint of A. E. M. Anderson-Morshead, *The Building of the Chauncy Maples* (London: UMCA, 1903), with Vera Garland, *After the Building a Life of Service: The M.V. Chauncy Maples on Lake Malawi 1902–1990*.

Arnold, David, ed. 1988. *Imperial Medicine and Indigenous Societies*. Manchester: Manchester University Press.

Balme, Harold. 1921. *China and Modern Medicine: A Study in Medical Missionary Development*. London: United Council for Missionary Education.

Barnes, Bertram H. 1933. *Johnson of Nyasaland: A Study of the Life and Work of William Percival Johnson, D.D*. London: Universities Mission to Central Africa.

Baumann, O. 1894. *Durch Massailand zur Nielquelle*. Berlin: D. Reimer.

Beck, Ann. 1981. *Medicine, Tradition, and Development in Kenya and Tanzania, 1920–1970.* Waltham, Mass.: Crossroads Press.

Beidelman, T. O. 1982. *Colonial Evangelism.* Bloomington: Indiana University Press.

Bennett, Norman R. 1970. "David Livingstone: Exploration for Christianity." In *Africa and Its Explorers: Motives, Methods, and Impact,* ed. R. Rotberg, 39–61. Cambridge: Harvard University Press, 1970.

Blaut, J. M. 1993. *The Colonizer's Model of the World: Geographical Diffusionism and Eurocentric History.* New York: Guilford Press.

Blood, A. G. 1957. *The History of the Universities' Mission to Central Africa.* Vol. 2: *1907–1932.* London: Universities' Mission to Central Africa.

———. 1962. *The History of the Universities' Mission to Central Africa.* Vol. 3: *1933–1957.* London: Universities' Mission to Central Africa.

Boeder, R. 1973. "The Effects of Labor Migration on Rural Life in Malawi." *Rural Africana* [Michigan State University], no. 20 (Spring): 37–46.

Bond, George C., and Diane M. Ciekawy. 2001. *Witchcraft Dialogues: Anthropological and Philosophical Exchanges.* Research in International Studies, Africa series, no. 76. Athens, Ohio: Ohio University Press.

Bone, D. S. 1982. "Islam in Malawi." *Journal of Religion in Africa* 12:126–38.

Bowen, T. J. 1857. *Central Africa: Adventures and Missionary Labors in the Several Countries in the Interior of Africa, from 1849 to 1856.* Charleston, S.C.: Southern Baptist Publication Society.

Bowman, James. 2000. "Whit Stillman: Poet of the Broken Branches." *Intercollegiate Review* 35, no. 2: 15–19.

Brown, P. S. 1985. "The Vicissitudes of Herbalism in Late Nineteenth and Early Twentieth-Century Britain." *Medical History* 29:71–92.

Browne, S. G., 1979. "The Contribution of Medical Missionaries to Tropical Medicine." *Transactions of the Royal Society for Tropical Medicine and Hygiene* 73, no. 4: 357–60.

Buchanan, John. 1885. *The Shire Highlands as Colony and Mission.* Edinburgh: Blackwood.

Budd, W. 1867. "Memorandum on the Nature and Mode of Propagation of Phthisis." *Lancet* 2:451–52.

Burkitt, D. 1970. "Geographical Distribution." In *Burkitt's Lymphoma,* ed. D. P. Burkitt and D. H. Wright, 186–97. Edinburgh: Livingstone.

Burton, R. F. 1860. *The Lake Regions of Central Africa.* 2 vols. London: Longmans.

Caldwell, J. 1985. "The Social Repercussions of Colonial Rule." In *General History of Africa,* vol. 7, *Africa under Colonial Domination, 1880–1935,* ed. A. Boahen, 458–86. London: Heinemann/UNESCO.

Cardew, C. A. 1955. "Nyasaland in the Nineties." *The Nyasaland Journal* 8 (January): 57–63.

Chavunduka, G. 1978. *Traditional Healers and the Shona patient.* Gwelo, Zimbabwe: Mambo Press.

Chernin, E. 1992. "The Early British and American Journals of Tropical Medicine and Hygiene: An Informal Survey." *Medical History* 36:70–83.

Child, C. *The Universities' Mission to Central Africa Atlas.* Westminster: UMCA, 1924.

Christie, James. 1876. *Cholera Epidemics in East Africa.* London: Macmillan.

Christopher, A. J. 1984. *Colonial Africa.* Totowa, N.J.: Barnes and Noble.

Ciekawy, Diane, and Peter Geschiere. 1998. "Containing Witchcraft: Conflicting Scenarios in Postcolonial Africa." *African Studies Review* 41, no. 3: 1–14.

Cole, A. H. 1960. "The Relations of Missionary Activity to Economic Development." *Economic Development and Cultural Change* 9, no. 2: 120–27.

Cole-King, P. A. [1971] 1987. *Lake Malawi Steamers*. Historical Guide no. 1, Dept. of Antiquities, Ministry of Education and Culture, Malawi Government. Limbe: Monfort Press. Enlarged in 1987 by M. O. Chipeta.

Coleman, G. 1973. "International Labour Migration from Malawi, 1875–1966." *Malawi Journal of Social Science* 2:47–60.

Colville, Olivia, and Arthur Colville. 1911. *One Thousand Miles in a Machila*. London: Walter Scott Pub. Co.

Comaroff, John, and Jean Comaroff, eds. 1993. *Modernity and Its Malcontents: Ritual and Power in Postcolonial Africa*. Chicago: University of Chicago Press.

Cook, Albert R. 1904. "Relapsing Fever in Uganda." *Journal of Tropical Medicine* 7:24–26.

Cook, P. J. 1971. "Cancer of the Oesophagus in Africa." *British Journal of Cancer* 25:853–80.

Coquery-Vidrovitch, C. 1988. *Africa: Endurance and Change South of the Sahara*. Berkeley: University of California Press.

Cox, Canon H. A. 1952. "Consulting the diviner." *Central Africa* 70:99–101, 107.

Crosby, A. W. 1972. *The Columbian Exchange*. Westport, Conn.: Greenwood Press.

Crosby, C. A. 1980. *A Historical Dictionary of Malawi*. London: The Scarecrow Press.

Cross, D. Kerr. 1897. *Health in Africa: A Medical Handbook for European Travellers and Residents, Embracing a Study of Malarial Fever as It Is Found in British Central Africa*. London: James Nisbett.

Curtin, Philip. 1975. *Economic Change in Pre-colonial Africa: Senegambia in the Era of the Slave Trade*. Madison: University of Wisconsin Press.

———. 1989. *Death by Migration: Europe's Encounter with the Tropical World in the Nineteenth Century*. Cambridge: Cambridge University Press.

Dale, Godfrey, ed. 1925. *Darkness or Light: Studies in the History of the Universities' Mission to Central Africa*. 3d ed. London: Universities' Mission to Central Africa.

Davies, J. N. P. 1956. "A History of Syphilis in Uganda." *Bulletin of the World Health Organization* 15:1041–55.

———. 1979. *Pestilence and Disease in the History of Africa*. Raymond Dart Lecture, no. 14. Johannesburg: Witwatersrand University Press.

Dawson, Marc. 1987. "The Social History of Africa in the Future: Medical-related Issues." *African Studies Review* 30, no. 2: 83–91.

Decle, Lionel. 1906. "The Development of Our British African Empire." *Proceedings of the Royal Colonial Institute* 36:311–36.

Deveaneaux, G. C. 1978. "The Frontier in Recent African History." *International Journal of African Historical Studies* 11:63–85.

Devisch, René. 1993. *Weaving the Threads of Life: The Khita Gyn-Eco-Logical Healing Cult among the Yaka*. Chicago: University of Chicago Press.

Diamond, Jared. 1999. *Guns, Germs, and Steel*. New York, W. W. Norton.

Douglas, Mary. 1950. *The Peoples of the Lake Nyasa Region*. London: Oxford University Press for the International African Institute.

Dutton, J. E., and J. Todd. 1905. "The Nature of Human Tick-fever in the Eastern Part of the Congo Free State." *Liverpool School of Tropical Medicine Memoir*, no. 17.

Ekechi, F. K. 1972. "The Holy Ghost Fathers in Eastern Nigeria, 1885–1920: Observations on Missionary Strategy." *African Studies Review* 15:217–39.

Elmslie, W. A. 1899. *Among the Wild Ngoni: Being Some Chapters in the History of the Livingstonia Mission in British Central Africa.* Edinburgh: Oliphhant, Anderson and Ferrier.

Elton, J. F. 1879. *Travels and Researches among the Lakes and Mountains of Eastern and Central Africa.* Edited by H. B. Cotterill. London: J. Murray.

Elston, Rev. P. 1972. "A Note of the Universities' Mission to Central Africa: 1859–1914." In *The Early History of Malawi,* ed. P. Pachai, 344–64. Evanston: Northwestern University Press.

Falola, T., and D. Ityavyar. 1992. "Health in Precolonial Africa." In *The Political Economy of Health in Africa.* Monographs in International Studies, Africa series, no. 60, 35–48. Athens, Ohio: Ohio University Center for International Studies.

Feierman, Steven. 1986. "Popular Control over the Institutions of Health: A Historical Study." In *The Professionalisation of African Medicine,* ed. Murray Last and G. Chavunduka, 206–20. Manchester: Manchester University Press.

———. 1990. *Peasant Intellecturals: Anthroplogy and History in Tanzania.* Madison: University of Wisconsin Press.

———. 1995. "Healing as Social Criticism in the Time of Conquest." *African Studies* 54:73–88.

Ford, John. 1971. *The Role of the Trypanosomiases in African Ecology.* Oxford: Oxford University Press.

Fountain, O. C. 1966. "Religion and Economy in Mission Station–Village Relationships." *Practical Anthropology* 13:49–58.

Gatrell, A. 2002. *Geographies of Health: An Introduction.* Oxford: Blackwell.

Gelfand, Michael. 1961. *Northern Rhodesia in the Days of Charter.* Oxford: Blackwell.

———. 1964. *Lakeside Pioneers: A Socio-medical Study of Nyasaland (1875–1920).* Oxford: Blackwell.

———. 1988. *Godly Medicine in Zimbabwe.* Gweru, Zimbabwe: Mambo Press.

Good, Charles M. 1978. "Man, Milieu, and the Disease Factor: Tick-borne Relapsing Fever in East Africa." In *Disease and African History,* ed. G. W. Hartwig and K. D. Patterson, 46–87. Durham, N.C.: Duke University Press.

———. 1987. *Ethnomedical Systems in Africa: Patterns of Traditional Medicine in Rural and Urban Kenya.* New York: Guilford Press.

———. 1988. *The Community in African Primary Health Care.* Studies in African Health and Medicine, vol. 2. Lewiston, N.Y., and Queenston, Ont.: The Edwin Mellen Press.

———. 1991. "Pioneer Medical Missions in Colonial Africa." *Social Science and Medicine* 32, no. 1: 1–10.

———. 2000. "Cultural and Medical Geography: Evolution, Convergence, and Innovation." In *Cultural Encounters with the Environment: Enduring and Evolving Geographic Themes,* ed. Alexander Murphy and Douglas Johnson, 219–38. Lanham, Md.: Rowman and Littlefield.

Gray, Richard. 1990. *Black Christians and White Missionaries.* New Haven: Yale University Press.

Greeley, E. H. 1988. "Planning for Population Change in Kenya: An Anthropological Perspective." In *The Anthropology of Development and Change in East Africa,* ed. D. Brokensha and P. Little, 201–16. Boulder, Colo.: Westview Press.

Green, Edward C. 1999. *Indigenous Theories of Contagious Disease*. Walnut Creek, Calif.: AltaMira Press/Sage.

Greenhill, Basil, and Ann Giffard. 1979. *Victorian and Edwardian Merchant Steamships from Old Photographs*. Annapolis: Naval Institute Press.

Gregory, J., and E. Mandala. 1987. "Dimensions of Conflict: Emigrant Labor from Colonial Malawi and Zambia, 1900–1945." In *African Population and Capitalism: Historical Perspectives*, ed. J. Gregory, and D. Dennis, 221–24. Boulder, Colo.: Westview Press.

Hailey, Lord. 1956. *An African Survey*. Oxford: Oxford University Press.

Hammond, Dorothy, and Alta Jablow. 1992. *The Africa that Never Was: Four Centuries of Writing about Africa*. Prospect Heights, Ill.: Waveland Press.

Hancock, K. 1942. *Survey of British Commonwealth Affairs*, vol. 2: *Problems of Economic Policy*. London.

Hanegraaf, T. A. 1974. "Population Based Studies of Endemic Goitre." In *Health and Disease in Kenya*, ed. L. Vogel et al., 395–401. Nairobi: East African Literature Bureau.

Hanna, A. J. 1956. *The Beginnings of Nyasaland and North-Eastern Rhodesia, 1859–95*. Oxford: The Clarendon Press.

Harlow, Vincent, E. M. Chilver, and A. Smith. 1965. *History of East Africa*, vol. 2. Oxford: Clarendon Press.

Hartwig, G. 1978. "Social Consequences of Epidemic Diseases." In *Disease in African History*, ed. G. Hartwig and K. D. Patterson, 25–45. Durham, N.C.: Duke University Press.

Hautvast, J., and M. Hautvast-Mertens. 1972. "Analysis of a Bantu Medical System: A Nyakyusa Case Study." *Tropical and Geographical Medicine* 24:406–16.

Hayes, G. D. 1964. "Lake Nyasa and the 1914–1918 War." *The Nyasaland Journal* 17 (July): 17–24.

Headrick, D. 1981. *Tools of Empire: Technology and European Imperialism in the Nineteenth Century*. New York: Oxford University Press.

———. 1988. *The Tentacles of Progress: Technology Transfer in the Age of Imperialism 1850–1940*. New York: Oxford University Press.

Headrick, Rita. 1994. *Colonialism, Health and Illness in French Equatorial Africa, 1885–1935*. Atlanta: African Studies Association Press.

Herbert, E. W. 1975. "Smallpox Inoculation in Africa." *Journal of African History* 16:539–59.

Hine, Bishop J. E. 1924. *Days Gone By*. London: Murray.

Hochschild, Adam. 1998. *King Leopold's Ghost: A Story of Greed, Terror, and Heroism in Colonial Africa*. Boston: Houghton-Mifflin.

Hodgkin, Henry T. 1915. *The Way of the Good Physcian*. London: Church Missionary Society.

Hopkins, J. M. 1980. "Theological Students and Witchcraft Beliefs." *Journal of Religion in Africa* 11:55–66.

Howard, Robert. 1904. *A Report to the Medical Board of the Universities' Mission on the Health of the European Missionaries in the Likoma Diocese*. London: Universities' Mission to Central Africa.

———. 1908. "Malaria Prophylaxis in Small Communities in British Central Africa." *Journal of Tropical Medicine and Hygiene* 11, no. 1: 1–16.

————. 1909. "Some Notes on the Surgery of Injuries from Wild Beasts." *Journal of Tropical Medicine and Hygiene* 12 (Novemebr 15): 334–36.

————. 1910. "General Description of the Diseases Encountered During Ten Years' Medical Work on the Shores of Lake Nyasa." *Journal of Tropical Medicine and Hygiene* 13 (March 1): 66–71.

Hunter, John, and M. O. Thomas. 1987. "Hypothesis of Leprosy, Tuberculosis and Urbanization in Africa." In *Health and Disease in Tropical Africa: Geographical and Medical Viewpoints*, ed. Rais Akhtar, 91–155. Chur, London: Harwood Academic Publishers.

Hutt, Michael. 1991. "Cancer and Cardiovascular Disease." In *Disease and Mortality in sub-Saharan Africa*, ed. Richard Feachem and D. Jamison, 221–40. Washington, D.C.: Oxford University Press for the World Bank.

Hyam, R. 1990. *Empire and Sexuality: The British Experience*. Manchester: Manchester University Press.

Iliffe, John. 1984. "The Poor in the Modern History of Malawi." In *Malawi: An Alternative Pattern of Development*, Centre of African Studies, University of Edinburgh, Seminar Proceedings no. 25, 24–25 May 1984, 243–92.

————. 1987. *The African Poor: A History*. Cambridge: Cambridge University Press.

Irvine, C. 1958. *How to Behave: Some Manners and Customs of Civilized People*. Nairobi: The Highway Press.

Isichei, Elizabeth. 1995. *A History of Christianity in Africa*. Grand Rapids, Mich.: W. B. Eerdmans.

Isaacman, A. F. 1989. "The Countries of the Zambesi Basin." In *General History of Africa*, vol. 6: *Africa in the Nineteenth Century until the 1880s*, ed. J. F. Ade Ajayi, 179–210. Paris: UNESCO/Heinemann International.

Ityavyar, D. 1992. "Health in Colonial Africa." In *The Political Economy of Health in Africa*, ed. T. Falola and D. Ityavyar, 35–48. Monographs in International Studies, Africa series, no. 60. Athens, Ohio: Ohio University Center for International Studies.

Janssens, P. G. 1971. "Old and New Dimensions in Medical Aid." *Transactions of the Royal Society of Tropical Medicine and Hygiene* 65:S2–S15.

Janzen, J. 1978. *The Quest for Therapy in Lower Zaire*. Berkeley: University of California Press.

Johnson, Hildegard B. 1967. "The Location of Christian Missions in Africa." *The Geographical Review* 57:168–202.

Johnson, William Percival. 1884. "Seven Years' Travels in the Region East of Lake Nyasa." *Proceedings of the Royal Geographical Society* 6:512–36.

————. 1922. *Nyasa the Great Water*. New York: Negro Universities Press.

————. 1926. *My African Reminiscences, 1876–1895*. London: Universities' Mission to Central Africa.

Johnston, H. H. 1897. *British Central Africa*. London: Methuen.

Kappa, P. 1980. "The Role of the Traditional Healer in Malawi and Zambia." *Curare* 3:205–8.

Kaspin, Deborah. 1993. "Chewa Visions and Revisions of Power: Transformations of the Nyau Dance in Central Malawi." In *Modernity and Its Malcontents: Ritual and Power in Postcolonial Africa*, ed. John and Jean Comaroff, 34–57. Chicago: University of Chicago Press.

Kimambo, I. N. 1989. "The East African Coast and Hinterland, 1845–80." In *General History of Africa*, vol. 6: *Africa in the Nineteenth Century until the 1880s*, ed. J. F. Ade Ajayi, 234–69. Paris, UNESCO/Heinemann International.

King, Michael, and Elspeth King. 1991. *The Story of Medicine and Disease in Malawi: The 130 Years since Livingstone*. Blantyre, Malawi: Montfort Press.

Kiple, Kenneth. 1993. "Diseases of sub-Saharan Africa to 1860." In *The Cambridge World History of Human Diseases*, ed. K. Kiple et al., 293–98. Cambridge: Cambridge University Press.

Kirk, Sir John. 1965. *Zambesi Journal and Letters, 1858–63*. Edited by Reginald Foskett. Edinburgh: Oliver and Boyd.

Kjekshus, H. 1977. *Ecology Control and Economic Development in East Africa*. London: Heinemann.

Kubicek, R. V. 1990. "The Colonial Steamer and the Occupation of West Africa by the Victorian State, 1840–1900." *Journal of Imperial and Commonwealth History* 18:9–32.

Kuczynski, Robert. 1949. *Demographic Survey of the British Colonial Empire*. 2 vols. London: Oxford University Press.

Langworthy, Harry W. 1971. "Swahili Influence in the Area Between Lake Malawi and the Luangwa River." *African Historical Studies* 4, no. 3: 575– 602.

Lankester, Herbert. 1897. "Medical Missions." *Mercy and Truth* 1:245–50, 255–57.

Last, Murray. 1986. "The Professionalisation of African Medicine." In *The Professionalisation of African Medicine*, 1–19. Manchester: Manchester University Press.

Latourette, Kenneth S. 1943. *A History of the Expansion of Christianity*. Vol. 5: *The Great Century in the Americas, Australsia, and Africa, A.D. 1800–A.D. 1914*. New York: Harper.

Laws, Robert. 1898. "Livingstonia Missionary Institution." *The Aurora* 2, no. 7: 1–12.

———. 1934. *Reminiscences of Livingstonia*. London: Oliver and Boyd.

Leys, Norman. 1926. *Kenya*. 3d ed. London: Hogarth Press.

Linden, Ian. 1974. *Catholics, Peasants, and Chewa Resistance in Nyasaland, 1889–1939*. Berkeley: University of California Press.

Livingstone, David. 1857. *Missionary Travels and Researches in South Africa*. London: Ward, Lock.

Livingstone, W. P. 1921. *Laws of Livingstonia*. London: Hodder and Stoughton.

Lonsdale, J. 1968. "European Attitudes and African Pressures: Missions and Government in Kenya between the Wars. *Race* (10 October): 141–51.

Lyons, M. 1988. "Sleeping Sickness, Colonial Medicine, and Imperialism: Some Connections in the Belgian Congo." In *Disease, Medicine, and Empire: Perspectives on Western Medicine and the Experience of Western Expansion*, ed. R. MacLeod and M. Lewis, 245–56. London: Routledge.

Maples, Chauncy. 1899. *The Journals and Papers of Chauncy Maples, Bishop of Likoma*. Edited by E. Maples. London: Longmans.

Marwick, M. 1950. "Another Modern Anti-witchcraft Movement in East Central Africa." *Africa* 20, no. 2 (1950): 100–12.

Mbiti, J. 1971. *New Testament Eschatology in an African Background*. London: Oxford University Press.

McCracken, John. 1977. "Underdevelopment in Malawi: The Missionary Contribution." *African Affairs* 76, no. 303 (April 1977): 195–209.

McKelvey, J. J. 1973. *Man against Africa: Struggle for Africa*. Ithaca, N.Y.: Cornell University Press.

McKinnon, M. 1977. "Commerce, Christianity, and the Gunboat: An Historical Study of Malawi Lake and River Transport, 1850–1914." Ph.D. diss., Michigan State University.

McNeill, William. 1976. *Plagues and Peoples.* Garden City, N.Y.: Anchor Books.

Meade, M., and R. Earickson, eds. 2000. *Medical Geography.* 2d ed. New York: Guilford Press.

Meinig, Donald. 1982. "Geographical Analysis of Imperial Expansion." In *Period and Place: Research Methods in Historical Geography,* ed. A. Baker and M. Billinge, 71–78. Cambridge: Cambridge University Press.

Miller, B. J., and C. B. Keane. 1987. *Encyclopedia and Dictionary of Medicine, Nursing, and Allied Health.* 4th ed. Philadelphia: W. B. Saunders.

Miller, Jon. 1994. *The Social Control of Religious Zeal: A Study of Organizational Contradictions.* New Brunswick, N.J.: Rutgers University Press.

Miller, Joseph. 1988. *Way of Death.* Madison: University of Wisconsin Press.

Mills, Dora S. Yarnton. 1911. *What We Do in Nyasaland.* London: Universities' Mission to Central Africa.

———. 1931. *A Hero Man: The Life and Adventures of William Percival Johnson, Archdeacon of Nyasa.* London: Universities' Mission to Central Africa.

Miracle, Marvin. 1966. *Maize in Africa.* Madison: University of Wisconsin Press.

Morris, Brian. 1986. "Herbalism and Divination in Southern Malawi." *Social Science and Medicine* 23, no. 4: 367–77.

———. 1989. "Medicines and Herbalism In Malawi." *Society of Malawi Journal* 42, no. 2: 34–54.

Msukwa, L. A. H. 1987. "The Role of the Churches in the Development of Malawi." *Religion in Malawi* 1, no. 1: 22–27.

Mudimbe, V. Y. 1988. *The Invention of Africa: Gnosis, Philosophy, and the Order of Knowledge.* Bloomington: Indiana University Press.

Mufuka, K. N. 1977. *Missions and Politics in Malawi.* Kingston, Ontario: The Limestone Press.

Munday, J. T. 1941. "Witchcraft in England and Central Africa." Parts 6, 9–11. *Central Africa* 59: 33–35, 45–46, and 99–101.

Murray, Nancy U. 1987. "The Need to Get There First: Staking a Missionary Claim in Kenya." *Journal of African Studies* 12, no. 4: 181–93.

Murray, S. S., compiler. 1922. *A Handbook of Nyasaland.* Zomba: Government of Nyasaland, Government Printer.

Mutungi. O. K. 1977. *The Legal Aspects of Witchcraft in East Africa.* Nairobi: East African Literature Bureau.

Nelson, H. D., et al. 1975. *Area Handbook for Malawi.* Washington, D.C.: U.S. Supt. of Documents.

Newman, James L. 1995. *The Peopling of Africa.* New Haven: Yale University Press.

Niddrie, D. 1954. "The Road to Work: A Survey of the Influences of Transport on Migrant Labour in Central Africa." *Rhodes-Livingstone Journal,* no. 15: 31–42.

Ofosu-Amah, S. 1980. "The African Experience." In *Changing Disease Patterns and Human Behavior,* ed. N. Stanley and R. Joske, 299–322. New York: Academic Press.

Oliver, Roland. 1952. *The Missionary Factor in East Africa.* London: Longmans.

Olumwalla, Osaak. 2002. *Dis-ease in the Colonial State: Medicine, Society, and Social Change among the AbaNyole of Western Kenya.* Westport, Conn.: Greenwood Press.

Pachai, B. 1972. "The State and the Churches in Malawi during the Early Protectorate Rule."*Journal of Social Science* 1:7–27.

Palmer, E. S., and E. Ashwin, *East Africa in Pictures: 102 Illustrations of the Work of the Universities' Mission to Central Africa.* London: UMCA, 1900.

Parrinder, G. 1963. *Witchcraft: European and African.* London: Faber and Faber.

Patterson, K. D. 1981. "The Demographic Impact of the 1918–19 Influenza Pandemic in sub-Saharan Africa: A Preliminary Assessment." In *African Historical Demography*, ed. C. Fyfe and D. McMaster, 2:403–31. Edinburgh: Edinburgh University Press.

―――. 1993. "Disease Ecologies of sub-Saharan Africa." In *Cambridge World History of Human Diseases*, ed. K. Kiple, 447–52. Cambridge: Cambridge University Press, Cambridge.

Peltzer, Kar. 1987. *Some Contributions of Traditional Healing Practices towards Psychosocial Health Care in Malawi.* Eschborn bei Frankfurt am Main: Fachbuchhandlung fur Psychology.

Pike, John G. 1968. *Malawi: A Political and Economic History.* London: Pall Mall.

Pike, John G., and G. T. Rimmington. 1965. *Malawi: A Geographical Study.* London: Oxford University Press.

Pollock, Norman, Jr. 1971. *Nyasaland and Northern Rhodesia: Corridor to the North.* Pittsburgh: Duquesne University Press.

Population Reference Bureau. 1998. *World Population Data Sheet, 1998.* Washington, D.C.: Population Reference Bureau.

Pretorius, J. L. 1972. "An Introduction to the History of the Dutch Reformed Church in Malawi, 1889–1914." In *The Early History of Malawi*, ed. B. Pachai, 365–71. Evanston, Ill.: Northwestern University Press.

Ranger, Terence. 1975. "Introduction." In *Themes in the Christian History of Central Africa*, ed. T. Ranger, 3–13. Berkeley: University of California Press.

―――. 1981. "Godly Medicine: The Ambiguities of Medical Mission in Southeast Tanzania, 1900–1945." *Social Science and Medicine* 15B: 261–77.

―――. 1982. "Medical Science and Pentecost: The Dilemma of Anglicanism in Africa." In *The Church and Healing*, ed. W. Sheils, 333–65. Oxford: Blackwell.

Ransford, Oliver. 1983. *'Bid the Sickness Cease': Disease in the History of Black Africa.* London: Murray.

Rawlinson, G. C. 1917. "Some Lessons from the Chilembwe Rebellion." *Central Africa* 35:61–66.

Read, M. 1942. "Migrant Labour and its Effects on Tribal Life." *International Labour Review* 24, no. 1 (1942): 605–31.

Reader, John. 1998. *Africa: A Biography of the Continent.* New York: Alfred A. Knopf.

Richards, A. 1935. "A Modern Movement of Witch-finders." *Africa* 8, no. 4: 448–61.

Richards, Paul. 1983. "Ecological Change and the Politics of African Land Use." *African Studies Review* 26, no. 1 (June): 1–72.

Rodriguez, L. C. 1991. "EPI Target Diseases: Measles, Tetanus, Polio." In *Disease and Mortality in sub-Saharan Africa*, ed. R. Feachem and D. Jamison, 173–89. Washington, D.C.: Oxford University Press for The World Bank.

Roome, William J. 1926. *A Great Emancipation: A Missionary Survey of Nyasaland, Central Africa.* London: World Dominion Press.

Ross, P. H., and A. D. Milne. 1904. "Tick Fever," *British Medical Journal* 2:1453–54.

Ross, R. 1902. *Mosquito Brigades and How to Organize Them*. London: Philip.

Rotberg, Robert. 1965. *The Rise of Nationalism in Central Africa: The Making of Malawi and Zambia, 1873–1964*. Cambridge: Harvard University Press.

Roundy, R. 1987. "Human Behavior and Disease Hazards in Ethiopia: Spatial Perspectives on Rural Health." In *Health and Disease in Tropical Africa: Geographical and Medical Viewpoints*, ed. Rais Akhtar, 261–78. Chur, Switzerland: Harwood Academic Publishers.

Rowley, Henry. [1867] 1969. *The Story of the Universities' Mission to Central Africa, from Its Commencement to Its Withdrawal from the Zambezi*. London. Rept. New York: Negro Universities Press.

Sandwith, F. M. 1907. "Hill Stations and Other Health Resorts in the British Tropics." *Journal of Tropical Medicine and Hygiene* 22, no. 10 (November 15): 361–70.

Schneider, H. K. 1981. *The Africans: An Ethnological Account*. Englewood Cliffs, N.J.: Prentice-Hall.

Schoffeleers. M. 1976. "The Nyau Societies." *The Society of Malawi Journal* 29:59–68.

Schram, R. 1968. "Notes on West African Public Health." In *Medicine and Science in the 1860s*, ed. F. N. Poynter, 253–65. London: Wellcome Institute of the History of Medicine.

Sharpe, Alfred. 1912. "The Geography of Economic Development of British Central Africa." *Geographical Journal* 39:1–24.

Shaw, Rosalind. 2002. *Memories of the Slave Trade: Ritual and the Historical Imagination in Sierra Leone*. Chicago: University of Chicago Press.

Shepperson, George. 1958. *Independent African: John Chilembwe and the Origins, Setting, and Significance of the Nyasaland Native Rising of 1915*. Edinburgh: Edinburgh University Press.

Simpkin, Alice 1926. *Nursing in Nyasaland*. London: Universities' Mission to Central Africa.

Sim, Arthur Fraser. 1897. *The Life and Letters of Arthur Fraser Sim*. London: Universities' Mission to Central Africa.

Sindima, H. J. 1992. *The Legacy of Scottish Missionaries in Malawi*. Lewiston, Maine: Edwin Mellen Press.

Smith, Edwin W. 1926. *The Christian Mission in Africa*. A study based on the work of The International Conference at Le Zoute, Belgium, Sept. 14 to 21. London: International Misionary Council.

Stanley, H. M. 1872. *How I Found Livingstone in Central Africa*. London: Sampson, Low.

Stewart, James. 1903. *Dawn in the Dark Continent*. Edinburgh: Oliphant.

Tapela, H. 1979. "Labour Migration in Southern Africa and the Origins of Underdevelopment in Nyasaland." *Journal of Southern African Affairs* 4:67–80.

Tindall, P. 1968. *A History of Central Africa*. New York: Praeger.

Thomas, H. B., and R. Scott. 1935. *Uganda*. London: Oxford University Press.

Thompson, J. M. 1992. "When the Fires Are Lit: The French Navy's Recruitment and Training of Senegalese Mechanics and Stokers, 1864–1887." *Canadian Journal of African Studies* 26, no. 2: 274–303.

Thomson, D. 1950. *England in the Nineteenth Century (1815–1914)*. London: Penguin Books.

Trimmingham, J. S. 1964. *Islam in East Africa*. Oxford: Clarendon Press.

Troup, J. R. 1890. *With Stanley's Rear Column*. London: Chapman and Hall.

Universities' Mission to Central Africa (UMCA). N.d. *Supplement to the History of the Universities' Mission to Central Africa, 1957–1965*. London: UMCA.

———. 1903. *UMCA Atlas*. London: UMCA.

van Velsen, J. 1960. "The Missionary Factor Among the Lakeside Tonga." *Journal of the Rhodes-Livingstone Institute* 26:1–22.

———. 1961. "Labor Migration as a Positive Factor in the Continuity of a Tonga Society." In *Social Change in Modern Africa*, ed. A. Southall, 230–41. London: Oxford University Press.

Vaughan, Megan. 1991. *Curing Their Ills: Colonial Power and African Illness*. Cambridge, England: Polity Press.

Vellut, J. L. 1989. "The Congo Basin and Angola." In *General History of Africa*, vol. 6: *Africa in the Nineteenth Century until the 1880s*, ed. J. F. Ade Ajayi, 294–324. Paris: UNESCO/Heinemann International.

Vogel, L. C., et al. 1974. *Health and Disease in Kenya*. Nairobi: East African Literature Bureau.

Wallis, J. P. R. 1956. *The Zambesi Expedition of David Livingstone*. London: Chatto and Windus.

Walls, A. F. 1982. "The Heavy Artillery of the Missionary Army: The Domestic Importance of the Nineteenth Century Medical Missionary." In *The Church and Healing*, ed. W. J. Shiels, 287–97. Oxford: Blackwell.

Warren, M. 1967. *Social History and Christian Mission*. London: SCM Press.

Welbourne, F. 1971. "Missionary Stimulus and African Response.' In *Colonialism in Africa 1870–1960*, ed. V. Turner, 3:310–45. Cambridge: Cambridge University Press.

White, L. 1987. *Magomero: Portrait of an African Village*. Cambridge: Cambridge University Press.

Williams, C. 1982. "Healing and Evangelism: the Place of Medicine in Later Victorian Protestant Missionary Thinking." In *The Church and Healing*, ed. W. J. Sheils, 271–85. *Studies in Church History*, vol. 19. Oxford: Blackwell.

Williams, S. G. 1958. "Some Old Steamships of Nyasaland." *The Nyasaland Journal* 11:42–56.

Wilson, G. H. 1920. *A Missionary's Life in Nyasaland*. London: Universities' Mission to Central Africa.

———. 1936. *The History of the Universities' Mission to Central Africa*. London: UMCA.

Wingate, P. 1976. *The Penguin Medical Encyclopedia*. 2d ed. Harmondsworth: Penguin Books.

Winspear, Frank. 1956. "A Short History of the Universities' Mission." *The Nyasaland Journal* 9 (Jan.): 11–50.

———. 1960. "Some Reminiscences of Nyasaland." *The Nyasaland Journal* 13 (July): 35–74.

Worboys, M. 1976. "The Emergence of Tropical Medicine: A Study in the Establishment of Scientific Specialty." In *Perspectives on the Emergence of Scientific Disciplines*, ed. G. Lemaine et al., 75–98. The Hague: Mouton.

Wright, Marcia, and Peter Lary. 1971. "Swahili Settlements in Northern Zambia and Malawi." *African Historical Studies* 4, no. 3: 547–73.

Yarborough, J. C., ed. 1888. *The Diary of a Working Man (William Bellingham) in Central Africa, December 1884 to October 1887.* London: Society for Promoting Christian Knowledge.

Young, E. D. 1868. *The Search after Livingstone.* Rev. by Horace Waller. London: Letts, Sons and Co.

———. 1877. *Nyassa: A Journal of Adventure.* 2d ed. London: John Murray.

Zelinsky, Wilbur. 1973. *The Cultural Geography of the United States.* Englewood Cliffs, N.J.: Prentice-Hall.

Index